Eating Disorders For Dummies®

5|08

Disordered Eating or Eating Disorder?

All of the following behaviors or beliefs are considered examples of *disordered eating*. Disordered eating means you don't necessarily have an eating disorder, but your approach to food and weight has some wrinkles in it *and* could be heading you for trouble. The more of these disordered eating behaviors or beliefs you have, the more likely you are to have a formal eating disorder:

- Skipping meals
- Fasting to lose weight
- Exercising to make up for overeating
- Cutting out a food group
- Trying every diet there is
- Regularly eating an amount of food that leaves you hungry
- Eating to manage emotions
- Binge-eating

- Using laxatives or diuretics for weight loss
- Vomiting for weight loss
- Believing the scales reveal your worth
- Being constantly preoccupied with food and weight
- Being extremely fearful of weight gain
- Believing you are fat even when everyone else tells you you're too thin

You can read Chapters 2–4 for specifics that will help you identify if you have one of the major eating disorders.

Where to Find Help

Check out the following online resources to find local eating disorder professionals, support groups, and residential treatment facilities:

Eating Disorder Referral and Information Center
Listings include therapists, nutritionists, and treatment facilities
www.edreferral.com

National Association of Anorexia Nervosa and Associated Disorders (ANAD)
Listings include therapists, nutritionists, support groups (free), and treatment facilities
www.ANAD.org

International Association of Eating Disorder Professionals (IAEDP)
Listings include therapists, nutritionists, and physicians
www.iaedp.com

National Eating Disorders Association
Listings include therapists, nutritionists, physicians, and free support groups
www.nationaleatingdisorders.org

Something Fishy
Listings include therapists, nutritionists, physicians, support groups, and treatment facilities
www.something-fishy.org

Bulimia.com (Web site for Gurze Books)
Listings include individual and group therapists and treatment facilities
www.bulimia.com or www.gurze.com

You can also call a local hospital or university and ask if they have an eating disorders program. Such a program will be able to give you referrals.

For more information about eating disorders, read this book (!)

For Dummies: Bestselling Book Series for Beginners

Eating Disorders For Dummies®

Things 1 Like about Myself That Aren't about Weight

One really important part of eating disorder recovery is learning to appreciate things about yourself that are attractive and worthwhile and *have nothing to do with your weight*. It's easy to lose track. With this list handy, you won't have to. I'll start you off with a few ideas. You can fill in from there with examples that are meaningful to you. (Hint: It's not cheating to get suggestions from other people!)

- ✔ I have great hair.
- ✔ I have a lot of natural physical strength.
- ✔ I'm very intuitive about people.
- ✔ I'm a great joke-teller.

_____

_____

_____

_____

_____

A Few Things to Remember when Eating Disorder Shame 1s Getting the Better of You

- ✔ Your eating disorder is the way you've coped. It's how you've survived. Survival is a *good* thing! (Read inside for some ideas on how to cope and survive that don't require an eating disorder.)

- ✔ Just by opening this book you've taken a step. That's *courage!*

- ✔ Most modern American women and an increasing number of men share in some kind of disordered thinking, feeling, or behavior when it comes to food, weight, and body image. Our culture makes it hard to avoid.

- ✔ The media want you to feel shame about yourself. That way you'll buy their products!

- ✔ You can make anyone binge by putting them on a diet long enough.

- ✔ Outside of this moment are things you feel proud of. List a few when you aren't feeling so shamed, so you'll have them handy next time you need them:

_____

_____

_____

_____

- ✔ There are a few key people you can count on to see your worth and remind you of it when you forget. You can list them here and think about them whenever you need to:

_____

_____

_____

For Dummies: Bestselling Book Series for Beginners

Eating Disorders

FOR

DUMMIES®

by Susan Schulherr

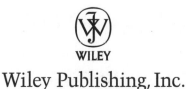

WILEY

Wiley Publishing, Inc.

Eating Disorders For Dummies®

Published by
Wiley Publishing, Inc.
111 River St.
Hoboken, NJ 07030-5774
www.wiley.com

WILEY

About the Author

Susan Schulherr, LCSW, is a licensed clinical social worker who has had a private psychotherapy practice in New York City for nearly 30 years. She has worked with people with eating disorders for over 20 of those years. Her chapter on treating binge eating disorder appears in the 2005 book, *EMDR Solutions: Pathways to Healing* (Shapiro, Norton). Her article, "The Binge–Diet Cycle: Shedding New Light, Finding New Exits," was published in *Eating Disorders: The Journal of Treatment and Prevention* (1998). She has presented workshops at the local and national level on eating disorders and on issues of weight and eating to both professional and nonprofessional audiences.

Ms. Schulherr is a trained family and couples therapist. She has extensive experience in the trauma specialty approaches of EMDR and Somatic Experiencing, each of which she has adapted for the treatment of eating disorders.

Author's Acknowledgments

I owe some particular thank you's now that this project that once felt so far off is a reality. For the collaborative outpouring that became the text of this book, my thanks to the indefatigable editorial staff at Wiley Publishing: Tracy Boggier, Stephen Clark, Christy Pingleton, and to Misty Rees for her technical review. For presenting me with the opportunity to participate in the first place, my special appreciation to literary agent Margot Maley Hutchison from Waterside Productions, Inc. For concept-to-completion professional feedback and moral support without which my part in this project would have been impossible, endless gratitude to Nancy J. Napier, LMFT.

I always wish to extend heartfelt thanks to the many clients and others who have shared their eating disorder stories and struggles with me over the years. All that you have taught me has made its way into this volume and inspired me with the possibilities for healing even in the most difficult situations.

Publisher's Acknowledgments

We're proud of this book; please send us your comments through our Dummies online registration form located at www.dummies.com/register/.

Some of the people who helped bring this book to market include the following:

Acquisitions, Editorial, and Media Development

Project Editor: Stephen R. Clark

Acquisitions Editor: Tracy Boggier

Copy Editor: Christy Pingleton

Editorial Program Coordinator: Erin Calligan Mooney

Technical Editors: Misty L. Rees, BS, CEDS, Program Director, Selah House, www.selahhouse.net

Editorial Manager: Christine Meloy Beck

Editorial Assistants: Joe Niesen, David Lutton

Cartoons: Rich Tennant (www.the5thwave.com)

Composition Services

Project Coordinator: Katie Key

Layout and Graphics: Reuben W. Davis, Alissa D. Ellet, Melissa K. Jester, Christine Williams

Proofreaders: Context Editorial Services, Inc., Cynthia Fields

Indexer: Potomac Indexing, LLC

Publishing and Editorial for Consumer Dummies

    Diane Graves Steele, Vice President and Publisher, Consumer Dummies

    Joyce Pepple, Acquisitions Director, Consumer Dummies

    Kristin A. Cocks, Product Development Director, Consumer Dummies

    Michael Spring, Vice President and Publisher, Travel

    Kelly Regan, Editorial Director, Travel

Publishing for Technology Dummies

    Andy Cummings, Vice President and Publisher, Dummies Technology/General User

Composition Services

    Gerry Fahey, Vice President of Production Services

    Debbie Stailey, Director of Composition Services

Contents at a Glance

Table of Contents

Introduction

Could this be you? You don't have much self-confidence (this applies most often to females, but males are not immune). You'd love to feel in charge of yourself, your emotions, your life. You'd do anything to be someone others love and admire. You don't feel any of these things are true — for you.

Add to this that you live in a culture that tells you the world is yours if you're thin. That you, or anyone, can become model-thin (or fat-free buff) if you just diet and exercise enough.

You may be a little precise or obsessive by nature. And you may have fewer of the natural brain hormones that buffer most people in life. You may even have a history of some kind of trauma that you have yet to resolve.

These characteristics are the ingredients for making an eating disorder. Because you feel vulnerable, an eating disorder is, above all else, the way you struggle against internal doubts, trying to cope. Dieting is how you try to put together a sense of control and self-esteem. Bingeing is how you comfort yourself or respond to the extremes of dieting. You have come to rely on your eating disorder symptoms so completely that the thought of surrendering them is terrifying — even when they begin to cause a lot of physical and emotional trouble.

If you recognize yourself — or someone you love — in this portrait, you've come to the right book! Although the culture offers plenty to keep an eating disorder going, the pages that follow supply you with lots of ingredients to counter those effects from the inside. Or to start you on that path. I describe the eating disorders from the inside out so you can make sense of what you or your loved one is experiencing. I tell you about what you need for recovery. I describe the process and personnel of treatment in detail. I advise you as a family member or other caring person how to help the person you care about and how to take care of yourself at the same time.

Eating disorders are treacherous. They destroy and even take lives, and they make sufferers doubt and hate themselves. But the happy news is that the majority of people who pitch into treatment and stay with it through recovery get better. They go on to think about and engage in other things, become successful and fulfilled, and leave their eating disorders behind. So can you.

About This Book

This book is aimed at helping you recover from your eating disorder (or helping someone you love recover). I build two big assumptions about what's necessary for recovery into the organization of the book:

If you're aiming at getting better, it helps to understand the nature of an eating disorder and how you get one.

The way you think about a problem determines how you try to solve it. For instance, if you think your eating disorder shows you don't have enough willpower to control your eating, you may search for bigger and better ways to put controls on yourself. If, on the other hand, you understand that your disorder reflects low self-esteem and problems handling emotions, you can go to work on improving your life in these areas.

I spend a lot of time going over the ways of thinking and looking at yourself that make you vulnerable to an eating disorder. I spend at least as much time describing ways of thinking and behaving that can build inner reserves and make an eating disorder much less likely. This building process can be exciting and gratifying at times. But it can be frustrating and slow-going at others. Knowing what you're doing and why can help you to keep plugging.

Studies show that people who stay in eating disorder treatment long enough to build up inner strengths, rather than just manage outer symptoms (like bingeing or starving), are more likely to get better and stay better.

Getting better means getting treatment.

For most people, recovering from an eating disorder isn't a self-help operation. (You can read about the exceptions to this rule in Chapter 12.) You need to hire experts and invest a lot of yourself and your time in your treatment. I devote a lot of space to taking you through the treatment process, step-by-step, from beginning to end. This includes understanding treatment options and when to choose them, selecting a therapist and other members of your treatment team, and understanding your own role in the treatment process. I want you to have the best possible chance of being successful.

If you're a family member, I go over in detail how to approach the person you love about treatment. I discuss your role in treatment and how to support recovery in day-to-day living.

I've written *Eating Disorders For Dummies* so that you can jump in wherever your interest takes you — you don't have to read this book from start to finish. Each section includes references to other parts of the book that have more information on the subject you're reading about.

Conventions Used in This Book

Many times in this book, particularly in the treatment sections, I use fictional people to illustrate a point I'm making. These people represent composites of people I've met and/or worked with over the years. In no case do they represent real people.

From time to time, I introduce new terms as I explain ideas important to your understanding of the eating disorders. Mostly I do this when you're likely to run into the term elsewhere and it may be helpful for you to know it. Each time I first use a new term, I *italicize* it, and usually follow it with an explanation.

Eating disorders are still primarily a female affair. So I make my life, and hopefully your reading, easier by using all female pronouns: *her, hers, she.* That doesn't mean I'm not aware that men can develop eating disorders, too. If you're a guy, your disorder is just as serious! (See Chapter 15.)

It would have made for easier language to refer to people with anorexia as *anorexics*, people with bulimia as *bulimics,* and so on. I avoid this streamlined language to make a crucial point: Saying you are a *person with an eating disorder* serves as a reminder that there's more to you, much more, than your eating disorder. Also, there's no reason to assume your disorder is a permanent part of your identity, the way you do when you say you're a woman, or a Latina, or American-born. Saying you're a person with an eating disorder is more like saying you have a major illness. Beating your eating disorder may be a big battle, but your eating disorder is not who you are.

What You're Not to Read

You're not to read anything that isn't crucial to understanding eating disorders and their treatment *if you don't feel like it.* Sometimes I add some extra information that's a little more in-depth but not essential. I mark all such in-depth detours with a Technical Stuff icon.

In the same spirit, along the way I offer extra nuggets of information on the subject you're reading about tucked away in gray boxes called *sidebars.* Read them. Don't read them. The choice is yours. It won't make a difference in your understanding of the subject at hand.

Foolish Assumptions

I assume if you're reading this, you're one of the following people:

✔ **You have or suspect you have an eating disorder:** You want to know there's hope, get a better handle on your problem, be pointed in the right direction for treatment, and get a preview of the recovery process.

✔ **You have a family member, friend, or roommate who has an eating disorder:** You want to understand her problem better, know how you can help, understand treatment options if you're the parent of a minor, and get some ideas about support for yourself.

✔ **You're a professional who works in some way with people with eating disorders:** You need a quick reference and overview to help you understand the problem and how you can help in your particular role.

If any of these descriptions sound like you, you've come to the right book!

How This Book Is Organized

Eating Disorder For Dummies is organized into 5 parts with 27 chapters. What follows is a description of what you can find in each part.

Part 1: Eating Disorders: An All-Consuming World of Their Own

Part I intends to help you really *get* what eating disorders are about. Chapter 1 gives you the big picture and previews what you find in the rest of the book. Chapters 2 to 4 introduce you to the three major eating disorders: *anorexia, bulimia,* and *binge eating disorder.* These chapters each come with a questionnaire so you can judge whether you're at risk for one of these disorders. Chapter 5 reviews the risk factors that make a person vulnerable to developing an eating disorder — genes, brain chemistry, family background, personality characteristics, trauma history, and dieting behavior. In Chapter 6 you can find out about the physical toll eating disordered behavior takes on your body. Finally, Chapter 7 describes other psychological disorders that typically accompany an eating disorder, such as anxiety, depression, addiction, and compulsive exercise.

Part II: Getting Well: Exploring Recovery and Treatment Options

Part II is your treatment handbook. I start you off with a map of recovery goals, so you know what you're aiming at. If you like, you can use the charts I provide to map yourself: Where are you now and what would you like to work on next in relation to each goal?

If you're just thinking about treatment or want to review the treatment you're in, Chapter 9 goes over all your treatment options. This includes treatment experts and facilities. It also includes a discussion of why you might make each choice. Chapter 10 helps you pick the approach to individual therapy that's right for you. It takes you right inside an imaginary session for each approach so you can get a feel for what it may be like. Chapters 11 and 12 explore additional options: family, couples, and group therapies; support groups; medication; and online treatments.

In Chapter 13 I help you think about your own role in using your treatment team and getting better. I follow this up with a chapter on managing early stage recovery successfully, including dealing with relapse.

Part III: Eating Disorders in Special Populations

This part focuses on special groups in the population who are at high risk for eating disorders or whose eating disorder risk has been under-recognized. I highlight special treatment considerations for each group. These groups include

- ✔ Men
- ✔ Athletes
- ✔ Dancers, models, and actors
- ✔ Children
- ✔ Middle-aged and elderly people
- ✔ People who are obese

Part IV: Advice and Help for Families and Others Who Care

Part IV is intended to help families and other people who care about someone with an eating disorder. I write as if you are a parent responsible for a minor child. But I stop along the way with special advice for others: siblings, partners, friends, roommates, and so on.

This is a how-to part, covering everything from getting informed to approaching someone for the first time about their eating disorder to managing life in recovery in a day-to-day way. The final chapter in Part IV focuses exclusively on your well-being and what services you may need to support it.

Part V: The Part of Tens

This is your at-a-glance part for quick ideas to inspire you or keep you on track in recovery. Ten don'ts remind you of recovery-interfering thoughts and behaviors. Ten do's give you the other side of the coin: ten thoughts and practices to keep your recovery cooking. Finally, I offer you a glimmer of benefits your recovery may hold in store that probably haven't occurred to you.

Icons Used in This Book

Throughout this book, I use figures in the margins — *icons*— to quickly point out the type of information you find in a particular paragraph. Here are the icons you see, along with a definition of what each one means:

This icon can mean one of two things. It can let you know I'm reviewing things I've gone over in more depth elsewhere. Or it can alert you that the paragraph contains some really valuable information for you to remember.

When you see the arrow in the target, you know the paragraph contains practical information for handling your eating disorder.

I place the warning icon next to any paragraph that tells you about situations or practices that may be harmful to you. I also use it when the paragraph informs you about ways you could be misled or other times you need to be on the alert.

This clever-looking guy tells you that the information in the paragraph gets a little technical, maybe providing a little more than you want or need to know. It's okay to skip this paragraph. Reading it isn't necessary to your understanding of the topic.

Where to Go from Here

Eating Disorders For Dummies is written so you can start wherever you want. You don't have to read the book in order. If you're urgent about getting treatment right now, you probably want to start with Chapters 9 to 11. If you're a family member, you may want to start with Part IV, which is written for you. Which chapter you choose depends on whether the person you love is already in eating disorder treatment or not. If you're still facing treatment choices, you're likely to find Chapter 9 a useful starting place.

Part I
Eating Disorders: An All-Consuming World of Their Own

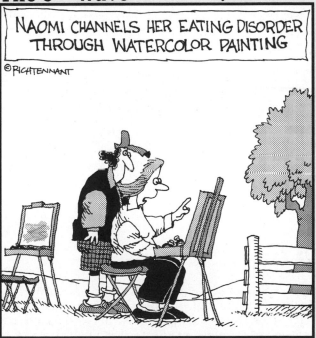

The 5th Wave   By Rich Tennant

NAOMI CHANNELS HER EATING DISORDER THROUGH WATERCOLOR PAINTING

©RICHTENNANT

"I'm working from the spicy side of the color wheel, blending ketchup red and cheddar cheese yellow to get the orange sorbet highlights on the hot dog colored barn."

In this part . . .

I introduce you to eating disorders and explain how they differ from less-worrisome eating problems. I describe how increasing pressures on women to achieve ideal bodies have contributed to a rise in eating disorders over the last 40 years. I go over the three major eating disorders — anorexia, bulimia, and binge eating disorder (BED) — in detail. I include tools to help you decide whether you may have one of these disorders or be at risk for developing one. I discuss the major risk factors that make a person vulnerable to developing an eating disorder, including genes, family style, cultural pressures, personality, and dieting behavior.

I include chapters that tell you how eating disordered behaviors harm your body and affect your thinking processes. I also review psychological and behavioral problems that commonly accompany eating disorders, such as addiction, compulsive exercise, depression, and suicidal tendencies. For all of these companion disorders, I provide tools to help you decide whether they apply to you (indicating you should seek evaluation and treatment).

Chapter 1

Understanding Eating Disorders

The term *eating disorder* sounds like something that refers to somebody who doesn't eat right. And, in one sense, it certainly does. Some people with eating disorders severely under-eat, to the point of risking their health or their lives. Others repeatedly overeat in extreme ways and may do risky things to get rid of the calories they've taken in. But what's not right about the eating is far more complicated than calories and nutrition.

In this chapter you get an overall sense of the eating disorders as physical and psychological syndromes: What do they look and feel like? Who gets them? What is an eating disorder doing in a person's life? How is getting an eating disorder driven by the culture, and how does that help us understand people with eating disorders better?

If you have an eating disorder, I tell you what you need to do to find treatment and get better. This previews Part II of this book, which covers treatments from soup to nuts. If you are a parent or caregiver to someone with an eating disorder, I discuss some of the difficulties of your situation. Part IV of this book, expanding on what I say here, is essentially a how-to section devoted to caregivers.

Getting a Sense of the Problem

People with eating disorders experience psychological issues and are compulsive in their eating habits. These play on each other over time, causing the eating disorder to become more entrenched. Some of the techniques used to try to drop a few pounds may lead to bad eating habits. However, if the concern about weight becomes obsessive, then the problem moves from simple dieting to an eating disorder.

Eating disorders involve the body and the mind. People with eating disorders express psychological problems through their behaviors with food. For example, someone who is struggling with self-esteem may decide that losing some weight would make them feel better and be a more appealing person. This person may try dieting, like many of her friends. But because she starts depending on dieting and weight loss for a sense of self-esteem, she can't let go of them. They become an obsessive focus, and the problem moves from simple dieting to an eating disorder. Psychological problems that existed before the eating disorder developed get worse, not better, as a result.

Eating disorders can't be separated from the culture in which they arise. In Western society, the overwhelming cultural message is that being thin is best. As people try to define themselves and what makes them valued members of the culture, the message to get or stay thin affects behavior such as eating, dieting, exercise, even cosmetic surgery. It may also affect self-image. I discuss in this section how these effects can lead to disordered eating habits even for a great many people who don't have formal eating disorders. For some people who are otherwise vulnerable (see "Seeing What's Behind the Symptoms" in this chapter and a discussion of risk factors for developing an eating disorder in Chapter 5), the message that thin is best provides the central principle for fixing their lives — and an eating disorder can soon follow. (Read "Understanding the Dramatic Rise in Eating Disorders," later in this chapter, to find out more about the development of the "culture of thin.")

In this section and throughout the book I give you a sense of what eating disorder symptoms are about in the belief that a solid understanding is necessary in order to arrive at the right kinds of solutions. I describe more about the cultural phenomenon of disordered eating practices, of which eating disorders represent the extreme end. I also give you a sense of who gets eating disorders and how many people have them.

Psyching yourself sick

For the person with an eating disorder, weight and eating develop into a *psychological* problem as well as a physical one. If you have an eating disorder you're constantly preoccupied with your weight and body shape. Your mood rises and falls with what you see on the scales. You judge your worth as a person by your weight and your success at dieting. What probably started out as ordinary dieting has developed into a rigid pattern that has gone seriously out of control. As time goes on, your eating disorder takes up more and more space while the rest of your life — friends, family, fun, future — takes up less and less.

Chances are good that you struggle with other psychological problems as well, such as depression, anxiety, obsessive-compulsive disorder, or alcohol or drug abuse problems. These problems, along with factors like personality type, family background, heredity, and biochemical make-up, may all contribute to the development of an eating disorder in a particular person.

Becoming more compulsive

The solution seems simple and obvious from the outside looking in. The person with anorexia *must* know she's not close to being fat and that she'll die if she keeps this up. The person who binges wants desperately to lose weight — so can't she just quit eating so much? A central quality of the eating disorder is the *compulsivity* of the symptoms and of the inner drive to be thin. Compulsions are behaviors that have an "I *have* to" urgency associated with them — to the point that the person often no longer feels they are a matter of voluntary control. (Ever tried to quit smoking?)

Eating disorders versus disordered eating

If you lined up all the people in the United States who eat, you'd have a spectrum ranging from Normal Eaters on one end to People with Eating Disorders on the other. The first thing you'd notice about this spectrum is that not very many people would be at the Normal Eaters end. Why? In this day and age we have more food than any society before us. At the same time, modern conveniences have cut the need for physical activity to nubbins. And the stresses of modern living often lead to eating patterns that are bound to make us tip the scales. Yet, despite all these trends pushing us to become heavier, as a culture we prefer a slim and fit look. It shouldn't be surprising that it all adds up to some strange relationships with food.

Who's in the middle? Most of the eating spectrum is taken up by people who don't have formal eating disorders but who have eating habits and beliefs that are *disordered*. Up to 60 percent of adult American women may be disordered eaters. Examples of disordered eating or beliefs include:

- ✔ Cutting out a food group to cut calories
- ✔ Eating to manage emotions
- ✔ Believing the scales reveal your worth

The more disordered eating behaviors and beliefs you have, the more at risk you are for developing an actual eating disorder. (You can read more about eating disorder risk factors in Chapter 5.)

Being at risk for an eating disorder

Precise figures for the numbers of people affected by eating disorders are hard to come by. People often deny or hide their disorder, and the symptoms that identify sufferers aren't always obvious, especially in the early stages.

Estimates indicate that between 5 and 8 million people in the United States are currently affected by some form of diagnosable eating disorder. Most of these people are young white women between the ages of 12 and 35 years. But this typical picture is beginning to shift in some ways:

- ✔ Both *younger girls* and *older women* are beginning to fill the ranks.
- ✔ More and more *men* are developing eating disorders, perhaps as many as a million currently in this country.
- ✔ *Minority girls and women* are showing eating disorder rates that often match those of their white peers.

According to statistics, as many as 70 million people worldwide suffer from eating disorders. Eating disorders occur at strikingly lower rates in non-Western, nonindustrialized countries than in Western industrialized ones. This tips us off that eating disorders have something to do with the culture.

Classifying the Eating Disorders

In upcoming chapters of this book, I go over the many ways an eating disorder can take shape in the lives of different people. However, three major eating disorders affect the most people, so they get the lion's share of attention. They are *anorexia nervosa* (usually just called *anorexia*), *bulimia nervosa* (usually called *bulimia*), and *binge eating disorder (BED)*.

Anorexia nervosa

Usually when people think of eating disorders, the first image that comes to mind is the emaciated face and body of the young woman with anorexia. Though actually the least prevalent of the major disorders — anorexia afflicts about 1 in every 100 people — it was the first to gain widespread public awareness. Anorexia also grabs our attention because it's the most dangerous eating disorder. According to the Academy for Eating Disorders, the risk of death for a person with anorexia is 12 times higher than that of someone without an eating disorder.

A person with anorexia is terrified of becoming fat — so terrified that the fear rules everything she does. She believes she's always on the verge of fatness, regardless of her actual weight or what anyone else tells her. To guard against the dreaded outcome, she refuses to eat. The resulting weight loss can put her health and life in jeopardy. A person with anorexia may also purge like the people with bulimia I discuss in the next section, and/or she may exercise compulsively to help her control her weight.

Bulimia nervosa

You could most easily identify the person with bulimia by the behaviors of bingeing and purging — that is, if you could witness them. These behaviors are almost always done in secret. *Bingeing* is eating *lots* of food in one sitting — sometimes tens of thousands of calories — often rapidly. *Purging* is what the person with bulimia does to get rid of these calories. She may do this by vomiting what she's just eaten, overusing laxatives or diuretics, exercising excessively, or other methods.

After binge episodes, a person with bulimia feels extremely shamed and worthless. She's as preoccupied with avoiding fat as the person with anorexia. Also like the person with anorexia, she believes her weight determines her worth. Unlike the person with anorexia, however, chances are good that the person with bulimia is also dealing with alcohol or drug abuse and with depression. As many as 3 or 4 in 100 young women in the United States have bulimia nervosa.

Binge eating disorder (BED)

People with binge eating disorder (BED) binge pretty much like people with bulimia. And they feel just as bad afterward. But they aren't driven toward purging behaviors. More likely, they become engaged in cycling between periods of bingeing and periods of rigid dieting. For some, this keeps their weight in a normal range. Other people with BED gain weight and may even become obese.

Estimates are that anywhere from 3 to 8 in 100 people in the United States have BED. According to a 1998 survey in the *Annals of Behavioral Medicine*, as many as 40 percent of the people with BED are men.

Seeing What's Behind the Symptoms

Eating disorder symptoms are very dramatic. But the real drama lies beneath the surface, in the hearts and minds of sufferers. While most people enjoy good food, those with eating disorders become obsessed over food-related issues. Eating isn't fun. Weight is the enemy. Strictly controlling eating and not eating is seen as a magical way to bring order to areas of life that feel out of control.

Food and weight as the visible focus

Think of the person with an eating disorder as a magician. The magician does his magic by getting us to look over *here*, while the real action is over *there*. The difference with the eating disorder is that the person who has it is as fixated on her food and weight symptoms as everyone else. And because her symptoms can cause anything from severe misery to outright physical danger, those who care have to keep at least one eye on them. But staying focused on food and weight means never getting to the heart of what an eating disorder is really about.

Eating disorders as "solutions"

Nobody has an eating disorder for the fun of it. If you've developed an eating disorder, it's because something hasn't been working in your life. You've turned to your eating disorder because it seems to help; never mind the terrible price you're paying for it.

Sadly, your eating disorder is a vote of no-confidence in your personal ability to solve problems, manage feelings, or create a life to be proud of. Depending on your disorder, you've discovered that weight loss brings admiration, dieting gives you a sense of control, bingeing provides temporary comfort, or purging offers a sense of release and relief. Each makes the eating disorder seem like a powerful and readily available ally.

The tricky thing about eating disorder symptoms is that the more they appear to solve for you, the more you ask them to solve — and the more you believe in them as problem-solvers. When a symptom seems to fix so much, it can achieve a very "dug-in" place in your life.

Seeing the Damage Eating Disorders Do

Eating disorders can take a terrible physical toll. They can also bog sufferers down in the self-defeating patterns of thinking and behavior that got them into their disorders in the first place. Having someone with an eating disorder in your life can leave you feeling helpless, angry, frightened, and exhausted.

Damage to the eating disorder sufferer

Eating disorders are physically dangerous. Anorexia and atypical disorders that include starving are the most dangerous. Starving can result in damage to the heart and other major organ systems. Death can follow. Anorexia has the highest mortality rate of any psychiatric disorder. Starving also impairs clear thinking and judgment.

Purging as part of bulimia or an atypical disorder can also damage the heart or other parts of the body. Though mortality rates are low compared to anorexia, the effects of purging can still be quite serious. (You can read in detail about the physical effects of the eating disorders in Chapter 6.)

Damage to those around the sufferer

From the time you realize someone you love has an eating disorder to the time she becomes ready to seek treatment can be a long journey. Those who care are often left to watch helplessly as the eating disorder sufferer gets drawn more deeply into her symptoms and potential danger. This is probably the worst part of caring about someone with an eating disorder. However, an eating disorder can affect the lives of those around the sufferer in a number of other ways as well, including:

- ✔ **Family functioning:** Eating disorder symptoms sometimes start to rule family life. Fear and worry can make it hard to find time for rest or fun.

- ✔ **Intimacy:** It often feels as if the person's relationship with her eating disorder takes priority over other relationships. Secrecy and deceit about symptoms interfere with feelings of closeness.

- ✔ **Personal rights and boundaries:** Stealing food or money for food and leaving a messy bathroom or kitchen are just a few of the ways eating disorder symptoms can infringe on others' rights.

You can read more about living with someone with an eating disorder in Chapter 23. Chapter 24 is all about getting help for yourself while you do.

Scoping the Rise in Eating Disorders

Before 1960, few people had heard of anorexia nervosa. By the end of the decade, it was taking the lives of a shocking number of young women. By the end of the next decade, bulimia and binge eating disorder were also taking a toll. At the same time, weight and eating preoccupations began increasing in the general population, mostly among women.

You might call the eating disorders the scary cousins of the more general cultural trends. Between the early '70s and the dawning of the new millennium, the number of women reporting dissatisfaction with their bodies went from just under 50 percent — bad enough — to nearly 90 percent.

How cultural forces have taken a toll

In many ways, it takes a village to create an eating disorder. By this I mean that cultural ideals about the best way to look can deeply affect a person's self-image and behavior. Achieving the ideal look is promoted in advertising and every form of entertainment as the way to purchase your ticket to many of the rewards society has to offer: admiration, a good mate, perhaps a better job.

In the last 40 years, the ideal look has come to mean, above all else, being thin and free of body fat. In fact, for women, it has meant becoming thinner and thinner. According to one study 45 years ago, models — who tell us what we should look like through media images — were just 8 percent slimmer than the average woman. Today, they're 23 percent slimmer than the rest of us.

How have women (and an increasing number of men) responded to these unreachable images? They've *dieted*. They've dieted alone, in groups, in secret, in public, with or without exercise, with supplements, with fasting . . . the list goes on. By now, for women, dieting is almost a cultural right of passage. For some women who don't feel okay about themselves or their worth, dieting seems like a solution. When you can't diet too much and the outcome of your dieting determines your sense of worth, you have the recipe for an eating disorder.

What makes eating disorders more likely

What happened to make us think that being thin is naturally superior? What happened to our tolerance for diversity and round edges? Two big things happened that the culture is still digesting: falling in love with youth and experiencing the women's movement.

The quest for youth

The baby boomers began to come of age in the 1960s. They were bound to have a big effect, if only because there were so darn many of them. Many believe the fashion trends of this era flowed from the boomers' new values, including street fashion over haute couture and a new waif-like look, embodied by the infamous model, Twiggy. The fashion industry took over the waif look and made it mainstream.

American society not only fell for the boomers' taste but it also fell for their youthful energy. If you couldn't be young, you could at least be *youthful-looking*.

Twiggy-style slimness came to stand for youthfulness. Dieting was the key to getting there. Fashion magazines began to report not just on clothing but on how women could perfect their bodies to fit the new trend and look good in more revealing styles.

Meanwhile, the belief that excess fat is also *unhealthy* exploded to a new level during the same period. Increasing weight was linked with increasing risk of heart disease. The ideal of fitness and its evil twin, fat phobia, became cemented into the mindset of the youth culture.

The belief developed that anyone who wanted it badly enough could achieve the new slimness. It sounds so democratic. You can't easily see the trap in it when no one is admitting that for many people — apparently the majority — the ideal is out of reach.

The women's movement

Up until recently, eating disorders have been mostly a women's affair. What's been different for women during the rise of weight obsessions and eating disorders? The biggest single development has been the women's movement and the social changes that followed.

Those who believe a connection exists between eating disorders and the women's movement point out that just as women began to break out of narrow roles and take up more space in society, the culture of thin told them they had to take up *less* space, not more. When women wanted to participate in the larger world, they were encouraged to become preoccupied with counting calories and the inches on their thighs.

Some see these developments as backlash by that other gender that had the most to lose as women gained power. They point out, for example, that the waif look made grown women appear childlike. No threat there. Others believe women also felt threatened. What if, for all they gained, they just ended up being rejected as unfeminine and unattractive?

Society still hasn't figured these issues out. Where are the guidelines for young women to follow? At a crossroads where neither the young nor the old have their footing, the path to success promised by the culture of thin remains seductively simple and clear.

How perceptions are beginning to shift

Are there any glimmers of hope in the 40-year march toward slimmer ideals, more dieting, and more disordered eating? A few. For example, the modeling world itself is beginning to look at the negative effect of too-thin standards on its models. Several manufacturers have started to present their products with average-sized women. (Read more about these trends in Chapter 17.) Prevention programs starting with the very young are popping up in classrooms and on TV. These programs counter messages that only thinness is acceptable with positive messages about a variety of body shapes and sizes.

Getting Better Is an Option

Eating disorders don't usually just go away on their own. But treatment is available and people get better. The process is neither quick nor easy. In fact, recovery usually takes a lot longer than people bargain for (though not forever!) For most this means a matter of years rather than weeks or months. The good news to keep in mind is that it's doable. And, contrary to what you may have heard, you don't need to think of your eating disorder as something you're stuck with for life once you have it. Full recovery from an eating disorder means leaving your symptoms behind and moving onto other things you'd rather focus on in life. For many, if not most, this is an achievable goal.

Getting help

The process of getting better is composed of two important parts. Engaging in both parts strongly improves your outlook for long-term recovery. The first part involves learning how to manage your eating disorder symptoms — starving, bingeing, purging, and/or dieting. The second part involves working on internal skills that can make you more effective in life and can help buffer you from eating disorder relapse in the future.

Your eating disorder affects your body, mind, and spirit. Getting better often includes some kind of healing work for all three. Creating a treatment team that includes medical, psychological, nutritional, and other experts to help you in your journey is typical. If your symptoms are severe or life-threatening, part of your treatment may need to take place in a protected environment, such as a hospital or residential treatment center.

Part II of this book is devoted to helping you through the maze of treatment choices. You can read about which steps you need to take first, who to contact, and how to choose among a variety of treatment approaches. I also include chapters on how to participate in treatment effectively and how to deal with relapse.

Emerging developments in treatment

In the early days of discovering anorexia, treatment focused on unraveling the hidden psychological dynamics holding the symptoms in place. Being able to see behind the curtain and make sense of things continues to be an important treatment option. But the last several decades have introduced treatments that allow you to work directly on reducing symptoms without having to reflect on their meaning. Cognitive Behavioral Therapy (CBT) was the first of these. Interpersonal therapy (IPT) and Thought Field Therapy (TFT) are two of the more recent additions. (I describe these and other therapies for eating disorders in detail in Chapter 10.)

Chapter 2

Getting Insight into Anorexia Nervosa

*L*ike the phantom in *The Phantom of the Opera,* anorexia nervosa has two domains: what's outside for everyone to see and what's inside, hidden not only from others but often even from the sufferer herself.

The visible behaviors and outcomes of anorexia are often shocking, except to people with the disorder. You can easily get lost in the focus on what's visible on the outside. But as you discover in this chapter, these behaviors are driven by an invisible engine of internal distress — and an astonishing level of determination to overcome that distress through thinness.

If you have anorexia, you may not agree with the part about distress or anything else in this chapter that describes your emotional reactions. You may feel that you're solving what's distressing in your life with your thinness and ability to control what you eat. Consider that, in fact, the genius of your anorexia is that it takes all that internal distress and turns it into one simple external issue: the daily challenge of avoiding fat and staying thin. Anorexia gives you a feeling of control when you otherwise feel helpless in life, and it makes you feel worthwhile when you so often doubt your worth.

This chapter reveals the key behaviors, psychological characteristics, and physical features that define anorexia. You can begin, if you like, by taking the questionnaire in the section "Determining Whether You Have Anorexia" at the end of this chapter, which taps anorexic characteristics.

Putting Anorexia Nervosa into Words

Anorexia is a severe emotional disorder that impacts your mind and damages your body through starvation. The hallmarks of anorexia are a fear of fatness and a refusal to eat. If you have anorexia, you've developed a fear of becoming fat that organizes your entire existence. You believe you're always on the verge of becoming fat, regardless of your actual weight or what anybody tells you about how thin you are. You take steps to manage your fear of fatness by refusing to eat. Food refusal also allows you to feel in control, which is of central importance to your sense of well-being. You may also binge and purge and may exercise compulsively to help control your weight.

Anorexia takes its toll on both your brain and your body. (For more information on the ways it affects your body, see Chapter 6.) The physical symptoms of anorexia are due to starvation. These symptoms include:

- ✔ Heart muscle damage
- ✔ Heartbeat irregularities
- ✔ Low blood pressure
- ✔ Kidney damage or failure
- ✔ Convulsions, seizures
- ✔ Liver damage or failure
- ✔ Loss of menstrual periods
- ✔ Loss of bone density
- ✔ Fertility problems

Anorexia nervosa is a *progressive* disorder, meaning that, without treatment, the disorder just gets worse and worse over time. The longer you have anorexia, the greater your risk of death. This progression is very likely due to the unique interaction between the mind and the body. The psychological and physical factors work together to create a tighter and tighter knot to untie, a prison of distorted thoughts and behaviors:

- ✔ **Distorted Behaviors:** You have psychological features that take on an increasingly addictive quality — probably feeling more and more vital for survival — as you become more deeply involved in your eating disorder and the rituals that accompany it. (See the section "Becoming ritualistic," later in this chapter, for more information on ritualistic behavior.)

- ✔ **Dangerous Thinking:** At some point, starvation begins to affect your brain and impair your thought processes. These effects actually change your emotions and the way you think. For instance, you may feel depressed or your need to be a perfectionist may increase. (I discuss these effects in more detail in Chapter 7.)

Anorexia defined by sufferers

If you have anorexia, it's desperately important to you to maintain control of your weight and eating — and, for that matter, anything else you can control about your life. You like to get everything *just right*. Being thin, being restrictive about eating, and being perfect are how you try to make your world feel safe. It feels less safe when you think of facing an unknown or hard-to-control future. Here is how those issues look among different people with anorexia:

> *Jenny* is 8 years old. Her parents are getting a divorce. Everything in her world is turning upside down. When she thinks about dieting, she's not so upset. She's found something she's in charge of — what she puts in her mouth!

> *Nicole* is 13. Her friends talk about nothing but boys, which she finds stupid and boring. Even though her friends say they're worried because she's so thin, she thinks they're actually jealous. After all, they've all been dieting, too.

> *Michelle* is 18. She's just getting out of the hospital where she went when her weight fell dangerously low. She's a straight-A student with an athletic scholarship in track and field, but her parents have told her she can't go away to college in the fall if she doesn't maintain her hospital discharge weight. She's had to limit practice to keep her weight up and is afraid she'll lose her scholarship.

> *Polly* is 54. Her husband left her last year for his secretary (age 22). Compulsive dieting and exercise are taking the place of the life she lost and the future she can't imagine. Besides, she likes picturing that she's thinner than her ex's new wife.

> *Marie* is 79. Her kids and doctor have just made her leave her home of 45 years and move to this assisted living place. Okay, they won that one, but they can't force her to eat the food!

Anorexia defined by professionals

Mental health professionals attempt to establish a basic working agreement with each other about what constitutes various psychological disorders, including eating disorders. Controversy abounds, but these agreements, to the extent that they exist, come together in the *Diagnostic and Statistical Manual of Mental Disorders,* 4th Edition (DSM-IV), published by the American Psychiatric Association.

Be sure to notice that, right off the bat, DSM-IV distinguishes anorexia from any involuntary form of weight loss — such as weight loss resulting from an illness like tuberculosis or cancer — with the language "*refusal* to maintain body weight."

The following list paraphrases the DSM-IV's definition of the characteristics of anorexia:

- **Refusal to maintain minimum body weight:** Weight loss (or failure to gain weight during a growth period) leading to a body weight that is less than 85 percent of the normal minimum weight expected in accordance with age and height.

- **Fat phobia:** Intense fear of gaining weight or becoming fat, even though you're underweight.

- **Body image disturbance:** Disturbance in the way in which you experience your body weight or shape, or basing your self-image on weight.

- **Body weight denial:** Denial of the seriousness of your current low body weight.

- **Loss of menstrual periods in women:** Amenorrhea (the absence of at least three consecutive menstrual cycles). *Note:* This criterion doesn't apply to girls who haven't started menstruating, but may still have anorexia.

The DSM-IV also breaks anorexia out into two basic types:

- **Restricting type:** During the current episode of anorexia nervosa, you have not regularly engaged in binge eating or purging behavior. In the restricting type of anorexia, you rely only on cutting calories, and probably exercising, to control weight.

- **Bingeing/purging type:** During the current episode of anorexia nervosa, you have regularly engaged in binge eating or purging behavior.

In both the restricting and bingeing/purging types of anorexia, starvation is a key component. But according to Anorexia Nervosa and Related Eating Disorders (ANRED), Inc. (www.anred.com), as many as half of those who attempt to starve themselves can't stick to the starvation regime (it does totally defy nature!) and become bulimic rather than anorexic. (See Chapter 3 for more on bulimia.)

Others remain anorexic, but add purging — that is, they remain underweight and continue to starve, but they also resort to the purging techniques more typically associated with bulimia in order to control their weight. Purging techniques include vomiting, laxative and diuretic abuse, and/or the use of enemas. This second group constitutes the binge/purge subtype of anorexia. Some may actually have binge episodes, but many purge any time they eat more than their bare-bones regimens allow.

Looking at Anorexia's Behavioral Traits

If you have anorexia, you probably engage in some or all of the following characteristic behaviors. Because anorexia is progressive, you can expect all of these behaviors to become more pronounced or frequent the longer you have the disorder and don't seek treatment.

Restricting food intake — severely

The hallmark of anorexia is your refusal to eat, even for basic nutritional needs, in spite of facing starvation and the risk of death. The official criteria consider refusal to eat as anorexia when your weight falls below 85 percent of what is normal for your age and height.

Your food restricting is mostly in the form of calorie counting. Intake of just a few hundred calories a day is not unusual. But you may also cut out entire food groups. Fats, of course, are out. Carbs — that is, starches and sweets — are almost always out. Anorexic restricting is not just dieting. It's dieting run amok.

Becoming ritualistic

As anorexia develops, your eating habits get a little more precise. Everything related to the food you eat (or don't eat) comes under the strictest control, and you practice certain rituals related to eating. For example:

- Only certain foods are eaten.
- Foods are eaten only in certain combinations, in a certain order, or in certain bite sizes.
- You eat on a schedule others find strange, and you usually eat in private.
- You focus excessively on calories. Food accompaniments like condiments and spices get elevated to food group status because of their low caloric value.

And, as quirky as it may seem, you are frequently the family chef. Your interest in food has become obsessive and may lead you to pore over recipes and to shop for and prepare gourmet meals for your family (excluding yourself, or course, except as a test of your willpower to abstain).

Exercising compulsively

In anorexia, your basic drive in life is toward thinness and away from fat. Restricting calories is one major means to this end. Burning them up is another. If you have the restricting type of anorexia, you're particularly likely to be obsessively devoted to your exercise routines *and any other extra motion or exertion that will burn up more calories*. You probably feel the same loss of control if you miss your exercise session as you do if you eat more than you meant to. And you probably exercise excessively, maybe for several hours a day, even if you're ill or injured, or your body is what others consider emaciated.

Feeling hyperactive

As anorexia progresses, you may show a kind of restlessness that seems to be driven from inside. It goes beyond your weight loss strategy and isn't something you can voluntarily control. Researchers think this form of hyperactivity is probably an outcome of starvation, either in the way starving affects body chemistry or the way it lowers your core body temperature. The hyperactivity is thought to be your body's instinctive response in an attempt to raise its temperature.

Bingeing — the big blowout

A binge isn't the amount you eat at the company picnic or even the tub of popcorn you go through while watching a movie. A bona fide binge involves taking in as much as 4 to 5 days' worth of calories within a short period of time — and feeling desperate about it afterward.

The notion that having anorexia means you're not hungry is a myth. In reality, you're likely to experience constant hunger (not surprisingly) — you're starving! What do you do with that hunger? At times, you may do exactly what your body is screaming at you to do — eat! Bingeing is a normal response to starvation.

Using laxatives or enemas to atone

In the purging form of anorexia, you take action to get rid of calories when you believe you've eaten too much. Use of laxatives, enemas, or diuretics (water pills) and self-induced vomiting are common practices.

Purging practices put a severe strain on your body, which is already stressed to its limits by starvation. The outlook for the purging type of anorexia is actually a lot hairier than that of restricting anorexia. Getting better is harder if you purge.

Seeing Anorexia's Psychological Traits

Your psychological world as a person with anorexia is a fiercely controlled mini-universe that has come to feel absolutely essential to your psychological survival. As a vulnerable person you arrive at anorexia's door feeling completely inadequate. You don't know who you are or how you are supposed to take on the challenges that lie ahead in life. Anorexia offers a retreat from that forbidding world. But at the same time you believe your control and discipline will command the world's admiration.

As anorexia progresses, you, the person with the disorder, become more and more obsessed with food and dieting. This obsession is part of creating that controlled mini-universe, a place you can always lose yourself in when real-life challenges seem overwhelming. In the mini-universe, the terms of success are pretty much under your control, if you can just keep managing your hunger. The preoccupations and processes I discuss in the following sections typically make up the anorexic psychological universe.

Body image disturbance

In crossing over the line from everyday dieting to anorexia, you lose the ability to see yourself accurately when it comes to weight and body fat. Body image disturbance is a small pocket of irrationality in an otherwise lucid human being.

Those who are not anorexic probably can't comprehend the extent of this delusion by comparing it to self-critical moments with their own bodies. Even the most scarily emaciated anorexic person looks in the mirror and sees fat. She can't be talked out of it.

Fat phobia

Having anorexia means you are *terrified* of gaining weight, even when on the brink of death from starvation. Your conscious thoughts are about how fat and disgusting you look — or will look, if you eat another forkful.

Just beneath the surface, as you see in a minute, is an enormous fear, in which you equate fat — any fat — with being out of control of your life altogether. A victory over fat is a victory over feeling powerless.

Self-image based on weight

Like others with eating disorders and, for that matter, a lot of the female population of this country, having anorexia, you confuse your weight with your worth. If you weigh more than you think you should, nothing else about you counts.

The difference between people with anorexia and others who sometimes have these feelings is that for you, the belief is so unshakable that you pursue dieting beyond any limits the rest of us impose, like starvation and the threat of death.

Denial of the existence of a problem

Anorexic denial is in that same pocket of irrationality as the body image disturbance, in which you can only see yourself as fat. You deny the existence of any risky, perhaps deadly, consequences of your condition or behaviors. Emaciation, chronic hunger, fatigue, numbness, dizziness, and a parade of other side effects of starvation either don't exist or don't matter.

Adolescents, the largest group of anorexic people, aren't great at seeing the consequences of their behavior anyway. The psychological urgency of anorexia and perhaps the physical effects of starvation on the brain just exaggerate this already risky life-stage tendency. The death rate for anorexia is higher than for any other psychological disorder. This is true not only for adolescents, but for people of all ages. In fact, the death rate from anorexia is even higher for older people. (See Chapter 19 for more on this.)

Preoccupation with personal control

If anorexia is about anything, it's about being in control. Or at least feeling in control. (Being in control and feeling in control are two different things.) As a person with anorexia, your empire is your body and you exercise your power by saying no to food and to anyone who wants to make you eat.

What is going on that makes the creation of such an empire feel so important? The need to create this kind of empire reflects your feeling of powerlessness, in part, because you don't feel in control of your external environment. Following are some common ways your external environment may leave you feeling you have too little control:

✔ Being a child in a family where parents hold the reins a bit too tight so it's hard to stretch and feel personal independence

✔ Finding yourself among peers who are raring to move on to the next stage in life and seem, magically, to know exactly how to do it, when you feel neither eager nor capable

✔ Being faced with other life transitions for which you feel unready (leaving home, graduating, becoming sexual, entering the work world, marriage, and so on)

Perfectionism

As a person with anorexia, you experience a need to get everything right in order to feel that you're okay. All of the eating disorders are characterized by this quality, but it may look a little different in you. In other eating disorders, perfectionism has more to do with trying to undo rampant feelings of shame. Although you are certainly struggling with limping self-worth, you have put your money on being thin and being in control. Your perfectionism is increasingly related to these efforts. Here are some examples:

Jillian has had a perfect day. She's had 50 calories plus water for breakfast, 50 calories plus water for lunch and 50 calories plus water for dinner. She's climbing up and down the stairs to the basement now to burn off dinner.

Elissa had a 4.0 average for her first two years in high school. If there were a way to record all her A+s, she'd have a 4.5 average.

Amanda is a model. She didn't get the last job she tried out for. She was sure it was because of her weight. (Amanda wears a size 2.) She fasted three days before she was next sent out, just to make sure.

Girls with anorexia, in particular, are well-known to have spent their pre-anorexic careers as the best of children. They are model students who do everything right. These girls concluded long ago that they have to perform at extraordinary levels to be valued. Discovering the "empire of thin" allows them to take their extraordinary powers to a place shared by few others. If they surrender — even for a moment — to mere human urges for food, it becomes a harsh reminder of how powerless and ineffective they feel without their symptoms.

Interestingly, researchers are finding some overlap between anorexic perfectionism and the traits of obsessive-compulsive disorder (OCD) — a syndrome of need for control, if ever there was one. (Read more about eating disorders and OCD in Chapter 7.)

Black-and-white thinking

Black-and-white thinking is another characteristic you find in just about everyone with an eating disorder. When experiences are processed in this manner, they must be either one way or another, with no gray area in between. For example, you may think like this:

- ✔ I get everything right, or I'm stupid and worthless.
- ✔ The first ounce of extra fat puts me on the road to obesity.
- ✔ I'm in perfect control of everything, or I'm totally out of control.

This thinking style meshes with your standards of perfection, but it makes life awfully difficult to live. If you think in this black-and-white way, chances are you learned it in a family where other members thought in a similar way.

Need for external approval

A constant need for the approval of others describes almost everyone with an eating disorder. In anorexia, this need often reflects growing up with the belief that you are valued more for what you *do* than who you *are,* or that you are valued most when you do what others want you to do.

People with these beliefs inevitably become focused outside themselves. That's where the information they need — what other people think or want —comes from. But this reliance on others comes at the expense of knowing themselves and their own needs. Believe it or not, people are not born with this ability to know themselves. For most people, it comes about as a result of being nurtured through the care and interest of others. The person with anorexia who lacks this nurturing fails to develop the ability to know herself, her needs, her feelings, her beliefs, and so on, and this void feeds the feelings of powerlessness she experiences.

Orthorexia nervosa

Orthorexia nervosa is a term coined by Colorado physician Steven Bratman to describe the patient who, like a person with anorexia, has made food and eating an obsession, but for a different reason. For the orthorexic person, the obsession is about health and the purity of the foods eaten rather than calories. As with anorexia, it can start innocently, usually as a health quest, and end up with the person's life and self-image being controlled by the rules of pure eating.

Determining Whether You Have Anorexia

If you're wondering whether your way of eating and thinking fits an anorexic pattern, you may want to try responding to the following statements.

Keep in mind that this questionnaire is only intended to jiggle your curiosity. **It in no way substitutes for getting a competent diagnosis from a qualified eating disorders professional.**

Instructions: Check each item that feels true or mainly true of you. I tell you how to score your responses at the end.

1. ❏ I've recently lost a lot of weight for no known medical cause.
2. ❏ I'm terrified of gaining weight.
3. ❏ I tend to want to go even lower when I reach a weight-loss goal.
4. ❏ I'm afraid that when I eat, I'll lose control and be unable to stop.
5. ❏ I think about food, weight, and calories almost all the time.
6. ❏ I keep calories to the minimum to lose weight or avoid gaining weight.
7. ❏ I sometimes rely on one or more of the following to lose weight or deal with overeating: laxatives, water pills, vomiting, or enemas.
8. ❏ I feel relieved or more in control when I starve.
9. ❏ I allow my weight to determine how I'm going to feel about myself on any given day.
10. ❏ I feel fat, no matter how much other people tell me I'm (too) thin.
11. ❏ I wear clothes that hide my weight.
12. ❏ I exercise so much to control my weight that some people consider my workouts to be excessive.
13. ❏ I feel anxious if I have to miss any part of my workout.
14. ❏ I get upset when people pressure me to eat more or gain weight.
15. ❏ I make up reasons to avoid eating with other people.
16. ❏ I love to cook for others, but of course I don't eat any of the food myself.
17. ❏ I have a secret food stash.
18. ❏ I've noticed one or more of the following physical symptoms:
    - ❏ Loss of menstrual periods
    - ❏ Weakness or fatigue

- ❑ Low blood pressure

- ❑ Dry skin, hair, or nails

- ❑ Irregular heartbeat

- ❑ Intolerance of cold, especially hands and feet

- ❑ Dizziness

- ❑ Bruising more easily

- ❑ Growth of fine body and facial hair; loss of head hair

19. ❑ I often feel I'm not good enough, or that something is missing inside.

20. ❑ I feel that getting everything perfect is very important.

21. ❑ I'm a "people-pleaser."

22. ❑ I'm very proud of being thin.

23. ❑ I'd like myself better — and others would like me better too — if I were thinner.

Scoring: Give yourself one point for every item you checked, including a point for each separate item you checked on Item 18.

If you score 12 points or more, you have reason to be concerned. Your feet are already on an anorexic path. Dealing with your symptoms now is *much* better than waiting until you're farther down the road, when all your symptoms are more entrenched and you're dealing with the physical effects of the disorder on your body.

If you score 20 points or more, you may well have already developed an anorexic pattern. Getting diagnosed and seeking out the best treatment options you can find without delay is extremely important for your health and emotional well-being. The treatment section of this book (Part II) helps you do that.

Chapter 3

Seeing Inside Bulimia Nervosa

· ·

In This Chapter

▶ Reviewing the patterns of a bulimic profile

▶ Identifying the signature behaviors of bulimia

▶ Associating some psychological features with bulimia

▶ Completing a questionnaire to assess your bulimic tendencies

· ·

*I*f you have bulimia, you may be a student, a homemaker, an athlete, an entertainer, an executive — or come from any other walk of life. You may come from the suburbs or come from the streets. Your life may appear well-under-control or be quite chaotic. Yet despite all the ways your life may look different from the lives of other people with bulimia, in one way your lives are strikingly similar: You conceal a secret life of bingeing and purging that constantly demoralizes you and drains you of energy and self-esteem.

In this chapter, I shed light on the secret life of bulimic behaviors so that you and the people who love you can better understand what you're dealing with. You get a handle not only on the behaviors themselves, but also on the psychological underpinnings that keep the condition going.

In order to allow you to check your pattern against a bulimic one, I provide a questionnaire at the end of the chapter.

Identifying the Many Faces Of Bulimia

As with just about any illness or disorder, bulimia has no simple black-and-white definition. It's a complicated disorder with various faces. To help you get familiar with the disorder and possibly start down the road to diagnosis, the following sections present both real-life situations and psychiatric definitions that deal with the disorder.

Bulimia is a treacherous disorder that takes its toll on the body and the spirit of sufferers. (Read more about the physical consequences of bulimia in Chapter 6.) With chronic purging behavior, the risks you take include the following:

- ✔ Damage to your heart or heart functioning
- ✔ Liver failure
- ✔ Kidney failure
- ✔ Damage to your esophagus
- ✔ Damage to the functioning of your gastrointestinal system (for example, bloating, constipation, diarrhea)
- ✔ Damage to your tooth enamel

Beyond the physical consequences of bulimia are its damaging emotional effects. Your attempts to calm and soothe yourself with food have turned into the monster of out-of-control bingeing. The more you try to bring your bingeing (and, thus, your weight) under control with purging, the more the binges seem to occur. These behaviors serve to exaggerate the already-heavy burden of shame you carry around about yourself and lower your self-esteem even further.

Bulimia expressed by sufferers

Each of the people you're about to meet represents a different face of bulimia. If you're bulimic (or think you may be), you know these people. You may not exhibit one of these exact behaviors, but you recognize the experience of a relationship to food that has gone out of control. Unlike the person with anorexia who denies that anything is wrong (see Chapter 2), you know something is dreadfully wrong. In fact, you feel utterly possessed by your feelings and urges.

> *Cassy* feels overwhelmed with self-loathing and hopelessness after a day in which she has binged and purged 22 times. The only thing she can think to do is get really drunk.

> *MaryAnn,* a suburban housewife, tries to scrape the layer of bug spray off the cake she threw in the garbage so she can eat it before her kids get home.

> *Nicky* has just vomited her dinner in the restaurant's bathroom, hoping none of her friends would follow her in. She's frantically searching her purse for those darn breath mints.

Bulimia expressed by professionals

Despite differences in lifestyle among people with bulimia, the disorder has some pretty clear and common characteristics that allow therapists to recognize and treat it. Experts rely on the presence of bingeing and purging behaviors to diagnose bulimia.

The *Diagnostic and Statistical Manual of Mental Disorders,* 4th Edition (DSM-IV), published by the American Psychiatric Association, provides guidelines that mental health professionals and insurance companies use to diagnose various psychological disorders. The following list paraphrases how the DSM-IV defines bulimia:

- **Bingeing episodes:** Recurrent episodes of binge eating. An episode of binge eating is characterized by both of the following:

  - Eating, in a discreet period of time (within any two-hour period, for instance), an amount of food that's definitely larger than most people would eat during a similar period of time and under similar circumstances

  - A sense of lack of control over eating during the episode (a feeling that you can't stop eating or control what or how much you're eating)

- **Purging episodes:** Recurrent compensatory behavior in order to prevent weight gain after the binge. Behaviors include the following:

  - Self-induced vomiting

  - Misuse of laxatives, diuretics, enemas, or other medications

  - Fasting

  - Excessive exercise

- **Frequency:** The binge eating and purging (or other compensatory behavior) both occur, on average, at least twice a week for three months.

- **Weight equated with worth:** Your self-evaluation is unduly influenced by body shape and weight.

- **Bingeing and purging are not related to anorexia:** The disturbance doesn't occur exclusively during episodes of anorexia nervosa. (You don't also meet the criteria for anorexia while engaging in bingeing and purging behaviors.)

The DSM-IV distinguishes between two types of bulimia. The difference between the two is that one involves purging, while the other doesn't:

> ✔ **Purging type:** During the current episode, you regularly engage in self-induced vomiting or the misuse of laxatives, diuretics, or enemas.

> ✔ **Non-purging type:** During the current episode, you use other inappropriate compensatory behaviors, such as fasting or excessive exercise, but you don't regularly engage in self-induced vomiting or the misuse of laxatives, diuretics, or enemas.

Recognizing Bulimia's Behavioral Traits

A person with anorexia is controlled — especially if she has the restricting type of anorexia (see Chapter 2). But as controlled as the person with anorexia is, that's how out of control a person with bulimia can feel and be. You struggle to manage your impulses on many fronts, not just with food. These areas of struggle can include drug abuse, self-injury, stealing (related to your bulimia), or missing priorities because of your symptoms (see Chapter 7 for more).

Despite the constant struggle against chaos, you may manage enough of your life quite well. No one may be the wiser to your condition because your symptoms are so well-hidden. Of course, the emotional price for this behavior is enormous. The following sections break down the behavioral features of bulimia and how the afflicted person can hide them as she spirals out of control.

Bingeing — not your ordinary overeating

The word "binge" has become a common expression for any kind of excess behavior. People talk about bingeing on eating, shopping, watching television, reading trashy romance novels, and so on. But if you have bulimia, you know that ordinary "overdoing it" has no resemblance to what happens when you enter a binge state, in terms of your behavior or your emotions. The following sections detail the binge state of mind and the patterns that develop out of it.

You may call it a "binge" any time you eat more than you mean to or eat some "forbidden" food, but I reserve the term for episodes where you take in unusually large amounts of food in a very short period of time. A single binge may involve tens of thousands of calories. In the binge state, you probably prefer carbs and sweets, but you'll eat anything. Whereas a person with anorexia may eat plain mustard because it has few calories, you eat it because you're up at 3:00 a.m. and that's all you have left in your fridge. Or perhaps you want to drive to the all-night deli farthest away from your home because you're too embarrassed to go back to the one where you dined earlier this evening.

I use the term *binge state* because many, if not most, people with bulimia describe being in some kind of altered state when bingeing. The following feelings are common in this state:

✔ You feel as if you're outside yourself, watching what's going on.

✔ You feel numb or anesthetized.

✔ You feel as if you're in a zone of unusual calm.

✔ You feel a constant drumbeat of internal pressure: "I *must* do this."

The common thread in these bingeing experiences is the sense that what you're doing is outside your voluntary control. You feel as if some other force has taken over while all your will and good intentions get left by the roadside. This "I have to" urgency doesn't come from the food or hunger (unless you've been starving yourself). It comes from what the food is supposed to do for you: to calm you down or cover up overwhelming emotions. (I go into this in detail in Chapter 5.)

The binge state probably lasts until your stomach is in pain. Most likely, you reach some kind of psychological tipping point and shift out of the altered state — at which time you readily feel the pain in your stomach.

If you're reading this in support of a bulimic person, you need to understand just how different out-of-control binge urgency feels from ordinary strong urges. The people who understand most readily are those with some kind of addiction — drugs, alcohol, gambling, and so on. In fact, many experts consider eating disorders to be addictions. Whether or not you agree, the urge to binge certainly has all the irresistible strength of addictive behavior. (To become more understanding and helpful, turn to Part IV.)

Purging to compensate

If you have bulimia, chances are you feel absolutely frantic and desperate when you shift out of the binge state. You have to do *something* about the food you just ate. Actually, not just something; you have to get rid of it! If you're a compulsive exerciser, you have your internal ledger cooking and it dictates how many miles you have to run or how long you have to spend on the stairmaster to burn off those calories.

More likely, though, you've discovered one of the purging techniques associated with bulimia (see the section "Bulimia expressed by professionals"). With these methods, you want to get the calories out of your system pronto. Here are the most common purge behaviors:

✔ **Vomiting:** Vomiting on purpose for the relief it gives you when you've binged is a form of purging. You may do this by sticking your fingers down your throat until you trigger a gag reflex. Or perhaps you use some kind of implement to achieve the same end. Many people with bulimia have engaged in the behavior long enough that they only have to lean over for the gag reflex to occur. And for all the years of warnings about the deadly dangers of ipecac syrup (warnings I happily repeat in Chapter 6), way too many people still rely on this poison to induce vomiting in order to purge.

✔ **Laxative and enema abuse:** Many people with bulimia prefer to induce rapid transit through and out of their bowels as a way to rid their bodies of excess calories. If you use this method, your thinking probably is, "If a little is good, more is better." Some bulimics have been known to use dozens to hundreds of doses a day of laxatives. (See the sidebar "What happens when you purge with laxatives?" for a rundown on how laxatives work in your system.)

✔ **Diuretic abuse:** Perhaps you take diuretics (water pills) to lose fluids by urinating more frequently to achieve the same effect as taking laxatives.

Your bingeing and purging behaviors may be a once-in-awhile thing. Perhaps you binge and purge predictably at times of stress or as a way to channel emotion. Or, maybe cycling between bingeing and purging has become part of your daily living routine.

For many people, bingeing and purging behaviors alternate with periods of dieting. Maybe you meet with varying success in your dieting efforts. Perhaps you're always a little underweight, but not enough to draw attention like a person with anorexia (see Chapter 2). Maybe you hover around an average weight or are somewhat above that. You purge when dieting isn't doing the job to keep you where you want to be, or isn't doing it fast enough.

Keeping your bulimia a secret

Unlike the person with anorexia who feels pride in her symptoms (see Chapter 2), when you have bulimia you feel the need for extreme secrecy:

✔ You hide both your bingeing and purging behaviors.

✔ You may hide your binge foods.

✔ You turn on water in the bathroom to cover up sounds of vomiting.

✔ You may have a bulimia diary or participate in secret chat rooms.

What happens when you purge with laxatives?

You may or may not be aware of the great irony of laxative abuse for calorie management: Laxatives take effect in your large intestine *well after* most calorie absorption has already occurred in your small intestine. Taking laxatives has almost no effect on the calories in your body. The laxatives remove water from your colon; any weight loss is the result of dehydration.

Knowing this, laxative abuse should be history, right? Unfortunately, you may continue because you like the feeling of a temporarily flattened tummy. Or perhaps you maintain a case of denial, the way sufferers of anorexia do, because you need to feel you can do *something* to gain a sense of control. In recovery, you learn skills that allow you to feel real control in your life. Head straight to the chapters of Part II to find out more.

Bulimic secrecy is driven by shame. If you're bulimic, you probably feel shame about not only your symptoms, but also the ordinary flaws you live with as a human being. To have your symptoms exposed to the world is beyond imagination. In recovery it will be a big relief to learn that everyone has the same secrets and you can actually talk about them. (See Chapters 10 and 11.)

Avoiding situations that involve food

After you've binged for awhile and have tried unsuccessfully to stop yourself, you begin to feel afraid of losing control in any tempting food situation. For this reason, you may begin to limit your social interactions. For instance, you may not attend parties or other social situations — graduation gatherings, company lunches, family reunions — that are likely to have goodies on hand that you find hard to handle.

This is too bad. If you have bulimia, you already don't tend to see other people as safe, so you're probably avoiding social situations enough as is. Avoiding them because of food only leaves you home alone more often, out of the normal social loop. And this leaves you more vulnerable to bingeing and purging and more secrecy.

Seeing Bulimia's Psychological Traits

If you have bulimia, you probably arrived at it with more psychological baggage than people with other eating disorders. Your personal history may involve a lot more disruption, perhaps even trauma. Your past may have left you without the basic resources you need to feel good about yourself or to manage your life. Many companion disorders tend to go with eating disorders, like depression, anxiety, and addiction (you can read more about these in Chapter 7). In addition, the following psychological features tend to show up over and over again in people with bulimia.

Perfectionism, black-and-white thinking, and a need for external approval not only are part of your bulimia now, but also probably are traits you had before you developed bulimia. In Chapter 5, you can read about how these and other qualities make a person especially vulnerable to developing an eating disorder. The reason these so-called "vulnerability traits" are important to know about and understand is that developing greater resiliency in these areas is a crucial part of your recovery from your eating disorder. I talk about this more in the chapters of Part II.

Feeling disgust and self-hatred

For almost all sufferers of bulimia, disgust and self-hatred are the predictable feelings during the aftermath of a binge. Your suffering can be terrible. You feel that others, if they knew, would be equally disgusted with you, and that you would be — and should be — excluded from polite society. You feel isolated and without comfort in your self-hatred.

Far too many people with bulimia walk around with these feelings all the time, not just when they binge. For a lot of people with bulimia, these feelings are the legacy of a history of abuse or neglect. Anything you do wrong threatens to bring the feelings from your background to the crushing foreground.

And here's a cruel twist: Perhaps you (unconsciously) "hired" your eating disorder to help keep feelings of disgust and self-hatred from the past at a distance. Tragically, your bulimic symptoms just end up producing more of these difficult feelings.

Equating weight with self-worth

Many people with rocky histories who doubt their own worth tend to grab on to the cultural promise of a brass ring for the slim like nobody's business. These people equate weight with self-worth. Maybe a demanding and unrealistic sports coach, dance instructor, or even parent nudged you along in this direction.

When you suffer from bulimia, at many times it feels like weight is the only thing even theoretically under your control — especially when it comes to trying to feel good about yourself. This trait shows up in the belief that nothing else about you matters if you're not the right weight, so you purge to manage your weight. Most people with this disorder live in mortal fear that if they poke around beneath the surface of weight, they'll find nothing of worth about themselves. Better, it seems, to stay focused on the weight, because there's always the hope of fixing that.

Seeking elusive perfection

In the scenario of bulimia, perfectionism — trying to get *everything* right — is an attempt at protecting your self-image that requires constant vigilance. When you're forever feeling worthless, perfectionism is an interesting thing. The word conjures up a society hostess putting the final touches on a gala dinner. Whatever it may appear like to others, to a person with bulimia, perfectionism is instead a matter of forever trying to dig out of a ditch of worthlessness.

See if you recognize yourself in either of the following examples:

> *Patti* was at a party last night — her last with this crowd, she was sure. Right in the middle of the dance floor, she slipped and fell in front of everyone. She didn't think she could face anyone again after such a humiliation.

> *Lindsey* had just been through the worst week of her life. She promised herself a quiet day on Saturday to catch up at home, nap, and do what she pleased. But when her good friend, Ana, called to say she was still blue about the breakup with her boyfriend and wanted company to go shopping, Lindsey felt she had no choice but to say yes. Aren't you always supposed to be available when your friends need you?

Aiming at perfection to achieve worth is a process that you feel you have to begin again every day. You never accumulate any self-worth capital with yourself, nor do you believe you do with others. Every moment in which you could make a mistake is one in which you could fall back into that ditch of worthlessness. In the bulimic scenario, perfectionism is a constant struggle.

Limiting your thinking to black and white

If you have a black-and-white thinking style, you tend to see things as all one way or all another, with no in-between. You experience events or people, including yourself, as all good or all bad, all hopeful or all discouraging, all worthwhile or all worthless, and so on. For example, if you eat more than you meant to, you've ruined everything (so you may as well go ahead and binge). If you make a mistake, you're obviously stupid or inept. If you recognize this rigid thinking style as your own, chances are you learned it in a family where other members also think in black-and-white ways.

As your eating disorder progresses, this black-and-white thinking style is an important part of what makes your condition worsen. It leaves you forever on a narrow ledge of self-esteem from which you can fall for any lapse. If something doesn't go exactly as planned (isn't perfect; see the section "Seeking elusive perfection"), your world (your emotions) can crumble. Here are some examples:

- ✔ I'm at my goal weight, or I'm gross and disgusting.
- ✔ I ate exactly what I intended, or I pigged out.
- ✔ My friends approve of me every moment or they hate me.
- ✔ I binged and purged again, so I'm worthless.

Needing others' approval

A need for external approval is a quality you share with many people who have eating disorders; although how you developed it may differ. In order to develop trust in your own views, two key ingredients should be present in childhood:

- ✔ **Your childhood environment must feel safe enough for you to relax and focus on yourself.** If your environment is in turmoil when you're young, coming to know your own thinking, feelings, and opinions is a luxury you can't afford. As a practical matter, your focus turns outward to make sure you're alert to what your environment may throw at you next.

- ✔ **Your caregivers must support your growing sense of your individual viewpoint.** If your caregivers don't help you learn to prize your own views, you don't learn to prize them either. In fact, you may quit noticing you even have them! Under these conditions, other people's opinions have to fill in for opinions you can't find or trust in yourself.

You need to feel solid and grounded in yourself as a person. Feeling secure as an individual can help you withstand social pressures to be thinner than your body is meant to be.

Feeling overwhelmed by the disorder

If you've been around the bulimia block for awhile, you probably feel like the prospects for ever living another way are remote. You feel exhausted and overwhelmed from the struggle.

Part of feeling so defeated comes from the sheer urgency behind the symptoms. The symptoms of bulimia (bingeing, purging, dieting) always feel urgent. They have developed to help you manage something that was threatening to overwhelm you, such as emotions, current problems, or a history of trauma. The pressure is bound to feel bigger than you, and that feeling may double if you bring the wrong game to confront your symptoms. Perhaps in the past you've tried to get the better of the symptoms with willpower — a strategy that never works with eating disorder symptoms. Unfortunately, you may think this failure is just more evidence of your inadequacy. It isn't!

Determining Whether You Have Bulimia

Perhaps you're wondering if your way of eating and thinking fit a bulimic pattern. Well, you can stop wondering and start acting by responding to the questions in the following list.

Keep in mind, **this questionnaire in no way substitutes for getting a competent diagnosis from a qualified eating disorders professional** (see Chapter 9).

Instructions: Check each item that's true or mainly true of you. I tell you how to score your responses at the end.

1. ❑ I think about food, weight, and calories almost all the time.
2. ❑ I allow my weight to determine how I feel about myself on any given day.
3. ❑ I frequently binge (eat huge quantities in a short time period).
4. ❑ I frequently binge when I feel bad or overwhelmed.
5. ❑ I feel worthless, disgusting, and hopeless after a binge.
6. ❑ I regularly use one or more of the following purging methods to lose weight or compensate for bingeing:
   - ❑ Laxatives
   - ❑ Ipecac syrup (to make myself vomit)
   - ❑ Enemas
   - ❑ Vomiting
   - ❑ Colonics
   - ❑ Water pills
7. ❑ I sometimes exercise excessively to avoid weight gain from a binge.
8. ❑ I go to great lengths to keep my bingeing and purging a secret.
9. ❑ I often diet or fast to try to manage my weight.
10. ❑ I've stolen money, food, laxatives, or diuretics for bingeing or purging.

11. ❏ I've missed school or work due to my bingeing and purging.

12. ❏ I have one or more of the following psychological symptoms:

    - ❏ Depression

    - ❏ Drug abuse (legal or illegal)

    - ❏ Anxiety or panic

    - ❏ Alcohol abuse

    - ❏ Bipolar disorder

    - ❏ Self-injuring behaviors

    - ❏ Episodes of feeling disconnected from myself

13. ❏ I've noticed one or more of the following physical symptoms:

    - ❏ Irregular menstrual periods

    - ❏ Weakness and fatigue

    - ❏ Low blood pressure

    - ❏ "Chipmunk cheeks"

    - ❏ Irregular heart beat

    - ❏ Eroded tooth enamel

    - ❏ Chronic diarrhea

    - ❏ Inflamed throat

14. ❏ I rarely feel that I'm good enough.

15. ❏ I'm a "people-pleaser."

16. ❏ I often feel others are judging me.

17. ❏ I'd like myself more — and others would like me better too — if I were thinner.

18. ❏ Bingeing and purging interfere with my relationships with others.

Scoring: Give yourself one point for every item you checked — including a point for each separate item you checked on Items 6, 12, and 13.

> **If you scored 16 points or more,** you have a lot of indicators of a potential bulimic pattern. Be advised: Treating the condition now is much easier than doing so later, when your symptoms have become entrenched.

> **If you scored 23 points or more,** you have strong reason to suspect bulimia — enough for you to get a sound diagnosis and follow through with any recommendations for treatment. You can find plenty of practical advice to get you started in Part II of this book.

Chapter 4

Understanding Binge Eating Disorder

In This Chapter

▶ Discovering what binge eating disorder really is

▶ Identifying the behavioral and psychological characteristics of people with BED

▶ Finding out whether you fit the profile for BED

*B*inge eating disorder (BED) is the most common of the eating disorders. BED has been around for quite awhile but has just been coming into its own for research and treatment in the last 15 to 20 years. The lines that define just who and what qualify for the disorder are still a little squishy around the edges. But the main lines, the ones important for you to know, are clear. And they're the subject of this chapter.

If you're one of the majority of moderate-weight people with BED, you may have no idea that your use of diets is a central part of your disorder. You find out how and why this is true in the pages ahead — and how the pattern is connected to other aspects of who you are that make you vulnerable to an eating disorder.

You also discover basic differences in the bingeing patterns of moderate-weight versus obese binge eaters. Taken together with the information you find about key psychological features of people with BED, you develop a basic map for what you must work on in recovery (the subject of Part II of this book).

Defining Binge Eating Disorder

Binge eating disorder (BED) is characterized by episodes of overeating, frequently to the point of physical pain. Some binge eaters control their weight by alternating periods of bingeing with dieting, while others gain weight and become obese. Although the underlying psychological problems and physical consequences of BED tend to be less severe than those with anorexia or bulimia, people with the disorder experience intense emotional suffering. They are as dissatisfied with their bodies as people with other eating disorders. And they suffer great anguish, including self-loathing and despair after binge episodes. In this section I fill out the picture of BED for you by providing snapshot profiles of individual sufferers and by going over the professional definition of the disorder.

Binge eating disorder defined by sufferers

If you have binge eating disorder, you may feel that many aspects of your life are basically in order (though you never feel you're doing well enough at any of them). If you could only deal once and for all with those pesky extra 15 to 20 pounds! Of course, that would probably mean controlling bingeing episodes, which you're sure you could if you just tried hard enough. It just never feels as if trying hard enough makes any difference. It actually feels as if you're totally out of control when you binge and you can't stop until the episode has somehow run its course. The disgust and remorse you feel after a binge is often only alleviated by going on a diet. Here are some profiles of people who suffer with binge eating disorder:

Joe is a college wrestler. He binges after matches, especially when he loses. In the off-season, he's started to binge in response to all kinds of disappointments.

Tara has been on every diet you ever heard of. She's the best dieter you can imagine — for about 2 weeks. Then something snaps and she binges. After she binges, she cries and calls herself "stupid" and "pig." At least there's always another diet.

Marge has been a weekend binger since she was 20. She grazes her way almost nonstop from Friday to Sunday night. Now at age 45, she has 50 extra pounds to show for it.

Binge eating disorder defined by professionals

The *Diagnostic and Statistical Manual of Mental Disorders,* 4th Edition (DSM-IV), published by the American Psychiatric Association, provides the guidelines used by mental health professionals and insurance companies to diagnose various psychological disorders.

For those of you who are interested in where binge eating disorder stands as an official diagnosis, DSM-IV currently stashes BED in a category of eating disorders called "not otherwise specified," while the people who decide these things are working on whether to give it equal status with anorexia and bulimia (the most likely outcome). The following list paraphrases how the DSM-IV defines binge eating disorder:

- **Bingeing:** Recurrent episodes of binge eating. An episode of binge eating is characterized by both of the following:

  - Eating, in a discrete period of time (for example, within any 2-hour period), an amount of food that is definitely larger than most people would eat in a similar period of time under similar circumstances

  - A sense of lack of control over your eating during the episode (for example, a feeling that you can't stop eating or control what or how much you're eating)

- **Typical aspects of a binge episode:** The binge eating episodes are associated with three or more of the following:

  - Eating much more rapidly than normal

  - Eating until you feel uncomfortably full

  - Eating large amounts of food when you're not feeling physically hungry

  - Eating alone because you're embarrassed by how much you're eating

  - Feeling disgusted with yourself, depressed, or very guilty after overeating

- **Unlike the anorexic person, the person with BED feels something is wrong:** Marked distress regarding binge eating is present.

- **Frequency:** The binge eating occurs, on average, at least 2 days per week for 6 months. (*Note:* Current research shows there's no difference between once-weekly bingers and those who meet this twice-weekly standard.)

- **The bingeing isn't part of anorexia or bulimia:** The binge eating is not associated with the regular use of inappropriate compensatory behaviors (for example, purging, fasting, or excessive exercise) and does not occur exclusively during the course of anorexia nervosa or bulimia nervosa.

Understanding the Behavioral Features of Binge Eating

From one point of view, describing the behavioral profile of your binge eating disorder is pretty simple. You binge eat, and you do it on a fairly regular basis. (You may want to read Chapter 3 for a more detailed description of the binge experience.) However, things are never as simple as they seem, certainly not with BED. In this section, you find that different sub-groups binge differently and that one of them bears a surprising connection to dieting.

Binge eating across the weight spectrum

An interesting thing happens when you zoom in on binge eaters as a group: Binge behavior looks different across the weight spectrum. Binge eaters can be divided into two groups based on weight: those who are of moderate weight, and those who are obese. Your binge behavior depends to some extent on which group you fit into:

- **How you get into the binge:** Dieting, an *inhibiting* trigger that makes you want to eat more because you've been denying yourself, affects mainly those in the moderate weight category. (I discuss dieting in greater detail in the next section.)

  Those in the obese category are more likely to be triggered by *disinhibitors,* that is, things that reduce inhibitions, like alcohol consumption, according to NIH researcher, Susan Yanovski, MD.

  Both groups — those who are of moderate weight and those who are obese — tend to lose control when confronted with lots of great-looking food.

- **What you do during the binge:** Those of moderate weight tend to have more time-limited bingeing episodes. The binge may last several hours, but then, like the bulimic person's binges, it ends.

  Yanovski's findings show that obese people who binge may make the binge last over the course of a day, "grazing" throughout. (Some people with bulimia do the same thing. Iron-clad boundaries rarely exist with eating disorder behaviors; just trends.)

- **What happens after the binge:** After a binge, those in the obese group tend to go on about their business. Moderate-weight binge eaters are more likely, sooner or later, to go on a diet.

The binge/diet cycle

Most of those in the moderate-weight group of people with BED, and perhaps a number of others all along the BED weight spectrum, get locked into a cycle between periods of binge eating and periods of dieting. You may not even notice the cyclic nature of your pattern. Clues to the cycle you may be aware of are resolutions like: "I have to be good this time" or the despairing feeling: "Why can't I be good?" when the diet ultimately fails. The binge/diet cycle is so central to your disorder that understanding it is valuable for you, those who care about you, and those who want to help you.

Binge/diet cycling is actually just an example of naturally occurring, self-correcting human cycles. These cycles are like a pendulum that swings all the way in one direction, then, in reaction, swings all the way in the other. For instance, in fashion, a period of short hemlines is followed by a period of long hemlines — and then is followed by another period of short hemlines. A couple, feeling too distant from one another, looks for ways to be more intimate — and then follows this with a period in which they need a little more distance. An individual holds in her emotions until one day she explodes, shocking everyone — leading her to be more careful about holding in her emotions.

The more the pendulum swings to an extreme in one direction, the more you correct for it with an extreme swing in the other direction. It's just human nature. In the case of bingeing and dieting, the first half of the cycle is usually pretty easy to see. You correct for the binge phase with a phase of dieting. Most likely, it takes a series of binges to accumulate the resolve to correct with a diet. (By way of contrast, the bulimic person's binge/purge cycle involves correcting each and every binge.) You may need to take a closer look to see the second half of the cycle: how bingeing corrects for dieting. I walk you through each phase, one at a time.

First, you may relate to the following thoughts that typically come up after a binge:

- ✔ I'm disgusting.
- ✔ I can't believe I did it again.
- ✔ I hate myself.
- ✔ I'll never get better.

Now, here are some typical thoughts you may have in conjunction with the resolve to start a diet after a period of bingeing:

- ✔ This time I'm really going to do it.
- ✔ I'm so excited; I'm going to be thin.
- ✔ I'm going to feel good again; I'm going to like myself again.
- ✔ I'm in control again.

Notice how the resolve itself, before the diet has even started, begins to repair your mood and spirit. (If you suspect there's more here to fix than a diet is capable of, even if dieting were the right remedy, you have a good instinct. See the next section on psychological features.)

At this point, the way that you diet is likely to match how extreme your bingeing feels. At first, the diet provides feelings of healing and hopefulness. You're fixing the damage you've done. But eventually, the diet feels oppressive. The results aren't fast enough. The results aren't enough, period. You think you should probably eat less. You project forward and can't imagine going on in this depriving way until you reach your goal weight. The diet that seemed like your salvation now feels like a tyrant.

The rebellion brews underground until you reach some tipping point. Perhaps some other kind of trigger (for example, your job, personal stress, or a disappointment) puts you over the top. Or maybe you just hit your own "I've had it!" threshold. The biggest point here is that the pressure you've been putting on yourself to "fix" yourself leaves another part of you screaming for relief. *This part of you experiences the dieting and your expectations of yourself as every bit as extreme as the binge.* So, knowing deep down that you'll end up back on a diet anyway, it "corrects" for the extreme of dieting with an extreme of bingeing: "For just a darn moment, I'll have whatever I want!" Your dieting has triggered your next binge!

As happens so often with eating disordered behavior, you probably stumbled on dieting innocently as a quick way to deal with a few excess pounds. After all, everybody else did it. But eventually, the self-correcting nature of the cycle took on a life of its own, making it very difficult to change.

Secrecy

Your secrecy about your bingeing behavior is very similar to that of the person with bulimia — you'd probably rather die than have anyone see you binge or guess that you're doing it. You feel so much shame — that is, a sense of personal worthlessness — in relation to your bingeing that you even try to keep strangers, such as food store owners and food delivery people, from knowing what you're up to.

Social withdrawal because of "feeling fat"

For people with bulimia, hiding out from social events to avoid food exposure is often part of a larger picture of more general social avoidance. This tends to be less true for people with BED. You may have a good social network. Your social avoidance has more to do with shame when you "feel fat." You may see your weight go up and down the scale and tend to isolate yourself during "up-the-scale" periods.

Part of your treatment involves determining very frankly whether social connection is scarier than you've been admitting to yourself. You may be more like the person with bulimia if periods of bingeing and weight gain have been operating to provide you with a reason to withdraw to safety.

Connecting BED with other psychological disorders

A study by eating disorder researchers at Yale University found that those with BED tended not to experience the same severity of underlying psychological issues as people with anorexia or bulimia, nor as many companion diagnoses, such as drug addiction or bipolar illness. (This is, of course, an individual matter.) However, fully one-third of BED participants showed higher rates of depression-related symptoms (low mood and low self-esteem), and right along with those symptoms, more severe eating disturbances.

Seeing BED's Psychological Traits

As is the case with all eating disorder sufferers, those with BED typically experience underlying psychological distress that contributes to the disorder. In the following sections, I discuss the psychological features commonly exhibited by those with BED. Recognizing those features that apply to you is essential to your recovery.

Disgust about the bingeing relieved by dieting

Of all the words people with BED use to describe their feelings about themselves following a binge, "disgust" is the most common. It captures the terrible sense of shame that goes with bingeing. If you have BED, these feelings of shame may also be too much a part of your life in general.

As I discuss in the previous section, "The binge/diet cycle," just the *plan* of going on a diet can feel purifying and relieving, and give you the sense that you're solidly back in control. Dieting seems like the perfect antidote for the wretched feelings of disgust you feel toward yourself after bingeing.

Despair about overcoming the disorder

Once you get a sense of that no-exit quality of the binge cycle, you may understandably feel that there's no way out of the disorder. And that's just the half of it! Just like everyone with an eating disorder, you rely on your symptoms to fix things that really do need fixing, such as managing your emotions.

The people who brought us something called Brief Therapy introduced the important idea that most people get stuck in their symptom patterns because they're also stuck pursuing wrong solutions — like food to fix your feelings and dieting to fix yourself! (Turn to Part II to get going with some better solutions!)

Self-worth depends on weight

Even though you invest so much in performing at an outstanding level and showing the best kind of personal character, when all is said and done, you still feel you don't measure up unless you're thin. You may have a sense of existing outside the bounds of human deservedness when you're above a desired weight — and you don't believe you'll be welcomed back in until you're thin.

Perfectionism

As a sufferer of BED, you're likely to be one of the most conscientious people around. But you hardly know it. You're so demanding of yourself that you tend to see mainly your mistakes and often see your successes as flukes. Part of being you includes needing to be perfect and expecting no less of yourself, yet never being confident that you're capable of meeting the mark — or certain that you want to keep making the effort! The following examples represent perfectionist ways of thinking or behaving:

> *Liz* is project manager on her job. Everybody is singing her praises for the last project. She feels like a phony because she knows all the things that could have been done to make it *really* good if they'd only had more time.

> *Carole's* stomach is in a knot. Tomorrow is Mike's birthday party and she has no idea what gift to get for him. She prides herself on always getting exactly the right thing. She can't stand thinking of Mike's lukewarm response (and everybody else's) to a gift that's not perfect.

Notice that the way you react to your body and weight is an extension of the way you live your life more generally. In Part II, you get some ideas on how you can work on traits such as perfectionism to give you greater immunity to your eating disorder.

Black-and-white thinking

Black-and-white thinking is a way of organizing your experiences by seeing them as all one way or another, with little room for any thoughts in-between.

This is a thinking style that tends to get handed down in families from one generation to the next. (Our families teach us how to think about things.) The following thoughts are examples of black-and-white thinking:

- ✔ I did a perfect job or I failed.
- ✔ I maintained my diet exactly or I blew it.
- ✔ I'm a perfect size 4 or I'm disgustingly fat.

This trait shows up in the profiles of those with anorexia and bulimia as well as those with BED (see Chapters 2 and 3). Black-and-white thinking is a trait that seems to set you up for the development of an eating disorder in the first place, meaning you probably thought in black-and-white ways before you developed BED. You can read more about this in Chapter 5. Finding "gray" is important to your recovery.

Need for external approval

This trait seems to pop up in just about everybody with an eating disorder. It means setting more store in what others think and want than in your own views and opinions. You aim to please, and you believe others will like you better if you mirror them or give preference to their wants. This way of thinking can reflect a lack of trust in your own internal guidance system, so that you rely on others to be sure you're doing the right thing. It may be a pattern you saw modeled in one or both parents.

You may already be thinking ahead to how this affects your view of your body. That's right — the culture gets to tells you how you should look. To feel secure in yourself and in your place with others, you feel you have to live up to the cultural standard of thinness.

Some people have called binge eating the "good girl's way to be bad." Given the powerful way bingeing expresses a voice of *I want*, you might also call it the people-pleaser's way to have a self.

Determining Whether You Have BED

The following questions can help you figure out whether your way of thinking and eating fits the profile for binge eating disorder.

Keep in mind, **this questionnaire in no way substitutes for getting a competent diagnosis from a qualified eating disorders professional.**

Instructions: Check each item that feels true or mainly true of you. I tell you how to score your responses at the end of the questionnaire.

1. ❑ I think about food, weight, and calories almost all the time.

2. ❑ I allow my weight to determine how I feel about myself on any given day.

3. ❑ I frequently binge eat (eat huge quantities of food in a short period of time).

4. ❑ When I binge, I feel as if I have no control over what I'm doing.

5. ❑ When I binge, I often feel as if I'm outside myself, watching myself, or in some other way not in my usual state of mind.

6. ❑ I frequently binge when I feel bad or overwhelmed or lonely.

7. ❑ I feel worthless, disgusting, and hopeless after a binge.

8. ❑ I go to great lengths to keep my bingeing secret from other people.

9. ❑ I've been on every diet there is.

10. ❑ My weight goes up and down frequently.

11. ❑ When I decide to start another diet, it makes me feel hopeful about being in control again and getting thin.

12. ❑ It's not unusual for me to start and stop dieting many times in the course of a year.

13. ❑ I'm either following my diet to the letter or I feel I've blown it.

14. ❑ At some point, every diet begins to feel unfairly difficult — the rewards are too few; the effort is too great.

15. ❑ I'm frequently depressed.

16. ❑ I rarely feel that I am good enough.

17. ❑ It's very important to me to get everything perfect.

18. ❑ I'm a "people-pleaser."

19. ❑ I often feel others are judging me and finding me wanting.

20. ❑ I'd like myself better — and others would like me better too — if I were thinner.

Scoring: Give yourself one point for every item you checked.

If you scored 12 or 13 points, you're showing many warning signs of BED. Maybe you're hovering around that line between disordered eating and an eating disorder. No time like the present to respond!

If you scored 15 points or more, this is strongly suggestive of the binge eating disorder pattern. Awareness about treating BED is growing. You can begin finding out about what to do to get well in Part II.

Chapter 5

Eating Disorder Risk Factors

- -

In This Chapter

▶ Factoring family traits into the eating disorder equation

▶ Seeing how emotions affect eating disorders

▶ Looking at hormonal influences

▶ Making the connection to cultural pressures

- -

*I*f just one thing caused eating disorders, they would probably be a lot easier to treat and to prevent. In reality, no single smoking gun exists. Instead, a variety of risk factors appear to come into play — physical, social, and psychological — that can pile up to make you increasingly vulnerable. In this chapter you find out what the most important risk factors are and how they set you up to develop an eating disorder.

Some of these factors may be familiar to you. You may already have an inkling that all those skinny images you see in fashion magazines are stoking your urgency to be thin. Or that an all-or-nothing way of thinking makes you extra hard on yourself when you diet. Other factors may come as a surprise. For instance, did you know your brain chemistry could influence you to starve or overeat?

Eating disorder risk factors range from those over which you have no control (your genes) to those over which you can develop increasing control (such as the way you react to your particular family environment or deal with your emotions). In Part II you get ideas about how to better manage those risk factors over which you can exercise some control.

Table 5-1 sums up all the risk factors for developing an eating disorder I discuss in this chapter. Notice that for each risk factor, I indicate whether it is or isn't a factor that's potentially under your control, at least partially or under certain circumstances. With your eating disorder recovery, as elsewhere in life, knowing what you can control and what you can't is extremely useful. That way you know where to put your energies for getting better!

Table 5-1	The Potential to Influence Eating Disorder Risk Factors	
Risk Factors for Eating Disorders	**Can You Influence This Factor In Treatment?**	
	No	**Yes**
Genes	✓	
Brain Chemistry		✓ Sometimes, through medication or as the result of treatment
Cultural pressures	✓ But you can learn to be less susceptible	
Family style		✓ If everybody pitches in
Trauma history	✓ But you can work on resolving it internally	
Individual characteristics:		
Need for emotion management skills		✓
Shame		✓
Perfectionism		✓
Black-and-white thinking		✓
Need for external approval		✓
Avoiding growing up		✓
Dieting		✓

Looking at Family Traits that May Influence Eating Disorders

Eating disorder gene studies are in their infancy. What's more, it's mighty hard to separate those personality traits that are inherited from those that can be attributed to environment — that is, traits that are genetic versus those you derive from living day-to-day with people who handle life's challenges in a particular way. There's no blood test to make it all clear.

Further complicating the matter is the fact that some traits appear to team up genetically, meaning that if you are predisposed to an eating disorder, you are also more likely to be susceptible to related conditions, such as depression or substance abuse. I discuss this in greater detail in the section, "Co-existing symptoms run in families," later in this chapter.

Why should you even care? Zeroing in on genetic contributions to the eating disorders puts researchers in a better position to develop useful medical treatments. Knowing which traits tend to team up genetically can put your eating disorder specialists on the lookout for related problems, like depression, that you may not notice or report. And, for generations after you, knowledge about heritability will lead to improved prevention strategies.

Finding out what runs in families

Your family tree may play a significant role in your eating disorder. Eating disorders have been found to run in families, as have the traits that make you more vulnerable to developing an eating disorder. Symptoms that are likely to co-exist with your eating disorder have family ties as well. I discuss each of these in more detail in the following sections.

Eating disorders run in families

Researchers have discovered that if somebody in your family has an eating disorder — or even some kind of disordered eating pattern — you are more likely to develop an eating disorder yourself. If that somebody is your mother or sister, your chances are even greater. These findings suggest that your genes comprise part of the risk picture for developing an eating disorder.

Research further indicates that the genetic connection is strongest for anorexia. This doesn't mean, however, that you can inherit anorexia. What you *can* inherit are traits that make you more vulnerable to certain eating disorders, like anorexia, as I explain in the next section.

Vulnerability traits run in families

Certain personality traits or psychological characteristics are more likely than others to trigger eating disorders. These characteristics are known as *vulnerability traits* because they make those who possess them more vulnerable to developing an eating disorder. These triggers may be personality traits such as perfectionism or anxiety (see the section "Looking at Your Individual Vulnerability Traits" for more on these), or hormonal factors that have a psychological impact, such as those that affect mood or appetite (I review these in the section "Zapping the Brain with Hormones").

Information from gene studies suggests that families may also show clusterings of the genes for these inherited vulnerability traits. Researchers from Harvard and Michigan State University see in the collective research evidence that anorexia and bulimia are two distinct disorders with different sets of contributing genes. For more on gene clusterings, see the sidebar "Environment shapes gene expression."

Co-existing symptoms run in families

Two sets of symptoms that commonly occur along with eating disorders are also highly likely to be found in the relatives of people with eating disorders:

- Major depression is more likely to be found in people with bulimia and their relatives than in the general population.

- Substance abuse occurs at an elevated rate among binge eaters and their relatives.

Co-existing symptoms like depression and substance abuse worsen eating disorders and make treatment more complicated. Just how these symptoms relate to the development of eating disorders is a subject I discuss further in Chapter 7.

Seeing family patterns that may feed eating disorders

Families don't cause eating disorders in their children any more than they cause their children to fail at math, write bad poetry, or have hangnails. That said, certain family styles may provide more fertile soil in which a budding eating disorder can take root.

Overorganized family style

In an overorganized family, members are likely to feel the safety of predictability and a strong sense of belonging and unity. The family motto is "All for one and one for all." However, the same conditions make it difficult to feel okay about personal opinions, feelings, or needs that are different from the rest of the family's. When compliance — going along to get along — is highly prized, gaining a sense of confidence or independence can be hard. Disagreements feel threatening to the family's harmonious view of itself, so members don't learn how to resolve conflicts. Conflicts remain buried, causing ripples beneath the unified exterior. Because emotions are not valued, family members don't discover how to know and express their unique inner worlds of opinion, desire, and need.

Although any of the eating disorders can emerge from an overorganized family, anorexia is the most likely. The anorexic child needs to find ways to balance the rewards of connection to her family — which she gets from being compliant and agreeable — with her needs for a private niche of her own in which she has final control. Often the symptoms of anorexia not only supply this private empire, but they also serve to distract everyone from troubles brewing in other parts of the family, which are more threatening to the family's view of itself (for instance, unaddressed marital conflict between the parents).

Overorganized families appear to subscribe to the following beliefs:

- ✔ We are one.
- ✔ We all do exactly what's expected of us.
- ✔ We never fight.
- ✔ We are a family of few words, emotionally speaking.

These beliefs describe a family that

- ✔ Prizes togetherness and being alike over privacy and individuality
- ✔ Controls members' behavior within a narrow range
- ✔ Strongly avoids conflict
- ✔ Discourages expression of emotion

Overorganized families often have difficulty with developmental transitions. Such transitions call on families to change the way they relate to each other to allow for a child's growing abilities. Transitions are not easy for any family. But they're particularly tough for overorganized families who tend to be rigid about their ways of doing things and are, in general, pretty change-phobic.

The transitions that see children into adolescence and into young adulthood — the very ones where eating disorders are most likely to pop up — are especially difficult because they emphasize greater autonomy and separation in families that have always put togetherness first. Other kinds of transitions that can strain overorganized families and trigger the onset of an eating disorder include

- ✔ Entering a new school
- ✔ Moving to a new neighborhood or city
- ✔ Changing of a parent's job status, for example, a new schedule, increased responsibilities, or job loss
- ✔ Changing of a parent's marital status through divorce or remarriage

Underorganized family style

Chaos and unpredictability are the hallmarks of an underorganized family style. Bulimia may develop as a pattern of coping in an underorganized family. The dieting that almost always comes first (see "Dieting as the

Gateway to Eating Disorders," later in this chapter) initially provides the reassurance of rules and structure where everything else is chaotic. Bingeing enters the scene as a source of predictable comfort and emotional soothing. When a parent suffers from an addiction, as is often the case in underorganized families, bingeing copies the coping strategy of the addicted parent; that is, to manage uncomfortable experiences and feelings with something you swallow.

Like overorganized families, underorganized families really don't know how to manage emotions. Eventually the binge/purge cycle replays the emotional chaos of the family, while at the same time providing a predictable rhythm to life. Here are some of the features that can help you recognize an *underorganized* family:

- **You never know what will happen next.** The underorganized family has too little in the way of structure, rules, or guidance. Members can't relax into any sense of safety or reliability about the fundamentals of family life.

- **Mom (dad) has her (his) own addiction to worry about.** One or both parents commonly have some kind of active addiction, which, of course, makes day-to-day life that much more unpredictable.

- **You roll from crisis to crisis.** Underorganized families aren't very good at predicting what's coming down the pike or preparing for it. This makes them more vulnerable to the development of crises and they are less equipped to handle them when they arise.

- **Conflict is right out in the open.** Lots of it. And underorganized families don't particularly know what to do with it, so nothing much gets resolved.

- **You can't tell who's in your corner.** Members of underorganized families have difficulty bridging the distance from one person to another. As a result, individuals find it hard to feel emotional support from their family. Life in an underorganized family can feel lonely.

Shame-based family style

Shame is a sense of personal worthlessness that judges the entire self. I provide a closer look at shame when I talk about traits of eating disorder–prone individuals a little later in this chapter (see the section "Experiencing shame"). But what about when whole families are organized around the principle of avoiding shame? These families believe that to make mistakes is to risk humiliation and to be worthless. Their simple strategy is to be perfect and to achieve highly. Every member is expected to contribute their fair share of perfection and high achievement in order to reflect well on themselves and the family as a whole. Features of the shame-based family are likely to include

- An emphasis on appearances or looking good to others
- Adherence to the belief that they need to be perfect

✔ Adherence to the belief that they are worthless if imperfect

✔ At least one family member with addictive behavior

✔ Cycling between phases of peace and phases of addictive loss of control

As you might imagine, these families tend to be pressure cookers. It's not unusual for a family member to develop an addiction, which expresses the impossibility of living up to standards of perfection. Tension-relieving, addictive breakouts from these standards are inevitable. People are, after all, only human. But since members of a shame-based family don't accept their flawed humanness, they must compensate for the addictive breakout with more perfect behavior. This sets the stage for the next breakout, and so the cycle continues. The dynamic is the same as that of the binge/diet cycle (see Chapter 4) and is common in shame-based families. Shame and perfectionism are key contributing factors in all of the eating disorders, so any one of them may develop in a shame-based family.

A few other family effects

A few other family characteristics have been found to make an eating disorder more likely. These characteristics may potentially appear in any of the family styles described in the preceding sections. They include

✔ A parent who is visibly overly concerned about her own weight and appearance

✔ A parent with disordered eating behavior

✔ Too much emphasis, especially negative, on a child's appearance or eating habits

✔ Urging a child to diet or otherwise lose weight

✔ Using food for reward or punishment

✔ "Sexualizing" of the family environment; for instance, inappropriate comments or disclosures

✔ Unclear boundaries between mother/father and daughter

Looking at Your Individual Vulnerability

No single risk factor causes an eating disorder. But each of the characteristics I discuss in this section can make a person more vulnerable to developing an eating disorder. Whereas the traits I discuss in the previous sections derive from families, the traits I cover in this section affect individual thought processes. The more of these individual characteristics you possess, the more vulnerable you are to eating disorders.

Managing emotions poorly

One of the primary purposes having an eating disorder serves in your life is that it helps you to manage emotions. Restricting has the capacity to make the restrictor feel in control and therefore calm and reassured. Bingeing can soothe, comfort, calm, and distract. Both restricting and bingeing can numb and suppress emotions.

Part of feeling sound and stable as an adult is having the confidence to handle whatever life brings your way. You especially want to know that you can manage the tough feelings life events might stir up, such as grief, rage, humiliation, or rejection, as well as the more day-to-day emotions like disappointment, anger, annoyance, worry, sadness, boredom, envy, and so on.

When you don't know how to stay on an even keel emotionally, you are constantly threatened with being overwhelmed. Being overwhelmed means crossing the line from a state of "I can manage" to a state of "I can't manage; this is too much for me." If you have constructive coping methods already built in, you can use these resources to avoid feeling overwhelmed. Positive coping methods can include

- ✔ Calling a friend
- ✔ Meditating or praying
- ✔ Breathing deeply
- ✔ Practicing yoga
- ✔ Using problem-solving skills

Those who don't have these skills at their disposal will do whatever it takes to lower the distress level, even if it's destructive and causes its own bad feelings — including restricting, bingeing, and purging behaviors. Eating disorders supply alternative emotional coping methods. If you haven't acquired sufficient skills for managing your emotions, you are at greater risk for developing an eating disorder.

Whatever treatment you choose as a way to work on your eating disorder, it's likely to include a big focus on developing emotion management skills. If you'd like to get a jump-start, turn to Chapter 14.

Having a history of trauma

Trauma refers to any experience that overwhelms a person's ability to cope at the time it occurs. Trauma shatters boundaries of self, along with any sense of personal effectiveness and control. An eating disorder later in life can reflect the effects of early trauma. Eating disorder symptoms may represent an attempt to establish a sense of boundaries and control that was lost in early trauma.

Because children have fewer coping resources than adults, disturbing life events can more easily tip them into trauma. If the trauma involves key caregivers, a child may lose her most important trauma-buffering resource. Trauma is deeply disruptive to the life course of the person who experiences it (see *Post-Traumatic Stress Disorder For Dummies* by Mark Goulston [Wiley]). When it occurs in childhood, it pulls the child out of her normal developmental track — an excess of energy is required for coping — so trauma can have especially far-reaching effects for children.

Researchers find that people with bulimia are the most likely among eating disordered people to have trauma histories. Those who suffer from bulimia are especially likely to come from underorganized families (see the earlier section, "Underorganized family style," for more information). These families are very crisis-prone and often ill-equipped to protect their members from trauma. They can't seem to stop potentially traumatic events from occurring, and, when traumatic events do occur, they can't support their members enough to buffer the traumatic effects.

Common types of trauma

The most common sources of trauma reported by bulimic people and those with other eating disorders include

- ✔ Sexual abuse, including incest
- ✔ Physical abuse
- ✔ Verbal and emotional abuse
- ✔ Neglect
- ✔ Catastrophic loss

Studies show that people with eating disorders report significantly higher levels of trauma history than the general population but not more than people with other psychological disorders. Trauma doesn't specifically predict an eating disorder; it increases vulnerability. Other factors, including genes, personality, and environment, help determine whether the vulnerability is expressed as an eating disorder.

Factors that affect the impact of trauma

How greatly will a traumatic experience affect you? It appears to depend on a number of factors existing at the time of the traumatic event, including

✔ Age (the younger you are, the fewer internal resources you have to help you respond)

✔ How well or poorly you were functioning when the trauma occurred

✔ How severe the trauma was

✔ Whether the trauma was a one-time event or ongoing

✔ Whether the trauma was inflicted by a family member (that is, someone you trusted and depended upon) or a stranger

✔ How well your support system responded if you reported abuse

If you have trauma in your history, you probably have to devote a lot of energy to keeping it in a separate compartment, out of awareness, so you can get on with your life without too much disruption. An eating disorder often serves this purpose. Food is not only comforting, but it also creates vivid sensations that help distract your attention. Preoccupation with dieting can do the same thing. You may be putting distance between yourself and unmanageable feelings related to trauma by entering the world of the obsessive behaviors, emotions, and beliefs that make up your eating disorder. At the same time, the symptoms are a continuing signal that something just doesn't feel right and needs fixing.

Experiencing shame

Most people with eating disorders are struggling with a lot of shame. Much of it is a reaction to the eating disorder symptoms themselves (such as vomiting and bingeing — almost always done in secret). But shame often predates the eating disorder and is one of those experiences that can help make a person a sitting duck for development of an eating disorder.

Living with shame means living with a chronic sense of personal inadequacy and chronic fear that your inadequacies will be exposed and that you'll be humiliated and unloved. In an actual moment of shame, you judge your total self and find it worthless. Shame is the state in which you wish the earth would open beneath you so you could disappear. It includes the belief that others will judge you the same way you've judged yourself, so in your imagination you have been excluded from society. Shame makes you feel alone and like an outcast.

If you live with a lot of shame, you probably grew up in a shame-based family (see the earlier section, "Shame-based family style") in which at least one other member, most likely a parent, struggled with shame and didn't know what to do with it.

Dissociation

If you binge or purge, you may very well experience a feeling of being somehow outside yourself, as if in some kind of numb, altered, or disconnected state, while the behavior goes on. A state in which, in one way or another, you have stepped outside your usual sense of self is a *dissociated* state.

Dissociation is a method of coping in which our mind reflexively heads for the awareness exits when something is coming that we think we can't stand. Dissociation is often associated with early abuse. It makes sense. The younger the child, the fewer other ways the child has of dealing with such an overwhelming experience. By adulthood, the mind can not only be avoiding reminders of the childhood trauma, but it can now also be using dissociation to avoid just about any experience that feels too intense to manage.

Johan Vanderlinden and Walter Vandereycken, a Belgian research team, have discovered that bulimic women who dissociate extensively are more likely to engage in some kind of self-injury behavior such as cutting or burning. Pain associated with these behaviors may serve any of the following purposes, depending on the woman:

- To distract or feel relief from emotional pain

- To cue entry into a dissociated state in order to avoid some overwhelming experience

- To stimulate body sensation when in a numb or dissociated state as a way to move out of the numbness

- To unconsciously reenact abuse or neglect, this time being in charge of the pain

- To be in charge of current pain, since it seems unavoidable

- To express body hatred or self-hatred

If you have dissociative symptoms, you need to work with an eating disorder specialist who is experienced in working with these symptoms. I describe this in more detail in Chapter 10.

Dieting, with its promise of making you just what society most admires, can be almost irresistible if you feel like a shamed outcast. Many eating disordered people say that being able to achieve the slim body most other people in the culture only dream of (or the prospect of achieving it) makes them feel special or out-of-the-ordinary. It's a perfect antidote for feeling worthless and inadequate. Dieting, taken to the *n*th degree to fix shame, is a well-traveled path to an eating disorder.

Seeking perfection

Perfectionism is often attempted as a "cure" for shame. You may go to extremes to get everything right or to avoid mistakes. Or maybe you put a big effort into keeping up appearances so that the you the world sees will cover the you underneath that feels so unworthy. The demands can be exhausting and endless. They can make for a joyless existence in which your personal needs and desires must take a back seat to your public image.

Shame versus guilt

Shame is different from guilt. When you feel guilt, some behavior, impulse, or thought gets put in the hot seat, but other parts of you are left off the hook. In other words, you still have a basically intact self to deal with guilty feelings. You can think of ways to set things right with whatever is making you feel guilty — you can apologize, fix what you broke, be kinder or more honest next time — and thus repair your image of yourself. With shame, your entire self is judged and found unworthy. That's much harder to fix.

The perfectionism "cure" raises some pretty basic questions about your life:

- Am I good enough as I am?
- Am I deserving, even when I'm imperfect?
- Do my own needs matter?

If you're at risk for an eating disorder, you can't struggle with these questions openly. A compliant part of you has already decided the answer to each question is "No." A big part of being perfect is dieting perfectly and being the perfect size (though people who binge have an interesting way of keeping protest alive, even if unacknowledged, on these matters. You can hear the protest in the binge voice of "I want!" You can read more about this in Chapter 4).

Thinking in black-and-white

With a black-and-white mind-set, there's no gray area or middle ground in which a mixture of feelings or experiences can exist, such as basic support and approval with a few criticisms, momentary gaffes in a basically capable person, or friends who still love you even if they can't always be available or if they disappoint you. Things are all either one way or another, so a drop of anything negative poisons what's otherwise fine.

For instance, what happens when you have a bad day? Perhaps your boss, who is usually supportive, points out some flaws in your work. You may feel devastated, but you're looking forward to getting some feedback (and comfort) about your day from your best friend. But then you find out that your friend isn't available, even though the two of you had talked about getting together. On the way home, the heel of your favorite pair of shoes breaks in the middle of traffic. Hobbling, you stop for an ice cream cone and then go home with the following thoughts going through your mind:

✔ My boss thinks I'm a loser. He'll never give me more responsibility.

✔ My friend is pulling away. Doesn't anyone want to spend time with me?

✔ I'll never be able to show my face on the corner where I broke my heel again. Everyone could see what a klutz I am!

✔ I had the stupid ice cream cone. I've blown it now. I'm such a glutton. I may as well eat all that ice cream in the freezer as well.

Notice how easily black-and-white thinking can end up in insulting conclusions about yourself. *I'm a loser. Nobody likes me. I'm a klutz. I'm a glutton.* This is extremely bad for your mental health! And these personality generalizations easily slide into black-and-white criticisms about your body — the kind that can lead to eating disorders. Extra fat on your thighs says everything there is to be said about your entire body, your looks in general, your personal discipline, and you as a person. *(How did that fat get there in the first place, and why haven't I gotten rid of it by now? I can't look the way I should. I'm gross. I'm worthless.)*

Needing external approval

Some people listen to their own internal guiding voice to make decisions and form opinions. These people are thought of as centered and self-confident. Others often don't seem to be aware of having an internal guiding voice. They achieve confidence only when they get a seal of approval from others. Their own voice, should they find it, is either untrustworthy or doesn't count. If you need a lot of external approval, here are some ways that pattern may have developed:

✔ Growing up in a family whose members are preoccupied with what others think

✔ Growing up without enough encouragement for your own opinions and feelings to be able to develop any confidence in them

✔ Growing up on a constant diet of criticism

✔ Growing up in an environment of abuse or neglect (pleasing others becomes a way to adapt)

Women in this culture receive the message practically from birth that society will reward them for achieving the correct body size and shape and will shun them for having the wrong shape.

If you are already vulnerable to trusting outside sources more than yourself to define what's right for you, contemporary culture is there to tell you how you should look and what priority to give it. The message is so strong that even centered, secure women struggle with it. For approval-seekers, the cultural message can be an irresistible road to an eating disorder.

Avoiding growing up

If you've developed an eating disorder as a girl or young woman, you may have fears about moving on to the next stage of life. Sometimes these are conscious fears; other times, not so much. Maybe you are nervous about social expectations you don't feel ready to tackle, such as peer relationships with less parental supervision, dealing with cliques, and so on. Maybe your fears focus on sexual development and dating. If you are an older teen or young woman, perhaps your challenges are about separating from your family and that which is familiar and taking on the responsibilities of the adult world.

The ability to put on the developmental brakes via an eating disorder is particularly obvious with anorexia. Anorexia can seem to roll back time by giving an anorexic girl a pre-pubertal body. However, even if less obvious, any of the eating disorders offers a world of more immediate stuff to think about and pushes the scary stuff of development farther down the road.

While you can certainly arrive at growing-up fears on your own steam, if you have them, you are probably also dealing with complications such as the following:

✔ Family members who are also anxious about you growing up and leaving

✔ A parent or sibling who had serious difficulties with the same transition

✔ A major loss or life change in the family's recent past that has reduced personal and/or family resources to help support this next stage of growth

Zapping the Brain with Hormones

As you read this, medical scientists are busy trying to figure out whether individual brain chemistry may help explain why some people develop eating disorders while others in the same environment do not. Some interesting quirks of our brains are showing up from this research, namely, that the very same brain mechanisms and chemicals that affect our eating and appetite also regulate the moods and behaviors typical of eating disorders.

If everyone planning on developing an eating disorder would just raise their hands, scientists could measure their brain chemicals now, before they have the disorder. They could then compare these with people who aren't planning on having an eating disorder. That way, they could see whether there are any brain chemicals that create greater risk for these disorders.

Because this kind of foresight exists only in fantasy, the best scientists can do is to measure brain chemicals of people who already have an eating disorder and measure them again when these same people are in recovery. This leaves to guesswork whether unusual levels found when the disorder is still "active" were there before, influencing the disorder's development, or whether the physiological changes produced by starvation, bingeing, purging, or severe or frequent weight fluctuations made the person's brain chemistry go haywire.

Tinkering with your mood and appetite: Serotonin

If you or anyone you know has been medicated for depression or anxiety, you probably know about *SSRIs*, the medications that allow more of your body's natural brain chemical, *serotonin*, to keep circulating in your system. The extra circulating serotonin seems to help combat both depression and chronic anxiety, as well as some other problems that frequently come up with eating disorders.

Serotonin is a particular kind of hormone called a *neurotransmitter*. Neurotransmitters are brain chemicals used by brain circuits to communicate with different parts of the brain and control our movements, thinking processes, moods, body states, and other human experiences. Brain circuits are made up of individual *neurons* that "talk" to each other by releasing neurotransmitters from one neuron to the next, thus communicating the circuit's intentions. When things go wrong in brain circuit communication, you experience symptoms. Often symptoms can be improved by influencing neurotransmitter activity with drugs like SSRIs.

Serotonin acts in circuits in many parts of the brain, with different effects depending upon where it's acting. Medical researchers at the University of Pittsburgh have shown a disruption in serotonin's activity in several groups of women with eating disorders:

- **Women with anorexia and bulimia showed low levels of serotonin activity.** Low serotonin levels, it turns out, are associated with impulsive behavior. In fact, the lower the serotonin levels of the bulimic women, the more likely they were to binge and purge.

- **Women *in recovery* from anorexia and bulimia showed the opposite serotonin abnormality.** Their serotonin levels were higher than normal. Higher serotonin levels are associated with anxiety, perfectionism, ritualistic behaviors, and obsessive thinking, characteristics of eating disordered people that these women still displayed.

His serotonin response vs. *her* serotonin response

According to findings at MIT's Clinical Research Center, women start off with lower serotonin levels in their brains than men. (I know; there's no justice.) When a woman goes on a diet, her serotonin-challenged brain now has to make do with even less, especially if she's on a low-carb diet. Without enough carbs, her body can't make tryptophan, and without tryptophan, her brain can't make more serotonin. What with serotonin's mood and appetite-regulating effects, this will leave her hungry and crabby at best, possibly depressed. And what about a guy on the same diet? His serotonin levels — and thus his mood — are relatively unscathed. This may be another piece of the puzzle explaining why women are so much more likely to develop eating disorders than men.

A couple of other things in addition to these findings make researchers think serotonin could play an important role in the development of eating disorders — and possibly in their cure:

- **SSRIs have been helpful in the treatment of bulimia** and, to a lesser extent, in the treatment of anorexia. This makes a pretty strong case for serotonin levels having something to do with eating disorder symptoms.

- **Several of the problems the SSRIs are known to help improve are also problems that are associated with the development of eating disorders**. I mentioned a few already: anxiety, perfectionism, impulsivity, and obsessive thinking. Others include depression and full-blown obsessive-compulsive disorder (OCD).

- **Serotonin suppresses appetite**. Abnormal serotonin levels may possibly contribute to restricting or bingeing behavior.

Carbohydrates, a favorite binge food, are the only suppliers of *tryptophan,* an essential building block used to create serotonin in your brain. One theory is that bingeing on carbs is your brain's effort to increase serotonin levels and thus treat itself for depression or anxiety.

Making it feel so rewarding: Dopamine

Dopamine is another neurotransmitter, that is, a chemical messenger in the brain. One of the many things dopamine does is to modify your experience of pleasure. Dopamine may shine a bright light on experiences that give you pleasurable feelings. If your brain pays attention and stores these experiences, you make better choices about what to repeat in the future.

Reward circuitry of the brain uses dopamine to highlight the experience of a food's tastiness. Your brain wants you to remember and do this again! When a food experience, enhanced by dopamine, makes your reward circuits light up, it can override signals telling you when you've had enough.

The same researchers who looked at serotonin in people with eating disorders have also found that dopamine is working overtime in women recovering from anorexia. This may sound like it should be a good thing. But in reality, two important anorexia-related qualities may be compromised by dopamine overactivity:

- ✔ **The reward experience of eating:** For previously anorexic women, the ability to take pleasure from eating is diminished.

- ✔ **Learning from experience:** Researchers think having dopamine activity levels popping in the brain may help explain the denial — that is, *not* learning from experience — that is so characteristic of anorexia.

Researchers at the Brookhaven National Laboratory in New York have shown that obese people have too few dopamine *receptors*, brain equipment dopamine needs to do its job properly. They suspect that obese people may be overeating in an effort to stimulate the reward experience that people who have their fair share of dopamine receptors get from a lesser amount of food. A logical question under investigation is whether eating-disordered bingeing also reflects having too few dopamine receptors. Of course, the really important question is: Can the research findings lead to improved treatment?

A Culture that Breeds Eating Disorders

Eating disorders don't occur at the same rate in all cultures everywhere. What ingredients are present in our current culture to make such a potent brew for the creation of eating disorders?

Succumbing to the media

Most people in the mainstream culture — where eating disorders tend to develop — get their ideas about how their bodies should look from the media: magazines, movies, TV, and the like. In particular, the female bodies they see are 15 to 25 percent smaller than the average woman's, not to mention that these bodies are airbrushed and sculpted to perfection by cosmetic surgery. The clothing that is on display is designed for model-thin bodies, so the average-sized woman is made to feel she is too big to wear what is fashionable. These images have special clout because they are with us everywhere and all the time, making these thoroughly abnormal body types seem ordinary and achievable.

Studies consistently find that interesting things happen when people are exposed to these images of perfection, besides making them cranky (yes, really!). Whether male or female, young or old, when people see media images of ideal-sized models, they are more likely to be unhappy with their own bodies, to feel distressed and insecure, and to become motivated to do whatever it takes (usually dieting and/or exercise) to make themselves look like these impossible images.

The media has done more than display slender images as the norm. Women's magazines, in particular, have actively sold the message that achieving a slimmer body will help you achieve a happier, more successful life. Just buy their magazine or the products inside, and that life is all yours.

Getting slim at any price

Women are especially affected by images of the slim standard because they know they will be judged by them. Researchers hear from both men and women that a woman will be sized up first and foremost by her appearance. Weight may affect a woman's ability to get a job or to get ahead in it, the amount of money she makes, or her ability to get a mate. Overwhelmingly, American women report that they are unhappy with their bodies.

At least when our great-grandmothers were dealing with the fashion in body shape, there were contraptions to do the job for them — stays, cinches, girdles. Not that these were a walk in the park. But a quirk of modern expectations for women is that the fashionable image is no longer a matter of hitching things in. The body itself is supposed to be made fashionable (that is, slim and fit) through personal effort. The result is that fashion is no longer just fashion; it has become a test that demonstrates an individual's discipline and moral character. Your body is supposedly a walking advertisement of your willingness and ability to be in control of your life generally. (Yikes!)

The marriage of fashion and health messages has only made the stakes higher. When medical experts advised the government that obesity was a disease — some claiming that even an extra 20 pounds could put your health at risk — a medical blessing was given to the idea that no sacrifice for slimness is too great.

Fearing cultural disapproval

Our culture not only saves its rewards and approval for the thin, it makes outcasts of the obese. Not only do obese people not look the way we think they should, but study after study shows we also assign all kinds of negative character traits to them: they have no will power and are lazy, morally weak, unintelligent, sloppy, emotionally immature, and sexually maladjusted.

Training begins very early. Even preschoolers report negative associations with overweight and obese people. By the time these children are adults, they are likely to graduate into the culture's extreme *fat phobia*. A Yale University study revealed the sacrifices ordinary adults would be prepared to make in order not to be fat. Almost half of the people who responded reported they'd give up a year of life. Another 15 percent would give up ten years. People would give up having children, eyesight, an arm, or a leg, or be depressed or alcoholic — any of these would be better than being fat.

After death and torture, the most powerful threat you can hold over anyone is the prospect of being a social outcast. If you have an eating disorder, you are likely to respond especially strongly to external standards for approval. As such, you tend to reflect and magnify the fat phobia of the mainstream culture and the thin-at-any-price thinking that goes with it. Although it may feel impossible to you now, developing ways to challenge the culture's extremes about body size is an important part of your recovery.

 If you have a daughter, she is absorbing media images and the eating disorder risk that goes with them, more so than boys. You can encourage her to think about what she's seeing, rather than just absorb it all uncritically. Depending on her age, you might ask her the following questions:

- Do the people look like other people she knows?
- What's the message about weight and appearance?
- Are there examples in her own life that are different from this message?
- Does somebody benefit from selling the message? Who?

By helping her think critically about what she's seeing and ask questions, you can help her develop internal buffering from a possible eating disorder in the future.

Dieting as the Gateway to Eating Disorders

Almost everybody with an eating disorder will tell you it all started with a diet. However, if you read the other parts of this chapter, you know that much has already gone on beneath the surface to make an eating disorder likely. Nevertheless, dieting still seems to be the most frequent "switch" for setting all the machinery of the disorder into motion.

Of all the risky things you can do, think, or feel, dieting is the one that most strongly predicts an eating disorder will follow. Keep a special alert out for this risk factor.

Dieting feels like control

Dieting provides the future anorexic person with feelings of personal control, perhaps for the first time in her life. For the binger, dieting provides "absolution" for the binge and a sense of regaining lost control. For both, dieting seems to be the promised road to gaining admiration for her appearance. What actually happens is that dieting simply leads to more and stricter dieting and eventual starvation for the person with anorexia. And it inevitably becomes part of the binge/purge cycle for the person with bulimia or the binge/diet cycle of the person with binge eating disorder.

Dieting increases the risk of eating disorders

Just like the other risk factors I discuss in this chapter, dieting doesn't, by itself, cause an eating disorder. It just makes it more likely — a lot more likely — to happen in an already vulnerable person. For example, Australian researchers, reporting their findings in the *British Medical Journal* in 1999, discovered that moderate dieters were five times more likely to develop an eating disorder than non-dieters; "severe" dieters were *eighteen* times more likely to develop an eating disorder.

If you are that "already vulnerable person" I refer to, it means you could be someone who stumbles onto dieting only to find that it seems to fit like a key in a lock, fixing other things in your personality or situation that feel bad. Anything that seems to solve what hurts in people's lives has enormous staying power.

The best possible advice is to avoid dieting if you haven't started and to stop immediately if you have. If you are dieting, or even just watching what you eat, here are some warning signs that you could be headed down the slippery slope toward an eating disorder:

✔ You are constantly preoccupied with thoughts about dieting.

✔ You constantly judge yourself by how well you are doing on the diet.

✔ You are spending less time with others and more time focusing on dieting.

✔ The goal posts keep shifting on how much is enough to lose.

Any of these could be signals that it's time to get into gear, read the chapters ahead on treatment, and find the help you need to stop your budding eating disorder in its tracks.

Chapter 6

Deconstructing Your Body with an Eating Disorder

You may think that your eating disorder only causes your body to be bigger or smaller. Unfortunately, that's not the case. Eating disorders give rise to a multitude of unpleasant and even downright harmful side effects. These can include the erosion of tooth enamel, the development of soft, downy hair called *lanugo* on your arms or stomach, or even heart failure.

The unhappy truth is that beyond the limits of what you can see, your eating disorder is having several physical effects on your body, and they aren't pretty. Some of these effects, like lanugo, are kind of shocking but not really dangerous. Others can severely harm your health and even put your life at risk. Some of the damage done heals as your eating disorder is managed. Other kinds of damage can cross the line of no-return, leaving you with lifelong impairments.

Why is it important to know these things? Awareness is one of your biggest allies in your recovery. Even a small increase in awareness about the reality of your disorder is a contribution to getting better.

In this chapter I go over the hazards associated with eating disorders and the damaging effects they have on your body. Until eating disorders come with warning labels, your safety depends on you understanding what you're doing to your body as you work toward making more self-caring choices.

Your health is more important than your weight

You may find it hard to believe that the toll your eating disorder takes on your body matters compared to losing weight — a response that's a symptom of your eating disorder! You may also find it hard to take a lot of the information in because it's scary, and you're still in the grips of your disorder. What to do? I invite you to do three things.

First, stop and imagine ways to support your reading with openness about how the information in this chapter may apply to you. Maybe you can recall some other time you stepped up when it was difficult to find out about something. Or you may find it helpful to think of a friend who always makes the tough stuff a little more bearable.

Next, use this as an opportunity to imagine how it might feel if you were to start believing your health matters as much as, or — dare I say it? — more than your appearance.

Finally, take in only as much as you can. You can always come back when you're ready to take in a little more.

Disordering Your Body from the Inside Out with Starvation

In a popular TV crime show, each episode includes a scene where the view zooms right inside a body so we can see what actually happened to bring about the victim's demise. If the cause of death were starvation, the view would have to zoom in on multiple sites within the body to reveal the full effect. So, let's take that close-up look!

Dehydration: Risking heart failure and more

Starving denies your body of more than just the solid food you think makes you fat; it also robs your body of essential liquid nourishment. All foods contain nutritious fluids that cannot be compensated for by drinking water alone. Severely limiting the intake of nutrients and fluids over time causes your body to become dehydrated. Severely restricting carbohydrates and fats can also result in dehydration. Dehydration disrupts and reduces the levels of important minerals called *electrolytes*, and it affects heart functioning.

Electrolytes are minerals (you recognize their names: sodium, calcium, potassium, and others) that dissolve in fluids, creating an electrical charge on themselves. This electrical charge allows them to act as conductors to help move materials in and out of body cells as needed. Electrolytes also conduct electrical impulses that stimulate muscles to action. Calcium and potassium are the electrolytes that are in charge of one of my personally favorite muscles, the heart, and are critical for stimulating a regular heartbeat.

Electrolyte imbalances can result in sudden cardiac arrest and permanent heart damage or death. An early symptom of dehydration and an electrolyte imbalance is irregular heart rhythm. Left untreated, deadly results can follow:

- **Heart muscle atrophy:** This is your heart wasting away! A weakened heart has trouble beating. When you rob your body of nutrients, your muscles can't rebuild themselves. The heart muscle gets no special treatment when it comes to starvation.

- **Low blood pressure:** The body just naturally shifts into a lower gear to try to conserve energy when you starve it.

- **Orthostatic hypotension:** You know how sometimes if you stand up too fast, you get dizzy? This involves a rapid decrease in blood pressure and in the heart's heft in pumping out blood. Electrolyte deficiencies affect the nervous system response that helps the body right itself. This is okay if you're otherwise healthy, but it can contribute to a deadly chain of events in an already weakened heart.

The heart is not the only part of your body that suffers from dehydration. Other dangerous effects of dehydration and electrolyte imbalances include

- Kidney damage or failure

- Convulsions, seizures

- Liver damage and failure

- Muscle paralysis (can range from weakness to immobility)

Dehydration is especially risky if you have type 1 or type 2 diabetes. Blood sugar levels can be thrown off by dehydration. Too much glucose in your system can have toxic effects on certain body tissues and eventually do damage to organs such as the eyes or kidneys. Also, because many of the medications used to control diabetes cause weight gain, diabetic people with anorexia are frequently tempted to cut back on their use — often with disastrous, even deadly, consequences.

Not all the effects of dehydration are life-threatening, but they reduce your quality of life and they're not pretty. Here are some of the nonlethal outcomes you can expect — or may already be experiencing — from cutting calories to the bone:

- Abdominal bloating

- Inability of your body to increase blood circulation during exercise

- Constipation

Re-feeding syndrome

Surprisingly, many of the physical risks of starvation can also be caused by its treatment. If you re-feed a very starved person too quickly, especially with a high carbohydrate load, their electrolytes and fluids can be thrown out of whack. This may result in problems for the heart, muscles, and lungs that can be fatal. The risks of too-rapid re-feeding were first discovered in treating starved war refugees. You can read more about re-feeding as a part of inpatient hospital care in Chapter 9.

- Dark circles under your eyes
- Headaches
- Leg cramps
- Swelling in legs and feet (*edema*)
- Very dry skin
- Weakness, fatigue

Malnutrition: Undermining your body's essential systems

When you deny your body the nutrition it needs through self-inflicted starvation, you make your body malnourished. Malnutrition results from deficiencies of essential protein, carbohydrates, fats, vitamins, and minerals in your diet. Even if you can make your body run on fumes for awhile, beneath the surface damage to systems and the seeds of breakdown are brewing, such as

- **Loss of menstrual periods (*amenorrhea*):** A starved body produces fewer of the hormones needed to stimulate menstrual periods. (Excessive exercise may also be a cause.)

- **Fertility problems:** You can't have a baby if you aren't having your periods.

- **Loss of bone minerals (*osteopenia*) or decreased bone density (*osteoporosis*):** This increases your risk of bone fracture, probably as a result of estrogen deficiency, calcium deficiency, or possibly through an excess of cortisol, the "stress" hormone. (If you binge and purge, bone loss is worse.)

- **Possible immune abnormalities:** Studies show that certain members of the body's immune "army" aren't present in starved bodies in the numbers needed for an adequate immune response to infectious invaders.

- **Multiple organ failure:** That's right; with enough deprivation, all the organs in your body can close up shop and quit functioning.

✔ **Stunting of height/growth:** The onset of anorexia while the body is still in the process of growth is of special concern. This is an effect that can have lifetime consequences.

✔ **Severe cold sensitivity; cold hands and feet:** Starvation throws off your body's temperature regulator. Also, lack of fat deprives you of the layer of warmth that's intended to protect you from cold.

✔ **Growth of down-like body hair (*lanugo*):** Your body is trying to give itself a coat to warm up! This occurs in almost a third of people with severe weight loss due to anorexia.

✔ **Easy bruising:** Your body can't heal itself as well as it should without certain vitamins. Low blood pressure and low weight make the effect worse.

✔ **Anemia and pale skin:** *Anemia* is a disorder in which you end up with too few of the blood cells that carry the oxygen you breathe to tissues that need it to fuel energy-making processes. Anemia is often caused by low iron levels.

✔ **Damage to hair, skin, and nails:** This is due to vitamin deficiencies which cause dry, brittle hair and nails; hair loss; and dry skin.

Wearing Your Body Down with Purging

Purging behaviors are the things you do to try to "undo" the calorie-accumulating effects of a binge or even ordinary eating. (See Chapter 3 for more on purging.) Purging behaviors include

✔ Vomiting

✔ Laxative abuse

✔ Use of enemas

✔ Use of diuretics (products that increase urination, also called water pills)

When you purge regularly, you dehydrate your body and you cause wear-and-tear on your body. Dehydration and body wear-and-tear, in turn, each lead to a host of harmful effects, which I go over in this section.

Robbing your body of fluids

You're dehydrated when your body takes in fewer fluids than it loses and can't function normally as a result. Starving is one way to become dehydrated, but it's not the only way. Purging behaviors rob your body of fluids and, along with them, essential minerals. Because of resulting mineral imbalances, you run the risk of a slowed heart rate, heart attack, or heart failure. You can read in detail about these and other effects of dehydration in the previous section, "Dehydration: Risking heart failure and more."

You need to be aware of the dangers of dehydration due to purging. First, because you are harming vital organs, some mortality risk is involved. Your risk isn't as high as that of the person who starves, but if it's your mortality, that probably doesn't matter to you. Even if your purging isn't fatal, you can still do serious damage to your body. Second, if you both purge *and* starve, you've got double trouble. Starvation weakens your body so it's less equipped to withstand the harmful effects of purging. You're at greater risk than the person who purges without starving.

Putting wear and tear on your body

Purging behaviors can also exert serious wear and tear on body parts. The effects worsen in accordance with how frequently and strenuously you purge and how weakened your body has become from other effects of your eating disorder. Some of the most common or worrisome wear-and-tear symptoms of purging are

- **Broken blood vessels in the eyes:** From straining to vomit.

- **Puffy face:** Due to swollen salivary glands.

- **Erosion of tooth enamel:** From repeated exposure to stomach acid.

- **Sore throat; damage to throat or choking:** From implements used to induce vomiting.

- **Inflamed, ulcerated, or ruptured esophagus:** Due to vomiting. (A torn esophagus causes shock; a ruptured one requires surgery.)

- **Reflux:** The valve-like muscle that joins the esophagus to the stomach can no longer prevent stomach acids from backing up into the esophagus. Regular contact with these acids causes heartburn and can damage the lining of the esophagus.

- **Stomach rupture, erosion, or bleeding:** From straining to vomit.

- **Inflamed pancreas (*pancreatitis*):** Caused by vomiting or excess laxative use. The pancreas swells, causing severe abdominal pain, distention, and fever.

- **Hiatal hernia:** From straining to vomit.

- **Chronic diarrhea; loss of normal bowel function:** From overuse of laxatives.

Bulimia creates reproductive mysteries

Two symptoms of the reproductive system, menstrual irregularity and a disorder called *polycystic ovary syndrome* (*PCOS*), are associated with bulimia for unknown reasons. Here's what's known and what's suspected in each case:

✔ **Menstrual irregularity:** As many as half of women with bulimia have irregular menstrual periods. A percentage of these women quit menstruating altogether. The reasons for this aren't as clear-cut as with anorexia. You need a minimum amount of fat to produce the hormones that regulate the menstrual cycle. It seems that, even though the bulimic woman isn't becoming emaciated, the amount of fat loss associated with frequent dieting, perhaps along with high stress levels, can be enough to throw reproductive hormones off balance.

✔ **Polycystic ovary syndrome:** PCOS is a disorder of the hormone system that occurs in 5 to 10 percent of women in their child-bearing years and is the most common cause of infertility. Imbalances of the female reproductive hormones, along with the presence of high levels of male hormones, cause the formation of cysts on the ovaries. Risk of PCOS appears to be higher if you have bulimia or BED. The big fluctuations of food intake that occur in these disorders may throw off reproductive hormone levels. Women with bulimia have also been found to have high blood insulin levels, which can affect PCOS. The good news is that as women with PCOS and bulimia or BED recover from their eating disorders, PCOS symptoms also improve.

 If you regularly use ipecac syrup to induce vomiting, you may be poisoning yourself. Ipecac is poisonous to muscle. If you take too much or take it frequently and it accumulates in your system, you run the risk of *cardiomyopathy* (that's wasting away of the heart muscle), cardiac arrest, seizure, coma, or shock. Just to be completely clear, ipecac can kill you, and suddenly.

Reversing the Effects with Recovery

Happily, most of the physical symptoms of starving yourself improve as your weight is restored and you return to sound eating and exercise habits. The unfortunate exceptions to this may be regaining regular menstrual periods and adequate bone density.

The two are related. Regular menstrual periods and the estrogen levels that go with them protect you against bone loss. Although most women with anorexia return to normal menstruation in recovery, about one-fourth of them do not. (Of course, this also spells potential fertility problems in the future.) Because of lacking the bone-protective effects of estrogen, adolescents may lose much bone density during the critical growth period that normally occurs at this stage of life. Weight gain does not restore lost bone. Medical scientists are searching for ways to address the problem as you read this.

Here's good news if you purge: Except for some of the dental damage caused by vomiting, your body mostly restores itself from the effects of purging as you find ways to manage your eating disordered symptoms.

Chapter 7

Sidekicks That Often Accompany Eating Disorders

*E*ating disorders rarely travel alone. One or two other disorders are likely to be hanging around and making trouble when you've already got your hands full with your eating disorder–related problems. Some of these other disorders, like the eating disorders themselves, involve compulsive behaviors, such as substance abuse. Others affect your mood, such as anxiety and depression. In this chapter you find out what the most common companion disorders are. You also find questionnaires to help you determine whether you may have a particular disorder, and I give you some ideas about where to turn for help.

You may be thinking that the presence of several problems at once means something is *really* wrong with you. On the contrary, mood disorders and addictions commonly accompany eating disorders — you're not alone. On the other hand, you may not even be aware of the significance of other problems like chronic anxiety or depression — they may just feel like background noise. The important thing to understand is that these disorders are treatable, just like your eating disorder.

Just how the eating disorders and co-existing disorders relate to each other is not completely understood. In this chapter I clarify what *is* known so you can see how the total picture of your symptoms makes sense. This also helps clarify why treatment is a total package, involving all the ways that things just aren't going right or don't feel right. Before you let that overwhelm you, let me share the good news: Many of the treatment approaches that help with your eating disorder also help with these companion disorders.

Altering Thoughts and Perceptions

Anorexia produces some effects on your thoughts and perceptions that don't occur among the other eating disorders. These effects have consequences: They make it harder to participate in both your daily life and your recovery.

An important feature of anorexia is that it's a *progressive* disorder, meaning that it gets worse over time. What makes it progressive? In large part it's the effects of starvation. I discuss the effects of starvation on your body in Chapter 6. But just as your body needs adequate nutrition to function properly, your brain does too!

With anorexia, you can't think straight!

When you starve your brain, the results show up in your thought processes. You probably attribute these effects to other causes, like personality, fatigue, depression, or anxiety. You may be surprised to discover that all of the following cognitive effects are common to starving brains:

- ✔ You're not as alert; your mind may feel a little dull.
- ✔ You have difficulty concentrating.
- ✔ You can't put your thoughts together quite as clearly as in the past.
- ✔ Your judgment isn't as sound.
- ✔ Your thinking is less creative and more rigid.

Your world centers on food and weight

When you have an eating disorder, your primary focus in life revolves around two things: your weight and food. It's hard to tell just where all the influences come from that lead you to focus so completely on weight and food in the early stages of your eating disorder. I consider some of the personality factors that come into play in Chapter 5. However when that focus leads you to the point of starvation, your obsession with food is more easily understandable.

A famous study at the University of Minnesota shows that preoccupations with food and weight are a predictable outcome of prolonged starvation, even in people without eating disorders. The study placed normal-eating World War II conscientious objectors on a diet of half their usual calories. After six months the subjects were

- ✔ Thinking and talking about food more or less constantly
- ✔ Developing strange food rituals and eating strange food combinations

> ✔ Hoarding food and other objects
>
> ✔ Withdrawing from social connections
>
> ✔ Feeling blah about much of anything besides food

In other words, after six months of semi-starvation, the subjects ended up in a food-focused world that looked just like that of the average person with anorexia. These negative effects can be reversed by providing the brain with the food it needs.

Recognizing Other Disorders That Require Treatment

If you have an eating disorder, you're very likely to have one or more companion psychological disorders. The presence of other psychological disorders makes your life more difficult and requires treatment in order for you to get better. Exactly how these companion disorders and eating disorders are related isn't known. Some may have slid in on the same genes. Some may have been there before your eating disorder and made you more vulnerable to developing it. (See Chapter 5 for more information on eating disorder risk factors.) It may be years or decades before the connections are understood. What's important for you to know now is that these disorders are treatable, and getting the proper diagnosis and treatment for any that you suffer from can speed your overall recovery.

Considering suicide

Suicide is often described as a permanent solution to a temporary problem. Many factors line up to make life's problems feel overwhelming and unendurable to certain people under certain conditions. Additional factors make some people more likely than others to act on these feelings. The temporary feelings that lead to suicide can be treated. But the at-risk person has to be identified in order for treatment to take place and for an unnecessary tragedy to be prevented.

If you think you may be at risk for becoming suicidal or are already having suicidal thoughts, take steps immediately to get help. See the sidebar, "Steps to take if you're feeling suicidal," for direction on where to turn.

Who's most at risk?

Suicidal feelings, attempts, and completed acts occur more frequently among some groups of people than others. If any of the following characteristics apply to you, you may be at greater risk:

✔ **You have a mood disorder.** Mood disorders, such as major depression, dysthymia (a less severe type of depression), other forms of depression, and bipolar disorder make you more susceptible to suicidal thoughts.

✔ **You're female.** This simple fact of gender means that you're more likely to attempt suicide (probably because women have a higher rate of mood disorders). Men, however, are more likely to succeed at their suicide attempts.

✔ **You're impulsive.** This often describes people with bulimia, bipolar disorder, and substance or alcohol abuse problems. Being impulsive means you're more likely to act on suicidal feelings.

✔ **You have a family history of depression and/or suicide.** This can include previous generations.

✔ **You have a personal history of suicide attempts**. Having made an attempt before seems to lower the threshold for making another attempt.

Suicide and eating disorders

Eating disorders don't, by themselves, cause you to become suicidal. Risk for suicidal thoughts and behavior are impossible to disentangle from your increased risk for depression and/or history of trauma. (You can read about depression later in this chapter in the section "Dealing with depression: Both cause and consequence." I discuss trauma effects in Chapter 5.) The most important thing for you to know is that if you have anorexia, your chances of surviving a suicide attempt may be diminished because of the way starvation weakens your body.

Moving toward suicide

People who are contemplating suicide tend to progress from lower to higher levels of commitment to the idea. (You can move up and down levels many times as well, depending on your circumstances.) With each increasing level of commitment comes a greater risk of suicide, so being frank with yourself is important in assessing your personal risk. The following are common stages of becoming suicidal, from lowest to highest in terms of risk:

1. **Passing thoughts or urges:** You may have fleeting thoughts of ending your own life, but you quickly dismiss them.

2. **Predisposing events and feelings:** Mood disorders like depression and/or anxiety may predispose you to suicidal thoughts. If a particularly negative event or string of events occurs to boot, such as a loss or a humiliating experience, your feelings may go from bad to unbearable. At this point, the mood disorder and the bad experiences may be making each other worse.

3. **More enduring thoughts or urges:** You may have obvious thoughts of ending your life or more direct ones, such as the belief that you're no good to anyone. Your feelings start to focus on the hopelessness of your situation — it seems as though nothing you or anyone else can do will make things better.

4. **Suicidal intention and planning:** You start doing things to let go of life: putting your affairs in order, leaving "goodbye" messages for people, giving away possessions. You also take action to give yourself the means to suicide, such as hoarding medication. This kind of thinking and planning begins to spin a kind of isolating cocoon around you. It's important to know that your thought processes and judgment are probably quite distorted by this stage.

5. **Passive suicidal activity:** Many people who either are unaware of their own suicidal intentions or are standing undecided at the threshold will engage in dangerous activities that could take the suicidal action for them. This may include reckless driving, having unprotected sex, or hanging out in dangerous places.

6. **Actual activity to carry out a plan:** You put your previous plan into motion and actually attempt to commit suicide.

Working on your suicidal feelings when your commitment to the idea is at a low level is less harrowing than when your risk is high. That makes it an excellent idea to acknowledge these feelings early on and take action to get treatment before things get worse. This is particularly true if you are in one or more of the risk categories listed above. The questionnaire in the following section may also help you determine whether you're at risk.

Questionnaire: Are you at risk for suicide?

Place a check mark in the boxes next to the statements in the following lists that reflect your feelings or apply to you. When you respond to the statements, keep the following in mind:

✔ Thought and action statements are listed according to increasing risk.

✔ Action statements indicate a higher level of risk than thought statements.

Risky thoughts and feelings:

❑ I can't stand the situation/pain/feelings I'm in any longer.

❑ I don't deserve to live.

❑ I see no hope for a better future.

❑ I feel my family and friends would be better off without me.

❑ My death will make them all sorry.

❑ Death feels like a welcome relief.

Risky actions:

❑ I've been withdrawing from social contact.

❑ I've been using alcohol or drugs more than usual.

❑ I've been engaging in reckless and dangerous activities.

❑ I've written a will or left other instructions about my death.

❑ I've been giving my belongings away.

❑ I've written a suicide note.

❑ I've acquired or begun to acquire the means to kill myself.

Overdoing it: OCD

Obsessive-compulsive disorder (OCD) is officially listed in the American Psychiatric Association's *Diagnostic and Statistical Manual of Mental Disorders* among anxiety disorders, but it has it has its own distinct profile and is more common in people with eating disorders. If you have OCD, you're plagued by repeated distressing thoughts and the need to repeat certain ritual behaviors. According to a study led by researchers from the Universities of Pennsylvania and Pittsburgh, 40 percent of people with eating disorders also have OCD. (In the general population, only about 2 to 3 percent of people have OCD.) A genetic link involving similar brain chemistry appears to exist between the two disorders.

Too much is never enough

OCD involves too much thinking — the *obsession* — and too much doing — the *compulsion*. Obsessive thoughts, images, or impulses intrude into everyday life despite your best efforts to ignore them or make them go away. Thoughts can involve doing harm to others, harming yourself (by way of injury, contamination, victimization), sexually distressing content, religious content, and so on. Obsessive content is senseless — which isn't news to you if you have obsessions. But this awareness doesn't get rid of them or make them any less upsetting to you.

Compulsions are behaviors (such as hand washing) or mental acts (such as counting) that you feel you must repeat to ward off the obsessive experience that you dread. Not being able to perform the compulsive activity is likely to make you feel very anxious.

Obsessions and compulsions tend to gobble up more and more of your life — sometimes hours a day — if OCD goes untreated. The symptoms serve to prevent awareness of real issues that may be too upsetting. Any time symptoms serve this purpose, they tend to get more and more elaborate over time — kind of like with an eating disorder.

Steps to take if you're feeling suicidal

Are you considering suicide? Here are the steps you need to take to protect yourself:

1. **Determine whether you feel confident that you can contain your suicidal thoughts and feelings without harming yourself.**

   If you have even a sliver of a doubt about this, call 911 or go straight to a hospital emergency room. Don't wait for the feelings to go away. Don't wait for your boyfriend to finish work. Get protection first and everything else can follow.

2. **If you feel you're in a suicidal crisis but are certain that, at least for now, you can stop yourself from acting on the impulses, reach out.**

Call a suicide hotline (a telephone operator can help you or you can call 1-800-SUICIDE / 1-800-784-2433); or call a friend or family member you trust. Don't be by yourself!

3. **Make arrangements for professional follow-up as soon as possible.**

   A hotline representative can direct you. You can also use any of the referral directories I recommend for eating disorder treatment in Chapter 10. Let the person know your situation is urgent.

4. **Keep the appointment, even if you're feeling better.**

OCD and anorexia: The perfect storm

If you have both anorexia and OCD, did the OCD come first and make you more vulnerable to developing anorexia later? This isn't clear-cut. What *is* known is that OCD just exaggerates anorexia symptoms. Both your thought processes and your behavior are likely to be farther off-track than those of people who have anorexia but not OCD. Many experts see an anorexic person's fear of fat as a perfect example of an OCD obsession.

Dieting and the numerous food rituals that go with it fit the description of OCD compulsions, including the intention to contain anxiety about the obsession (fat). What's more, people with anorexia and people with OCD are known to share certain personality characteristics: precision, perfectionism, and — what shall we call it? — a certain devotion to keeping things in a chosen order (think of Jack Nicholson in *As Good As It Gets*). From this viewpoint, it would seem that everyone with anorexia also has OCD. But more likely, you have two separate disorders with important similarities, so you get that perfect storm when they occur in the same person. As you may guess, getting better is harder work if you have both.

OCD and other eating disorders

The rate of OCD among people with bulimia, binge eating disorder, and the nonspecific eating disorders is very high compared to the general population. Research shows that in most people, OCD develops earlier than the eating disorder. OCD is likely to make a person more vulnerable to the perfectionist tendencies associated with eating disorders and to compulsive symptoms like bingeing and purging. Both the OCD and the eating disorder need to be treated to ensure an effective outcome.

Questionnaire: Might you have OCD?

Consider your responses to the following questions to see if you may have OCD. Place a check mark in the box next to each question that you answer with a "yes." OCD and other disorders can be confused with one another, so it's important that even if you answer "yes" to half or more of these questions, you get a good professional diagnosis.

❑ Do you have thoughts, images, or impulses you can't get rid of that upset, frighten, or repel you?

❑ If you have such impulses, do you worry that you won't be able to stop yourself from acting on them?

❑ Do you have certain behaviors or thoughts that you feel you must enact to be okay or to ward off some dreaded outcome?

❑ Do these thoughts or activities take up an hour or more of your time each day?

❑ Do these thoughts or activities interfere with your relationships or other things you need to be doing?

❑ Does a part of you see your thoughts or activities as excessive, even if you can't stop?

OCD rarely disappears on its own, and its symptoms may last for years if they aren't treated properly. OCD usually is treated with a combination of psychotherapy and medications.

Worrying too much: Anxiety disorders

If you have an eating disorder, your chances of having some kind of anxiety disorder as well are very good. Certain kinds of anxiety disorders, which I go over in this section, are typical of people with eating disorders. Anxiety disorders are not your everyday worries. The fears involved are exaggerated, irrational, and out-of-hand. Having an anxiety disorder makes your eating disorder symptoms that much worse. Here are three anxiety disorders that are common to those with eating disorders:

✔ **Generalized anxiety disorder (GAD):** If you have GAD, that which sets you apart from people without the disorder is not so much the things you worry about, but rather how much and how often you worry: a lot and all the time. You worry so much that it makes you exhausted and perhaps physically ill. And your worrying distracts you from other, more constructive things you might be thinking about and doing.

✔ **Panic disorder:** The beginning event of panic disorder is a *panic attack*. When you have a panic attack, you've crossed the line from manageable anxiety to what feels like unmanageable anxiety. Among other effects, your heart races wildly, things feel unreal, and you can no longer think straight. People having panic attacks commonly fear that they are having a heart attack or going crazy. You've developed panic disorder when you've not only had one or more panic attacks but also have one or more of the following symptoms:

- You (understandably) worry constantly about having another one.

- You worry about what could be wrong with you to have caused the attack in the first place.

- You avoid anything you think might set off another attack.

✔ **Social phobia:** If you have a *phobia*, your fear is focused on a specific object (like a snake) or situation (like driving). If you have a *social* phobia, situations in which you expect to be observed and judged negatively terrify you. Public speaking is a common social phobia. Social situations — meeting other people, using public facilities, being in groups — produce this fear in many people (thus, the name of the disorder). Those who are experiencing bulimia seem especially prone to social phobia.

Soothing anxiety with food

Your emotions, mind, and body all get into the act when you are anxious. Your emotions may range from low-grade worry to fear to outright panic. Your thoughts are consumed with dreaded possibilities. Meanwhile, your nervous system is treating you to jolts of adrenaline — the threat hormone that makes your heart beat faster, your palms sweat, and your stomach fill with butterflies. Most people are motivated to do something — anything — to make all those uncomfortable feelings go away.

For lack of a more constructive alternative, those with eating disorders use what they have: food. Many people find certain foods, like carbohydrates and sweets, inherently soothing. Maybe your family taught you to use food as an emotional soother, or maybe you discovered it on your own. One way or another, the first time food had a comforting effect on your feelings, it made you likely to return to it the next time you needed comfort . . .and the next and the next.

Questionnaire: Has your anxiety gone beyond everyday worrying?

If you are experiencing any of the first four symptoms that follow (psychological signs of anxiety) and one or more of the remaining four symptoms (physical signs that may indicate anxiety), it may be evidence of one of the anxiety disorders:

❑ Uncontrolled worrying

❑ Constant agitation

❑ Unmanageable fear

❑ Avoidance of feared situations

❑ Physical sensations accompanying irrational fears

  • Shortness of breath, rapid breathing

  • Dizziness

  • Pounding heart

  • Nausea

❑ Fatigue

❑ Difficulty sleeping

❑ Unexplained body aches

Getting a good diagnosis for symptoms that feel like an anxiety disorder is really smart for several reasons, including the following:

✔ Your symptoms might actually be explained by something else, like a medication side effect or a physical illness.

✔ If you have an anxiety disorder, it needs to be treated properly to help you recover from your eating disorder.

✔ People get better when they get treatment. You don't have to feel like this!

Check first with your doctor to rule out medical causes. If you determine that there are no physical reasons for your symptoms, the next step is to seek an evaluation for psychological causes. Eating disorder therapists you find through the Resource Guide at the back of this book should be able to offer you a competent evaluation for anxiety symptoms. For more hands-on help, check out *Overcoming Anxiety For Dummies* by Charles H. Elliott and Laura L. Smith (Wiley) and *Anxiety & Depression Workbook For Dummies* by the same authors (Wiley).

Dealing with depression: Both cause and consequence

If you have an eating disorder, chances are you've met depression both coming and going. More of you have some form of depression to start with than do people without eating disorders. This is especially true if you are bulimic. Depression probably made you more likely to develop an eating disorder in the first place.

Having an eating disorder is also depressing! Because the mind and body are not separate — what affects one affects the other — it can be hard to tell whether depression is the result of the physical effects of food restricting or the emotional consequence of so much effort with so much failure and so many bad feelings about yourself.

You don't get a diagnosis of depression for a fleeting blue mood, an experience that is normal at one time or another for all of us. Nor is depression the same as grieving a loss. If you have depression, you feel hopelessly despairing about who you are and your prospects for the future. Depression disrupts your sleep and your ability to concentrate. It robs life of all color and meaning.

Major depression is a term reserved for the staying-in-bed-with-the-covers-over-your-head kind of depression. Major depression interferes with so much of your functioning that it tends to really stop you in your tracks.

If your symptoms don't quite seem to measure up to the standards of major depression but you feel that what you're experiencing is more than just a typical blue mood, you may have a less severe form of depression known as dysthymia.

Dysthymia (chronic depression) refers to the walking wounded among the depressed. If you are dysthymic, you have most of the same symptoms as people with major depression but not in ways that paralyze you. Living with dysthymia is more like going through your daily paces with lead weights; you can get things done, it just takes much more time and effort.

With dysthymia, you are incredibly vulnerable to failures, slights, or other assaults on your self-image. These can trigger deeper feelings of depression. But you are probably more responsive than the person with major depression to injections of positive experience that support your self-image and improve your mood, at least temporarily. Dysthymia is also known as *chronic depression* because it lasts a long time, often years. Untreated, dysthymia can develop into major depression.

Soothing and distracting yourself with food

Just as food works to self-medicate for anxiety, that is, to comfort and tamp down the experience of dread and agitation, it can work just as well to medicate and take your mind off the emotional discomforts of depression. Everyone would stand up and cheer for such a result if it weren't so temporary and didn't have so many bad effects. (I talk more about how using food to manage emotions makes you vulnerable to an eating disorder in Chapter 5. I provide ideas about managing emotions without food in Chapter 8 and tell you about therapies that are especially helpful for emotion management in Chapter 10.)

Feeling bad when everything depends on weight

Your eating disorder is practically a recipe for depression. Since you are aiming at a cultural ideal of slimness very few bodies are actually equipped to achieve, you're more than likely to be disappointed. Either you can't achieve your goal at all, or you get there but can't stay there. You start from the position that achieving your weight goal is the only way for you to be okay, for you to like yourself. Body weight, which is not nearly as much under your conscious control as you might like to believe, is a highly undependable hook on which to hang self-worth. Low self-worth is a central feature of depression. Constantly doubting your worth because of your weight can help tip you into an episode of depression.

Seeing no light at the end of the tunnel

Despair is another central feature of depression — and of eating disorders, particularly bulimia and binge eating disorder. Each of these disorders involves being caught in a form of the following endless cycle: eating in an uncontrolled way; then taking steps to control eating that only increase the chances of eating in an uncontrolled way again. (You can read about this cycle in detail in Chapter 4.) Being unable to exit the cycle creates feelings of helplessness and hopelessness — ingredients that, in time, tend to lead to depression.

Questionnaire: Is what you're feeling depression?

The following statements are typical of what a person with major depression experiences. Place a check mark in the box next to those statements that you agree with. Checking any of the boxes is cause for concern and a reason to seek help. (You may be suffering from dysthymia, a less severe form of depression.) Checking off a handful or more could indicate major depression.

- ❑ I feel worthless about myself most of the time.
- ❑ I've lost interest in everything, even things that used to give me pleasure.
- ❑ I find it's really hard to focus or make decisions.
- ❑ I'm unusually irritable.
- ❑ I'm constantly tired; everything I need to do seems like too much.
- ❑ I sleep a lot more than usual.
- ❑ My sleep is very disrupted.
- ❑ I feel a lot of aches and pains that are not caused by physical illness.
- ❑ I have frequent thoughts of suicide.

Probably half of you with anorexia have experienced major depression. At least that many of you with bulimia have experienced the disorder, probably a good many more. Depression is also extremely common among people with binge eating disorder. Major depression is dangerous because it can lead to suicide if untreated. Take a look at the previous section, "Considering suicide," and the sidebar, "Steps to take if you're feeling suicidal," if you are feeling in any way suicidal.

Apart from suicide risk, major depression takes a major bite out of your life. It makes your eating disorder worse and harder to treat. But depression *is* treatable, and treating it can be a critical part of your recovery. Seek out the help of a reputable therapist, and be sure to check out *Depression For Dummies,* by

Laura L. Smith and Charles H. Elliott, and the _Anxiety & Depression Workbook For Dummies_ by Elliott, Smith, and Aaron T. Beck (both from Wiley) to get yourself started in the right direction.

Bouncing up and down: Bipolar disorder

Bipolar disorder, formerly known as _manic-depressive illness_, is a mood disorder that involves a lot more than being moody. Depending on severity, bipolar disorder can take you through anything from mild to wild cycling between high and low energy states. The "high" or manic states often involve inflated feelings about yourself and your abilities. They feel like a great ride, at least in the early stages, and seem to bother everybody else more than they do you. The "low" phases, on the other hand, are not fun at any stage. They are pretty well described by the depressive states I reviewed in the preceding section, "Depression: Both cause and consequence."

Studies find that bipolar disorder is much more common among people with anorexia, bulimia, and binge eating disorder than it is among people without eating disorders. Having bipolar disorder will make your eating disorder symptoms worse. They will also make it harder for you to get better. Likewise, your eating disorder symptoms can complicate the treatment of your bipolar illness. The message here is that both need to be treated.

Three great reasons for early evaluation and treatment

Of course you want the best evaluation you can get for any disorder you may have. But there are some particularly compelling reasons to get a sound evaluation for possible bipolar disorder, and to get it early:

- ✔ It appears that having manic episodes may trigger more and worse manic episodes in the future. Treatment to stop this snowballing process is a good idea.

- ✔ Many people whose bipolar disorders go undiagnosed are given antidepressants for their depressed phases. Antidepressants tend to trigger manic episodes. Not the effect you're looking for.

- ✔ Suicide is a very big risk in untreated bipolar disorder.

Questionnaire: Could your "up" moods be manic episodes?

Place a check mark in the box next to those items in the list that you feel reflect the way you feel. Checking even one of these boxes is at least a flag for bipolar disorder. The more you check, the greater the possibility that you may be experiencing manic episodes.

- ❑ I have more energy than I know what to do with.

- ❑ I hardly seem to need any sleep.

❑ I never felt so good, like I could do or be anything.

❑ I have so many ideas, I don't know which one to pursue next.

❑ My creative powers are amazing.

❑ Other people don't seem to share my excitement about myself or my plans.

❑ I can barely hold my thoughts still, one follows another so rapidly.

❑ I find it hard to concentrate.

❑ Sometimes I talk so fast, other people find it hard to follow my thoughts.

❑ I'm quite irritable.

❑ I've been spending a lot more money than usual, maybe money I don't have.

Note: If you feel that some of the statements would be true of you if they were a little less extreme, you may be experiencing a less severe form of the manic state known as *hypomania*. For example, while the person in a manic state may feel they can barely hold their thoughts still, you may feel a pleasurable sense of increased flow in your thoughts. Others may be impressed with this flow of thoughts, but probably won't find them hard to follow, as they would the thoughts of someone in a manic state. Though not as disruptive, hypomania still requires treatment. The nature of all forms of bipolar disorder is to grow worse over time if not treated.

The questionnaire for depression in the previous section also provides good indicators for the presence of the depressive states you find in bipolar disorder. If you haven't already taken this questionnaire, now may be a good time to do so if you think you may have bipolar disorder.

To get more information about bipolar disorder and its treatment, check out *Bipolar Disorder For Dummies* by Candida Fink and Joe Kraynak (Wiley). If you believe you may have bipolar disorder, ask your doctor to refer you to a therapist who can evaluate and treat your symptoms. You can find a local support group at the Depression and Bipolar Support Alliance (www.dbs alliance.org) or at the National Alliance on Mental Illness (NAMI www.nami.org). If you have a child or teen with bipolar disorder, you can find online or local in-person support groups for parents at the Child and Adolescent Bipolar Foundation (www.bpkids.org).

Even though bipolar disorder usually develops in the late teen years or early adulthood, it can show up in childhood and in the early teens as well. If you're a parent who thinks that your child may have bipolar disorder, it may be helpful to know that in children, "manic" symptoms often appear less as extreme happiness or excitement, and more in the form of irritability or tantrums. Several other disorders can look the same way, so you need a professional evaluation. Early treatment is so important with bipolar disorder that you want to have your child checked for any signs that concern you. You can find out more about recognizing possible bipolar illness in your child or young teen and getting help from the Web site of the Child and Adolescent Bipolar Foundation at www.cabf.org.

Adding Addictions to Your Eating Disorder

People who haven't had the chance to discover how to manage emotions constructively may engage in many other destructive behaviors besides their eating disorders to cope. Among the other destructive behaviors people use to cope with their emotions are addictions. While the intent is to feel better, the result is double trouble — more problems to solve when you're trying to recover from your eating disorder. Substance and alcohol abuse and exercise addiction are particularly common among people with eating disorders.

Abusing drugs and alcohol

If you have an eating disorder, you're up to five times more likely to abuse alcohol or illegal drugs than people without eating disorders. These were the findings of a three-year study on the relationship between eating disorders and substance abuse conducted by The National Center on Addiction and Substance Abuse (CASA) at Columbia University.

The connection starts early and involves not only young people with eating disorders but also those merely demonstrating risky eating symptoms, such as dieting, bingeing, or purging. For example, the CASA study found that if you're a young woman, the more severe your dieting behavior is, the more likely you are to drink heavily and to use illegal drugs. If you're a high school student with eating disorder symptoms, on average you're twice as likely to drink, including binge drinking, and to use marijuana, cocaine, and other illegal drugs.

Realizing it's most common when bingeing

Although alcohol and substance abuse can be found across the eating disorder spectrum, it shows up most among those who binge — whether in the context of bulimia, binge eating disorder, or binge/purge anorexia. Rarely is it associated with the restrictive type of anorexia.

By far the highest rates of alcohol and drug use occur among bulimic women. Bulimic women are known to abuse a wide variety of drugs, including amphetamines, prescription stimulants, barbiturates, cocaine, heroine, marijuana, and tranquilizers.

A study of mortality rates among people with eating disorders presented in the *International Journal of Eating Disorders* (July, 2000) showed that people with the bingeing/purging type of anorexia were 12 times more likely to die than their non–eating disordered peers and that alcohol abuse was one of the strongest predictors of death in this group. The researchers believed that alcoholism combined with malnutrition due to anorexia work together to increase chances of fatal cardiac arrhythmias, seizures, alcohol poisoning, and cirrhosis (liver disease). What's more, even weight-restored people with anorexia who were alcoholic showed elevated death rates, apparently due to alcohol's capacity to lower the threshold for suicidal impulses. Even though people with anorexia are less likely to drink alcoholically than people with other eating disorders, when they do, it's more likely to be fatal.

Thinking it will control mood and appetite issues

Depression, as I discuss in the earlier section "Depression: Both cause and consequence," is extremely common among people with eating disorders. People with bulimia are particularly hard-hit. Anxiety is another frequent problem. A widely-accepted explanation for the high rate of co-occurring eating disorders and substance and alcohol abuse is that both represent an attempt to deal with emotions that are swamping the sufferer. The picture you get is of somebody flailing — trying one symptom for relief and then another — just to feel better.

If you binge and then purge to get rid of calories, you're more likely to take amphetamines, cocaine, or heroin to suppress your appetite and increase your metabolism to lose weight. The problem is that your body simply isn't equipped to keep up with the physical wear-and-tear of these activities.

Questionnaire: Do you have a problem with drugs or alcohol?

In the following list, place a check mark in the boxes next to those statements that you answer with a "yes." Positive responses to the following questions may signal that your drug or alcohol use has become a problem, or even an addiction. The more boxes you check, the more serious the problem.

❑ Is your job or school performance suffering because of your use of drugs or alcohol?

❑ Have your relationships with others suffered due to your use of drugs or alcohol?

❑ Have you ever lied to a doctor to obtain prescription drugs?

❑ Have you ever stolen drugs or alcohol or risked your safety to obtain them?

❑ Have you ever used drugs or alcohol to manage emotional pain or stress?

❑ Does the thought of dealing with certain situations without drugs or alcohol, or running out period, terrify you?

❑ Have you ever overdosed?

❑ Do you continue to use drugs or alcohol despite negative consequences?

To find resources for drug and alcohol treatment, check out Drugnet at www.drugnet.net and DrugHelp at www.drughelp.org. Be sure to take a look at *Addiction & Recovery For Dummies* by Brian F. Shaw, Paul Ritvo, Jane Irvine, and M. David Lewis (Wiley) for some great ideas on how to get help with your drug or alcohol problem. In Part II of this book I talk about sorting out the order for treatment when you have alcohol or substance abuse problems along with your eating disorder.

Exercising excessively

Exercise addiction . . . compulsive exercise . . . exercise disorder . . . overexercising syndrome . . . obligatory exercise . . . exercise bulimia . . . all these are names for a pattern of exercise in which you no longer feel like you have a choice in the matter. Exercising excessively is so common among people with eating disorders that some people think it ought to be included in the definition of the disorders.

Thinking it's necessary

If you have an eating disorder, a master motivator for all your huffing and puffing is weight control (and, more recently, body sculpting, that is, shaping and toning your muscles through exercise). Anything that reduces your terror of fat can become essential for daily living. This includes use of exercise as a *compensatory behavior,* that is, behavior to even up the bookkeeping when you think you've taken in too many calories (or *any* calories).

Another big reason why many of you exercise excessively is the same reason you're doing a lot of things excessively (for example, watching your weight, bingeing or purging, trying to be perfect at school or in your job, and so forth): to try to manage emotions or to distract yourself from difficult experiences. Also, like successful dieting, exercise may increase your feelings of being in control and being effective.

Anything you do that serves the purpose of helping you manage your emotions or improve your self-image is likely to take on some serious staying power or even to become an addiction. This is because it starts feeling necessary to your survival.

If you're an addictive exerciser, chances are you feel guilty, out-of-sorts, and/or anxious when you can't exercise. You're not exercising for the fun of it or for the health benefits.

Ignoring the consequences

One of the signs that you may be exercising addictively is the price you are willing to pay for your workout. You may be willing to endure

- ✔ **Exhaustion:** Exercising beyond your physical limits; missing sleep to get your workout

- ✔ **Skeletal injury or damage:** Stress fractures, shin splints, bone fractures, degenerative arthritis, osteoporosis

- ✔ **Internal problems:** Dehydration, heart problems, loss of menstrual periods, infertility

- ✔ **Not showing up:** Cutting class, not going to work, or missing social events so you can exercise

- ✔ **Damaging relationships:** Not being there for friends, family, or your partner because you're putting your workout first

According to Anorexia Nervosa and Related Eating Disorders (ANRED), Inc. (www.anred.com), exercise that consumes more than 3,500 calories per week leads to decreased physical benefits and increased risk of injury.

Questionnaire: Are you exercising addictively?

Place a check mark in the boxes next to those statements that apply to you. Agreement with one or more of the following statements could indicate an exercise addiction.

- ❑ I'll make time to exercise no matter what the cost to myself, including exhaustion or injury.

- ❑ My feelings about myself are affected by how much I work out on a particular day.

- ❑ I've neglected my responsibilities (such as job or school) in order to exercise.

- ❑ Working out has taken the place of much of my social life.

- ❑ I'm likely to feel guilty, anxious, or angry if I can't exercise.

- ❑ It's nearly impossible for me to take a day off from exercise, even if I'm injured or sick.

Part II
Getting Well: Exploring Recovery and Treatment Options

The 5th Wave   By Rich Tennant

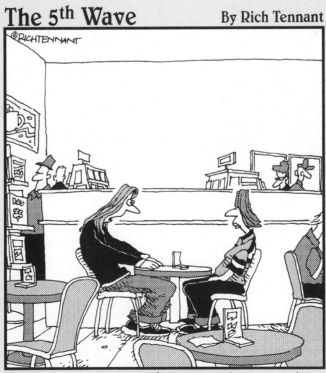

"I'd tell my parents that anorexia counseling wouldn't do me any good, but I'm afraid they'd make me eat my words."

In this part . . .

1 start you off with a rundown of what getting better looks like. Specifically, I detail the physical, behavioral, and emotional landmarks that signal recovery. For each of these landmarks I provide you with a chart so you can track where you are in your own recovery and what you want to work on next.

The meat of Part II is a detailed description of the choices you need to make when you decide to get treatment for your eating disorder. I go over in-patient and out-patient options, individual versus group or family therapies, and various kinds of alternative treatments. I provide guidelines for choosing one kind of treatment over another. I describe different forms of individual therapy in detail. I also review medications used to treat eating disorders.

I round out Part II with a discussion of the ways you can help your own treatment along, including management of early recovery and relapse. I help you recognize when your approach to treatment may be interfering with your progress and describe ways to turn such moments into opportunities to move forward.

Chapter 8

Seeing What Recovery Looks Like

....

In This Chapter

▶ Reviewing markers of renewed physical health

▶ Previewing life without your eating disorder symptoms

▶ Getting a take on healthy eating and exercise

▶ Discovering how to manage relationships, emotions, and self-image in a healthy recovery

....

*R*ecovery means getting over your eating disorder and being healthy. Some define recovery as returning to a normal state, one in which you no longer binge, purge, or starve. By these standards, the majority of people who get treated for an eating disorder get better.

But for most sufferers of an eating disorder, becoming free of symptoms is not enough. In order to emerge into recovery and stay there, you have to come out of your eating disorder better, stronger, wiser, and more skilled at coping with life than you were before. What are the markers of the long-term health you are aiming for? What milestones and accomplishments of recovery land you on a more solid shore in which relapse is less likely? This chapter maps them out for you. It provides a glimpse into your future, the one you'll achieve with a reliable treatment team and your own steady efforts.

Finding Balance in Recovery

As you familiarize yourself with the markers of recovery in this chapter, notice one big idea that weaves its way through most of them. The idea is that finding and maintaining *balance* is the key to your recovery. Balance is the middle ground that lies centered between the extreme ways you've been experiencing life through your eating disorder. If you take away just one idea from this chapter, the idea of finding that balance is the one I recommend.

After several sections you find examples of worksheets that you can adapt to chart your success during recovery. You fill these worksheets in by identifying the progress you've made to date on the recovery marker just discussed and what you need to do next to achieve a specific goal related to that marker. When these worksheets are complete, they become useful recovery tools.

Recovering from your eating disorder may take longer than you want it to. Most people measure the process in years, not weeks or months. On the other hand, those of you who stick with your treatment plan to achieve the strengths and skills I cover in this chapter will gain two invaluable benefits. You'll acquire a lot of insurance against eating disorder relapse, and you'll develop some great resiliency to take you through life's unpredictabilities!

Maintaining a Healthy Weight

Maintaining a certain weight range is a sign of recovery mainly if you've had anorexia. Being too thin is central to your disorder. Being underweight causes a lot of your symptoms or makes them worse. Achieving a healthy weight is essential to recovering physically and psychologically.

No weight standards apply to people recovering from bulimia or binge eating disorder. For these two disorders, healthy recovery has more to do with stabilizing your weight — a predictable outcome of ending the cycling between binging and purging and dieting. You may find this new focus disappointing if you still believe that to get better you must get thinner, but achieving a healthy, stable weight is the real goal. Take a look at the next section, "Finding your healthy weight," to find out how to determine what a healthy weight is for you.

Finding your healthy weight

A healthy weight is one at which all of your body's systems — organs, hormones, brain, the works — are able to get the nutritional support they need to function normally. When you achieve a healthy weight, your body can carry you through the physical, mental, and emotional demands of your day and your life.

Did you know you are living with the world's leading expert on exactly the right body weight for you? That expert is your body itself! Your body lets you know what weight range is right for you in two important ways: It sends distress signals when your weight falls too low, and it has a tendency to settle at and maintain a *setpoint,* the weight at which your body functions at its best.

When your weight goes too low

Your body signals you with distressing symptoms when your weight falls too low. Developing an awareness of these symptoms is important because they alert you when your weight falls below a healthy level. You find out more about these symptoms in Chapter 6, but in short, visible symptoms to be on the lookout for include:

✔ Dry, brittle hair and nails, hair loss, dry skin

✔ Severe cold sensitivity; cold hands and feet

✔ Easy bruising

While most of these symptoms occur only with significant weight loss, some earlier warning signals, perhaps specific to you, can also alert you to a potential problem. Consider the following:

✔ Do you feel a little less energetic when your weight falls below your optimum range?

✔ Do you feel a bit less alert?

✔ Does your mood start to tumble?

Changes in your mood and energy level may be signs that you need to either increase your food intake or reduce your energy output until your weight returns to a level that supports good health.

When your weight is just right for you

Your body tells you about its best weight range through the mechanism of *setpoint*. Your setpoint is the weight your body keeps returning to when you're eating in a healthy way and not doing anything in particular to control your weight (that is, you're not dieting, purging, or exercising compulsively). According to setpoint theory, this is your body's natural weight, the one that makes it happiest. When you try to drive your weight below your setpoint by dieting, your body eventually rebels and you see all your dieting efforts undone. Gaining weight to reach your setpoint may be upsetting, especially if your setpoint appears to be above your desired weight or cultural ideals of slimness. The payoff for accepting an outcome higher than your ideal is ending a state of warfare with your body. This kind of acceptance may take *lots* of work to achieve, but the outcome is well worth it.

Skirting the pitfalls of keeping track

When you've had an eating disorder, you need to move away from an obsessive focus on weight as part of your recovery. You should no longer concern yourself with the number on the scales. However, if you've been severely anorexic, the medical consequences of weight loss are too risky to be treated casually. In this case, *someone* needs to keep track of your weight during your recovery period; that someone just shouldn't be *you*. Most likely your nutritionist or doctor will be the one to track your weight. You'll probably be asked to agree to be weighed in his or her office and to be informed only of whether you're staying in your goal range (as opposed to knowing your exact weight).

For those of you recovering from milder cases of anorexia, or from bulimia or binge eating disorder, the goal is getting the greatest weight stability with the least focus. Letting your body find its setpoint is the easiest way to put your system on cruise control so you can pay less attention. (See the preceding section, "When your weight is just right for you.") Instead of focusing on calories and pounds, the idea is to focus on your health. When you eat and exercise in a healthy way (see the sections "Eating Healthfully with No Forbidden Foods" and "Exercising in a Healthy Way" later in this chapter), your body tells you how much you need to eat to maintain a weight that's right for you. Hearing it has just been extremely hard to do through all the cultural and eating disorder chatter.

Menstruating Normally

For a long time, disruption of menstrual cycles was thought to be a symptom only women with anorexia needed to worry about. Furthermore, the return of normal cycles was considered proof-positive that the weight of the woman with anorexia had returned to a safe range. More recently, exceptions to these rules seem to turn up all over the place. For instance:

- About half of women with bulimia have disrupted cycles for reasons not yet clear to researchers.
- Some women with anorexia who are still in weight jeopardy get their periods back anyway.
- Some women with anorexia fail to regain their periods at weights where they should have.

Despite the existence of these exceptions to the rule, if you are recovering from anorexia, normal menstruation without the help of birth control pills is still going to be one of the most important signs your physician looks for to make sure your physical recovery is on track.

Getting to normal periods

Being able to produce a menstrual period is about having enough body weight and enough body fat. Your body has to have a minimum of both to make estrogen and related reproductive hormones. No estrogen, no menstrual cycle.

As researchers take a closer look, other body systems and hormones seem to be important to menstrual balance as well — which ones are just not yet clear! Possibly a part of the brain called the *hypothalamus* is involved. The hypothalamus regulates metabolism and many other basic body systems. The series of hormonal events that tells your ovaries to produce estrogen is also linked to the hypothalamus. The stress hormone cortisol may also play a role.

Your body's systems need a healthy balance in your weight, nutrition, exercise, and emotional life in order to work properly. When you supply your body's systems with these basic needs, in most instances your body responds by supplying you with regular menstrual cycles.

Losing your periods

Fertility is a concern for many women in recovery from anorexia. The chain of hormonal events that controls your menstrual cycle results in *ovulation* — the release of an egg that might get fertilized and thus result in a pregnancy. If you're not menstruating, you can't get pregnant. Fertility problems can hang around for years after your disorder, depending on how long you had it. Fertility problems are mainly treatable.

Having your periods tells you that your estrogen production is back on line. Being able to become pregnant isn't the only positive outcome. Estrogen is a multitasking hormone, doing good in many parts of your body. Here are three of estrogen's most valuable effects:

✔ Keeping your bones strong. (You may have to work with your treatment team to undo bone loss that occurred during the worst of your disorder.)

✔ Protecting your heart and blood vessels.

✔ Improving your cholesterol levels.

Seeing Bingeing or Purging Symptoms Subside

If you're recovering from the binge/purge type of anorexia or from bulimia, a sound recovery means a significant reduction in bingeing and purging symptoms. If you suffer from binge eating disorder, recovery equates to a reduction in bingeing.

Recovery is not an all-or-nothing affair in which you either stop your symptoms 100 percent or you fail and remain disordered. In recovery, you're invited to explore the middle ground. A good recovery in terms of bingeing and purging symptoms means

✔ **You get a handle on what triggers your symptoms.** For example, you may figure out that the single biggest reason for your bingeing is trying to calm down when you become swamped with emotions. Anger and fear of abandonment are two triggers that get to you every time.

✔ **You develop constructive alternatives for handling your emotions.** For instance, maybe you find ways to speak up more directly and effectively when you're angry. Maybe you trace your abandonment fears to early losses in your childhood and turn your focus in therapy to comforting and reassuring yourself in ways that don't involve food.

✔ **You use constructive alternatives more often than you use your symptoms to manage your emotions.** Improvement is mostly a matter of practice, practice, practice — like getting to Carnegie Hall. And, yes, many people do, in time, leave their symptoms behind altogether.

Dieting is a key trigger for bingeing and many other aspects of your eating disorder. Talking about a sound recovery in which you are still dieting is not realistic.

Recovery isn't all or nothing

You may be wondering if success means that your bingeing and purging symptoms have to be done and gone forever. No! Your symptoms aren't likely to be gone for good for a very long time. Eating disorder recovery usually takes place over a number of years, not weeks or months. You're more likely to see a gradual shift that reflects not only your practice in using symptom alternatives, but also your growth in other related areas: increased self-esteem, improvement in mood, development of skills that allow you to feel more competent, and so forth.

A slip isn't a failure

Slip-ups happen. Visiting an old neighborhood doesn't mean you're going to live there again! Here is yet another great opportunity to explore the possibilities of living in middle ground. In middle ground, mistakes don't ruin things. First, you don't have to be mistake-free to be worthwhile or to be just fine. Second, mistakes aren't shameful black marks on your record. They're part of the human condition. What's more, they present opportunities to learn and make course corrections. To find out more about growing from your slip-ups, be sure to read the section on handling relapse in Chapter 14.

To measure your progress regarding slip-ups, you can use a worksheet like the example shown in Table 8-1.

Table 8-1	Bingeing Recovery Marker
What I've Already Achieved	*What to Work on Next*
Example: I'm aware my worst bingeing is when I'm feeling lonely. I'm trying to reach out to others more. I'm experimenting with journaling my feelings.	**Example:** Figure out more of my binge triggers and some ways to handle them.

Getting Thinking Processes Normal

Disordered thinking is an important part of the engine that keeps an eating disorder going. Here's a sampler of some typical disordered thoughts:

- ✔ I'll feel better when I'm thinner.
- ✔ Everything will be better when I'm thin.
- ✔ Things are all one way or another (so-called *black-and-white thinking*).
- ✔ I have to be perfect to be okay.

When you have anorexia, your thinking distortions include not only all the above, but also denial of your thin body state and the consequences of starving yourself.

Your thinking processes return to normal when you land solidly on ground where thin doesn't rule. A lot more important things determine what make you and other people worthwhile or likable. And life's problems aren't solved by being thin.

Middle ground is no longer just a theory; it's a place where you've established some real estate. You know how to find your way back there when you find you've slipped into the old extremes. For example, you know how to translate a negative thought like "I ate too much — I blew it" into more productive thinking like: "Wait a minute. I ate more than I meant to tonight. But that's part of a normal eating pattern. I just need to take a minute to think about whether it means I was stressed about something and didn't realize it."

De-stinking your thinking

If you've had anorexia, restoring your weight will go far toward improving the rigidities in your thinking. That's because many of your distorted thoughts are an actual effect of starvation on your brain. (You can read more about the effects of starvation in Chapter 7.)

Apart from clearing up anorexia's starvation effects, most of the rest of the improvement for all eating disordered people comes from participating in a therapeutic process that invites you to challenge your distortions — what the 12-step people call "stinkin' thinkin'." This process can take place in individual therapy, group therapy, a therapeutic community, Overeaters Anonymous (OA), or what have you — just so long as you have the chance to examine these disordered thinking processes and to replace them with healthier ones.

Enjoying better thinking

Your thinking processes have arrived in healthy territory when your basic self-esteem and sense of security are no longer threatened by the fact or the possibility of

- ✔ Weight gain
- ✔ Overeating
- ✔ Making a mistake or failing
- ✔ Disappointing someone
- ✔ Making someone angry

To measure your progress regarding improved thinking, you can use a worksheet like the example shown in Table 8-2.

Table 8-2	Thinking Process Recovery Marker
What I've Already Achieved	*What to Work on Next*
Example: I'm beginning to see how black-and-white thinking applies to all parts of my life, not just food.	**Example:** Practice looking for those gray areas about weight, food, everything!

Eating Well with No Forbidden Foods

I hesitate to use the word *diet* because it has had such toxic meanings for you. By diet I mean your *way of eating*. I am certainly not referring to restricting your food or calories in any form. As you recover from your eating disorder, you develop a way of eating that *includes* rather than *excludes* foods — an eating pattern that's about health and enjoyment, not pounds and performance.

Establishing a healthy eating pattern is as difficult as anything you accomplish in recovery. It means creating a whole new relationship with food and eating — one in which you aren't at war with each other! Imagine thinking of food as being on your side, supporting you in what you're trying to accomplish each day. Imagine that, at times, food can be there for pure pleasure, adding to the fun or ritual of a social event, or just enhancing a pleasant night at home. When food and hunger have taken their places as natural rhythms in your life, not enemies to be defeated, all these things can happen. (You find ideas on how to start developing a better relationship with food in Chapter 14.)

Understanding healthy eating

A healthy and varied way of eating means you get the nutritional value from your food that your body needs in order to function and thrive. It actually takes a wide variety of foods to supply all your nutritional needs: grains (including whole grains), proteins, vegetables, fruits. You don't have to achieve a perfect balance of the food groups with all vitamins and minerals represented every day. Nutritionists say that balance is something you figure out more on a weekly basis than a daily one.

Here's a really neat thing to look forward to in recovery. Once your practice is to partner with your body's nutritional needs rather than be at war with them, your body begins to let you know when you're running low on something by sending you urges for it. Sometimes the urges are for the fun stuff; sometimes they're for the stuff that makes your engines run. I know what you're thinking: "*Urges* for broccoli? No way! And what's that about urges for the fun stuff?" Read on . . . .

Including forbidden foods

You're probably thinking, "She can't mean onion rings. Or banana splits or corn dogs." Yes, actually, I do. This may come as a real shocker. As soon as you start making any food the enemy, you make it more desirable, and you're back in that contest of wills that's part of your eating disorder. In recovery, the idea of middle ground is there once again to guide you. Where do foods belong in your way of eating when they have no nutritionally redeeming value but they just taste so darn good? Probably not daily on a lettuce leaf for lunch, any more than you'd make weekly trips to Istanbul to see that guy you flirted with in the Grand Bazaar. But including these adventures once in awhile sure adds some important spice to life!

To measure your progress regarding healthy eating, you can use a worksheet like the example shown in Table 8-3.

Table 8-3	Healthy Eating Recovery Marker
What I've Already Achieved	*What to Work on Next*
Example: Tolerating small amounts of fat without freaking out. Learning about healthy fats.	**Example:** Having binge foods when I'm not bingeing

Exercising in a Healthy Way

Repeat after me: *Exercise is not for the purpose of burning off dinner or punishment for that candy bar I just ate.* Then what's left? I'm glad you asked! The following list includes some of the really great benefits you get when you exercise in a healthy way:

- ✔ **Physical benefits (just some of them!):**
  - Strengthens your bones (provided you weigh enough)
  - Improves your heart health
  - Strengthens your immune function
  - Protects you against diabetes and other metabolic disorders
  - Improves your sleeping
  - Increases your stamina
- ✔ **Psychological benefits:**
  - Reduces stress
  - Relieves anxiety
  - Improves your mood
- ✔ **Pleasure in movement:** You have an opportunity to discover all the ways your body can move through space and how it most likes to do so (see the section "Exploring physical activity for pleasure").

Exercising too much or too hard robs you of these benefits. Current government guidelines suggest about 30 minutes of moderate exercise most days of the week (that's *most*, not *every*) in order to maintain good health.

Determining what healthy exercise is

Exercising in a healthy way means, above all, remaining tuned in to your body. Being tuned in means staying alert for signals about how your body's doing with what you are asking of it. Assuming you're not an athlete in training (if you are, you may want to read Chapter 16, "Athletes and Eating Disorders"), during healthy exercise ask yourself the following questions:

- ✔ **What's happening with your breathing and your heart rate?** You shouldn't be wheezing nor should your heart be pounding out of your chest.

- ✔ **How do your muscles feel?** Hint: "Going for the burn" is a great way to get injured.

- ✔ **Are there any other sources of pain?** Remember, pain has a purpose: It signals you when something is wrong that needs fixing.

- ✔ **Has your workout left you feeling invigorated or wrung out like a dishrag?** Healthy exercise is supposed to give you energy, not take it away!

The point of all this tuning in, besides just knowing yourself, is to enable you to make necessary course corrections based on the information you get. If you meant to jog for 30 minutes but your body's screaming for the showers at 20, you can stop. Since you're exercising for health and enjoyment, not for size reduction, you're free to make a choice like this that puts your well-being before calories burned.

Being tuned in helps you make healthy day-to-day choices. It also guides you in the longer term. Do you find that six days a week of aerobic workouts regularly leaves you fatigued but four days feels about right? Are you sick or injured? Do you need to knock off your routine for a few days or even a few weeks so exercise won't make you worse? Were you sure you had to be a jogger to be okay, but find your joints telling you that they really prefer swimming? By being responsive, you form a partnership with your body, much as you do with food. This partnership ensures that you are fit and that your body is able to carry you through the activities you need and want it to in life.

Exploring physical activity for pleasure

Exercise shouldn't be drudgery. And it certainly shouldn't be your penance for eating too much. Dropping the focus on calorie burning while getting tuned in to your body opens up a whole new possibility: choosing exercise or physical activity because it feels good! The idea is to find an activity that appeals to your tastes and preferences, one that you really enjoy doing.

In recovery you have the freedom to experiment and discover what kinds of movement you like best. Do you like freestyle dancing? Aerobic dance? Yoga? Swimming? Soccer? Walking? Does your body prefer to exercise first thing in the morning or not until you've been moving around all day? Do you have the best time when you exercise in a class, on a team, or by yourself? Do you like lots of variety? Does the need for special skills get your engines going or get in your way? When you take the time to choose physical activity that gives you pleasure, you discover that your body can do a lot better things for you than get you skinny.

To measure your progress regarding exercising in a healthy way, you can use a worksheet like the example shown in Table 8-4.

Table 8-4	Healthy Exercise Recovery Marker
What I've Already Achieved	*What to Work on Next*
Example: I'm practicing being *in* my body when I exercise, so I'm aware of how my body is responding.	**Example:** Try dancercise. I hate jogging.

Creating Healthy Relationships

In recovery, you feel safe in knowing that you need other people. You don't have to rely on food as a poor substitute for human connection. You develop a range of skills that help you to get along with others and to keep the relationships you prize and make them better.

Sound relationships in recovery reflect the two sides of living in a world of other people: autonomy, separateness, and individuality on the one hand, and attachment and connection on the other. In other words, the *me* and the *we*. Healthy relating recognizes the fundamental importance of each and doesn't ask that, on the whole, either one be sacrificed for the other. This doesn't mean that one or the other doesn't get put on the back burner from time to time while the other is emphasized. That's just life. But overall, for any of us to thrive, the *me* and the *we* parts of our lives need to be equally well developed and expressed.

Setting appropriate boundaries

Boundaries reflect how an individual is treated in a particular relationship. Healthy boundaries respect individual rights, abilities, and opinions. (This doesn't always mean getting your way, although, of course, in a just universe it would.) Here's where the rubber meets the road. Not everyone you relate to is going to live up to these standards. That means your own boundaries must be clear enough to allow you to ask the other person to change or to allow you to set limits on the boundary violation.

Here are some examples of boundaries being crossed:

- ✔ Your roommate goes into your closet and borrows clothes without asking.

- ✔ Your father feels free to interrupt your every opinion and tell you what you should be thinking.

- ✔ Your sister tells her friends about something that happened with your boyfriend, even though you asked her to keep it a secret.

- ✔ Your boss calls you at home on Saturday about a matter that could have easily waited until Monday.

- ✔ Aunt Agatha can't resist fixing the way you decorated a cake or rearranging where you've put your new rug.

- ✔ Mom writes your report for class. She knows you've got the basic ideas; she just knows how to put them a little better.

- ✔ Your husband acts as if you are betraying him if you have friends or activities you don't want the two of you to share.

In order to set a limit and establish a clear personal boundary in any of these situations, you need the following qualities, skills, and beliefs:

- ✔ **You need a clear sense of self.** You need to know that a separate you exists in order to recognize boundary violations and to insist on your rights.

- ✔ **You have to know you are entitled to respect for your individual rights.** This comes from understanding healthy boundaries.

- ✔ **You have to *feel* or trust you are entitled to respect for your individual rights.** This comes from self-esteem.

- ✔ **You need to be able to say no to what the other person wants or expects when it isn't right for you.** This means trusting it won't kill them, it won't kill you, and, if the relationship is healthy enough, it won't kill the relationship.

The ability to say no when you need to, along with other skills of boundary-making, is so crucial to feeling you will be safe and won't lose yourself in relationships that it has led to a therapy maxim: *You have to be able to say* no *in order to be able to say* yes. *Yes* means agreeing to be in a relationship in the first place and being okay with the times when it seems right to put your needs second and compromise. In other words, before there can be a safe *we*, there has to be a secure, solid *me*.

Here's what healthy boundary-making might look like in a few of the preceding situations:

✔ Your roommate goes into your closet and borrows clothes without asking.

First you need to decide what's okay with you. Can she borrow if she asks ahead of time? Can she borrow some things, but not others? Maybe you don't like lending your clothes at all. Whatever you decide is all right. You might then say: "I noticed you borrowed my pink sweater last night. I don't mind. I just like to know ahead of time." Or: "I noticed you borrowed my sweater. I know some people are comfortable with sharing clothes, but I prefer not to."

✔ Your father feels free to interrupt your every opinion and tell you what you should be thinking.

Using what couples therapists call an *I-statement* (in which you focus on how someone's behavior makes you feel instead of attacking the person), you might say something like: "Dad, when you keep interrupting me and telling me what I'm supposed to think, it makes it too hard to be in the conversation with you. I just feel frustrated and unheard. It makes me feel like what I think doesn't matter. We have to change this pattern if we're going to talk to each other."

✔ Your sister tells her friends about something that happened with your boyfriend, even though you asked her to keep it a secret.

Using an I-statement again, you might tell your sister you feel really let down by her failure to honor your secrets. "It means I don't feel safe now confiding in you, which is a big loss to me. That makes me feel hurt and sad and angry."

Allowing appropriate intimacy

Intimacy is a quality of closeness and connection that describes family relationships, friendships, or romantic partnerships. In recovery, healthy intimacy includes

✔ **Knowing and being known.** Feeling safe in letting people know the inner you — your thoughts, hopes, fears, failings, secret ambitions — is the opposite of shame. Feeling safe requires you to trust that others will see your worth in spite of any negative qualities. The flip side is trusting that you can do the same for others, that an ability to see the whole package, including plusses and minuses, is replacing your old black-and-white thinking. When you develop a sense of trust, you feel safe enough to really get to know another person. Whatever you discover that's disappointing isn't likely to spoil what you value in them.

✔ **Relating in an interdependent way.** *Interdependence* is a word professionals use usually to describe an ongoing partnership. It means that each partner knows they can rely on the other for the commitment, emotional connection, and task-sharing that make the relationship work. If your history involves traumatic boundary violation, neglect, or abandonment, an interdependent relationship will reflect a lot of healing.

✔ **Resting your weight fully on the other person as a safe "sometimes" thing in which you don't have to lose yourself.** Perhaps you're sick, you're sad, you're stressed, or you just want a little babying. Indulging yourself is okay because you are confident that you can go back to the independent you when you've gotten your fill.

✔ **Disagreeing and fighting safely.** This means you are developing skills for being in conflict with another person and for resolving conflict successfully. It includes the skills of compromise, in which each person's needs are honored. Like saying no, it means trusting that anger and disagreement won't do either of you or the relationship in.

✔ **Figuring out how to repair damage when it's done.** This is the part where, among other things, you each acknowledge the other's wounds and say "I'm sorry."

✔ **Ensuring that sexual relationships include respect for your needs as well as your partner's.** This includes knowing your needs, being able to talk about them, feeling entitled to ask to have them met, and trusting your partner to respond with respect.

Your relationship with your therapist or members of a therapy group is a safe place to find out about and practice healthy relationship skills, including those of boundary-making and intimate connection.

To measure your progress regarding developing healthy relationships, you can use a worksheet like the example shown in Table 8-5.

Table 8-5	Healthy Relationships Recovery Marker
What I've Already Achieved	*What to Work on Next*
Example: I told my boyfriend it doesn't work for me when he makes decisions for the two of us.	**Example:** Trusting he'll still want to be with me if I continue to speak up.

Tolerating Your Emotions

Your eating disorder has served as a means of managing uncomfortable, and sometimes overwhelming, emotions. The good news is that it helped you survive when you didn't know what else to do. The bad news is that repeatedly turning to food or restricting convinced you that you couldn't tolerate difficult feelings. In recovery, you discover that you can!

Acknowledging the feelings of life experiences doesn't make life itself easier. But it does smooth out the self-inflicted hardships that come from dodging and weaving to avoid feeling. Maybe your eating disorder has been your main buffer. Or maybe you've also relied on the use of substances, alcohol, or other addictive behaviors. You may protect yourself with the emotional disconnection allowed by dissociation. Or you may resort to workaholism. Whatever stops you from knowing your emotional experience of events is bound to make trouble for you in some way. You're also likely to be left with a sense of emptiness, as if a dimension of you or your life is missing.

Being able to tolerate your feelings means you don't have to do anything to get rid of them. Even the most upsetting ones are safe to acknowledge, in spite of the fact that they may be uncomfortable. Grief, disappointment, anger, humiliation, rejection . . . these emotions remain as yucky-feeling as ever. What changes is that you discover that you can manage them; you can tolerate being uncomfortable. And the more you work at it, the more discomfort you can handle, like the way your lungs expand when you've been working out regularly.

Allowing and assessing feelings

While it may be hard to imagine now, in recovery you gain confidence in your ability to manage your emotions without resorting to your eating disorder. You don't fear being overwhelmed by your feelings because you have increased your toleration for them and you've developed more skills for coping with them (like self-soothing). People who are confident about managing their emotions do two things:

- ✔ They stay in awareness long enough to know what they're feeling and what those feelings are about.

- ✔ They take steps to feel better.

Being aware of your feelings

Staying in awareness means knowing what you're feeling in the present moment. The better you get at it and the more confidence you develop that you can tolerate whatever comes up, the more precise you are in what you're aware of. For example, in the past you may just have had a vague sense of "I feel bad." As you increase your ability to stay focused and aware of what you're feeling, you're better able to discover the all-important details: "I feel upset with myself because I snapped at Dad last night. He was only trying to help. There's just something about the way he puts things — like if I'd only listened to him — that makes me furious so I can't listen." Here's an example:

> *Mindy* spent the entire day with a cloud over her head. Something didn't feel right. In her eating disordered days, she would have binged when she got home to dispel the cloud. In recovery, she used the quiet of being home to really tune in to the feelings creating the cloud. She recognized that pit in her stomach: She felt *guilt*, mixed with a little anger and a little fear. By staying with the feelings, Mindy was able to trace them back to their source.
>
> Mindy's friend, Alison, had asked her to go to a party Saturday night. Mindy had been looking forward to some downtime for herself. Also, she wasn't comfortable with the crowd she knew would be at the party. It had taken a lot of courage to tell Alison no, something Mindy couldn't have done in the past. Alison's disappointment was obvious, even though she said it was okay.
>
> Mindy tuned in to her thoughts about what happened: "Shouldn't I have just gone to the party? I know there's this guy Alison wants to meet who's going to be there." (There's the guilt: "I'm a bad friend.") "Couldn't Alison have cut me some slack? She knows how hard I've been working." (Whoops. Now we've got the anger.) "What if Alison decides other people are just more fun and drops me?" (And now we've got the fear.) Read on to find out how Mindy resolves these feelings.

Addressing what feels bad

Any problem in life is easier to address if you know exactly what's wrong. Silence on the other end of the line because your cell phone needs recharging requires a different remedy than a silence that occurs when you've just shocked or angered your friend into speechlessness! Trying to address your feelings without knowing what they are is like stumbling around in a dark room. In recovery you find ways to feel more confident about knowing all your feelings. Knowing what your feelings are about means identifying

- ✔ **The emotion that's coming up:** Anger, sadness, fear, frustration, shame, disappointment, and so on.

- ✔ **The trigger for (source of) the emotion:** A person (including yourself), an event or behavior that happened (she dissed you, you tripped in front of everyone, your parents argued), an event or behavior that didn't happen (he didn't call, you didn't make honor roll).

- ✔ **The cause of the emotion:** The reason the trigger had the impact it did. For instance, the person that dissed you is your ex's new girlfriend. Your parents' arguing has been happening more frequently and is getting more severe. He didn't call even though he promised he would and it was your birthday. You didn't make the honor roll and the whole family was counting on you for it.

In the example in the preceding section, Mindy tuned in to what went on and how it affected her emotionally. This allowed her to take steps to make herself feel better. Instead of burying the feelings, she figured out what made her feel bad in the first place. For instance, she reminded herself of all the ways she'd been a good friend to Alison and that this one event didn't change that. But she also decided she'd been a little sharp with Alison, so she called her and said so. She also suggested they have lunch. Even though Mindy didn't want to go to the party, Alison still wanted to see her. Finally, Mindy decided she'd probably overreacted to the episode because she was so exhausted. She used this signal to make sure she got to her yoga class on Saturday. Yoga always seemed to have a soothing effect on her when she was frazzled.

Making better choices through awareness

You may wonder, "Isn't thinking about what's upsetting me just wallowing in my feelings?" It all depends on how you use it. *The point about awareness is that it allows you to make choices.* I suppose you could wallow, if that felt right to you. But you can also use awareness to make positive choices when you feel an emotional cloud hanging over your day. Any number of constructive possibilities becomes available once you know what's going on.

Not all emotional clouds are dispelled as easily as others. Some are more complicated because they invite in old, unresolved emotional wounds or trauma. Others involve ongoing situations in which you have to live with threat or uncertainty, such as waiting for the results of a medical test or knowing your job could be cut. Sometimes in recovery the most valuable discoveries turn out to be those things which simply soothe you without causing you harm. Even in the most difficult circumstances, awareness gives you the gift of choice and, where needed, the possibility of healing. (I go into more detail about developing emotion management skills in Chapter 14.)

To measure your progress with emotion management skills, you can use a worksheet like the example shown in Table 8-6.

Table 8-6	Healthy Emotions Recovery Marker
What I've Already Achieved	*What to Work on Next*
Example: If I've binged and purged, I stop to figure out what I was feeling that triggered the episode.	**Example:** Stopping to think about what I'm feeling *before* I binge and purge.

Maintaining a Healthy Self-Image

Creating a positive self-image that isn't based on your weight is a challenge of recovery that requires you to be better, or smarter anyway, than your culture. Keeping that image usually means tuning out many of the unhealthy aspects of the culture when it comes to its emphasis on weight. Even women who've never had a formal eating disorder (and an increasing number of men) struggle with this one.

A healthy recovery means you quit turning to your weight to find out if you're okay or whether you're likable or worthwhile. In recovery, you take your worth as a given. You don't have to earn it each day on the scales, or anywhere else.

Seeing your worth beyond your weight

You spent your eating disordered years so focused on your weight that you forgot to notice all the other terrific things about yourself. These will be the new basis of your positive self-image in recovery. You don't have to wait! Start making a list of your non-weight–related assets right now. Make sure you only include answers that actually feel meaningful to you.

- ✔ What do you like about yourself?
- ✔ What do you think of as your strengths?
- ✔ What accomplishments are you proud of?
- ✔ What compliments do you frequently get that have nothing to do with body size?
- ✔ What qualities do people tell you they appreciate in you?

Answers to questions like these will provide you with an anchor when you feel the pull of your own weight-based judgments in the future. You aren't required to stick with your old responses. You can begin to build new ones.

Deflating weight obsession

In recovery it becomes your reflex to move weight to the back burner of your attention, partly because you know that to focus on your weight is to risk fueling your eating disorder. But it also becomes your habit as a result of practicing. You may not be able to stop weight thoughts from coming into your mind. But as long as you're walking in the land of awareness, you can make choices about what you do with those thoughts when they pop up.

Here are some strategies that may help you keep your weight on the back burner:

- ✔ **Look in the mirror *once* before you leave home** — you don't want an uneven hemline or mismatched socks — but then get out of there. Don't dwell.

- ✔ **Take a friend without an eating disorder clothes shopping with you.** She'll see you more clearly than you see yourself.

- ✔ **Purchase accessories you love that don't have anything to do with body size.** Best are items that emphasize physical qualities you like, such as a scarf that shows off your dazzling eye color.

- ✔ **Always have in mind that list of all the qualities you like about yourself.** These may be physical or personal traits or both — whichever most effectively pulls you out of that weight-centered universe.

- ✔ **Think about something else.** Sometimes it's okay not to be in awareness!

- ✔ **Practice movement for pleasure** (see the section "Exercising in a Healthy Way," earlier in this chapter). It adds the dimension of appreciating your body from the inside out in ways that have nothing to do with weight.

- ✔ **Regularly update your list of other things you like about yourself, the things that really matter about you.** It keeps your eye on the ball where it belongs.

To measure your progress regarding regaining a positive image, you can use a worksheet like the example shown in Table 8-7.

Table 8-7	Positive Image Recovery Marker
What I've Already Achieved	*What to Work on Next*
Example: I've thrown away my scales. I've started my list of assets. They include physical agility, great eyes, a good sense of humor, and being a supportive friend and partner.	**Example:** Expand asset list. Keep copy on fridge and closet door. No more body size talk with friends.

Chapter 9

Deciding the Who, What, and Where for Treatment

Hospital? Residential treatment? Outpatient care? Once you accept the idea that you need treatment for your eating disorder, you're faced with a dizzying array of choices. What's the right setting for your treatment? How do you know? What experts do you need to include? In what order? How do you go about choosing them?

In this chapter I walk you through those first decisions you need to make. To make the best early treatment decisions, you need to determine how severe your eating disorder is. I go over how to match the severity of your symptoms with the treatment options out there. I explain who you can work with to help you figure this out. I also give you the information you need to find the professionals who'll make up your treatment team and suggestions for selecting the ones who are right for you.

Finding the Right Therapist

No matter how many people end up being involved in your recovery, getting better begins with you and an individual therapist. (See the section "Assembling Your Team" to find out about the different kinds of therapists.) The two of you are going to be doing some heavy lifting together, focusing on who you are, how you can get better, and how you can reach your fullest potential. If you're going to do this kind of intimate work with a person, you want to make sure she's someone you trust and feel comfortable with. How do you decide that? How do you find such a person in the first place? I address these questions in this section. In fact, most of what I discuss applies equally well to choosing any member of your treatment team with whom you'll need to work intensely and intimately during the recovery process.

Finding an eating disorder therapist

The first order of business is to find therapists who specialize in working with eating disorders. The following resources can get you started:

- ✔ **This book's "Resource Guide":** A great place to start your search for a therapist who specializes in eating disorders is the "Resource Guide" at the back of this book. There you find Web sites for a number of eating disorder organizations that keep lists of such therapists.

- ✔ **Online chat rooms:** Chat rooms are becoming more common as sources for eating disorder therapy recommendations. Everything I just said about needing to check credentials applies to names you get from chat rooms. But chat rooms provide an unusual opportunity to get feedback from people who've been in your shoes.

- ✔ **Eating disorder programs:** Another good potential source of eating disorder specialists is any program that treats or studies eating disorders. This may be a nearby university, hospital, or residential treatment facility.

- ✔ **People within eating disorder professional networks:** If you've already located any other members of your treatment team — for example, a nutritionist or a primary care provider (PCP) who treats eating disorders — these people are likely to be working with therapists and can probably recommend some they like. Even if you're just starting to assemble your team, your family's PCP probably has a pretty good file on hand of specialists, which just may include an eating disorder therapist.

- ✔ **School guidance counselors or college student health centers:** Chances are they've made eating disorder referrals before.

- ✔ **Word-of-mouth:** Do you have a friend who likes her therapist? Maybe he knows an eating disorder specialist. Does your neighbor's kid have an eating disorder? You may want to ask him for a recommendation.

Checking credentials

Credentials usually refer to professional degrees and state licensure to practice. These days you can get most of this kind of information about a prospective therapist from the Internet — and more and more people do just that. You can also ask directly. Any therapist you're interviewing should be ready, willing, and able to explain his credentials.

In addition to credentials, you want to know about this therapist's experience. You may want to ask the following questions:

- How long has he been in practice?
- How long has he been treating eating disorders?
- Has he had any special training in eating disorders?
- Does he treat all eating disorders or just some?
- What proportion of his practice is devoted to eating disorders?

You are entitled to ask questions. You need to know about the qualifications of someone who may be taking on a crucial and demanding role in your life. If the therapist you're interviewing makes you feel uncomfortable for asking about qualifications, he's probably not the person for you.

Knowing what you can expect

Some qualities that you should expect from any therapist go beyond training and expertise. Call them the human touch. Ask yourself the following questions:

- Does he listen?
- Does he seem interested in me and my situation?
- Does he seem to "get" me?
- Is he willing to work with other people on my treatment team?
- Is he respectful when discussing issues like fees and scheduling appointments?
- Does he respond respectfully to any doubts I express?
- Does he understand professional boundaries, in particular, that my therapy is not the place for him to get his personal needs met?

If you answer "no" to all or most of the items on this list about a particular therapist, consider restarting your search. On the other hand, if just one or two things trouble you about the therapist, bring them up. You may feel reassured by what he has to say. You'll also find out if this therapist is willing to discuss your concerns about him. A successful resolution means you've already become stronger as a team. (I talk more about building the therapy partnership through discussing disappointments and making repairs in Chapter 13.)

Determining goodness-of-fit

A therapist can have the best of credentials and training. She can be the best thing since sliced bread in the eyes of the friend who referred her. She can even respond pretty well to the basic questions I list in the preceding section. But that doesn't necessarily mean she's the right therapist for you. Intangibles, just like the chemistry you have with a good friend or partner, determine how you feel about working with a particular therapist.

A good "fit" is important when you're deciding on a therapist. You may be tempted to try to make do even though something just doesn't feel right. Frankly, if this is the only eating disorder therapist within a hundred-mile radius, making do probably makes sense until something changes to increase your options. But assuming more choices are available to you now, your uncomfortable feelings matter.

Recognizing a good fit can be tricky. Having an eating disorder may make you feel uncomfortable with a lot of people. Being close to someone who seems to understand you may make you uncomfortable if you feel undeserving. Or you may feel that people always let you down, no matter how nice they seem. If you're feeling uncomfortable with a therapist, you may want to start by asking yourself if this is a really familiar feeling for you. If the answer is "yes," it may be worthwhile to stick around a little longer, talk your feelings over with the therapist, and see whether doing so makes a difference.

Intangibles are, by definition, hard to put into words. But you may notice a few of the following qualities regarding the therapist's style and personality that may affect your feelings about goodness-of-fit:

- How she balances talking and listening. (This may also reflect the style of treatment. For example, an analyst talks less than a behaviorist.)

- How she expresses herself and gives feedback.

- How energetic she is.

- What her sense of humor is like.

- How well she expresses warmth.

- What choices she makes regarding self-disclosure.

Most people have a range in terms of what they can live with along these dimensions. If you really respect a therapist's work and think she can help you, it may be worth stretching a little, even if her laugh makes you grind your teeth. But you may want to think long and hard about the therapist whose style is a regular distraction or who makes it hard for you to settle in comfortably to focus on the work at hand — that is, you and your recovery.

Assembling Your Team

Eating disorders cover a lot of territory in the people they afflict. If you have an eating disorder, you know only too well that your body, mind, and spirit are all affected. Getting better usually means involving several experts to cover all the bases (Chapter 11 discusses including nonprofessionals, such as family, in your recovery). You want the best treatment team you can assemble to meet your individual needs. In this section I go over the experts you can choose from to create your team.

The size of your treatment team depends on the severity of your symptoms and the number of companion disorders (such as depression or alcohol addiction) you bring to treatment. Speaking very generally, people with anorexia usually require a larger team at the beginning due to their more serious medical situations. As treatment progresses and physical symptoms improve, the team may grow smaller. On the other end of the spectrum, people with binge eating disorder (BED) tend to have few medical complications and present less dire circumstances. A treatment team for someone with BED can be pretty minimal. Somewhere in the middle are the team needs of people with bulimia. Of course, your own team needs depend on your particular situation.

Addressing psychological and emotional health

An eating disorder springs from the way you think and feel about yourself, and subsequently affects your behavior and relationships. All these elements — thoughts, feelings, behaviors, and relationships — are the domain of the psychological and emotional experts on your eating disorder recovery team. The following experts are typical members of the psychological and emotional part of an eating disorder treatment team.

The therapist's role for each form of therapy

Therapy for eating disorders typically falls into four major categories: individual therapy, family therapy, couples therapy, and group therapy. You may benefit from participating in one or more of these types of therapy as part of your eating disorder treatment, depending on your personal needs. Following is a brief rundown of the role of the therapist in each type of therapy:

✔ **Individual therapist:** Your individual therapist is your team expert about the psychological and behavioral aspects of your eating disorder. She helps you reduce your eating disorder symptoms and build a strong recovery. (In Chapter 10, I outline a number of different approaches individual therapists use with eating disorders.) She should have specialized training in working with eating disorders and in her particular approach

to treatment. Your individual therapist serves as your guide and cheer-
leader throughout the treatment process and helps you understand your
role in getting better. If you have a trauma history, your best choice is a
therapist who's experienced in trauma treatment. That's one fewer part
of your therapy that will eventually have to be farmed out to someone else.

- **Family therapist:** People of any age may decide to include their family in
  their eating disorder treatment. But for children and young teenagers,
  some kind of family involvement is a must. (You can read about reasons
  for choosing family treatment in Chapter 11.) A family therapist works
  with the entire family to help the person with the eating disorder. He
  helps the family change any patterns that unintentionally contribute to
  the problem. These therapists usually have specialized training in family
  therapy.

- **Couples therapist:** If you have an eating disorder and you have a partner, chances are the two interact with each other in some way. And this
  may not be helpful to either your recovery or your partnership! Couples
  therapists often are added to the treatment team to help disentangle
  things. Couples therapists usually don't need specialized training in
  eating disorders. (You can read more about couples therapy for people
  with eating disorders in Chapter 11.)

- **Group therapist:** A group therapist has specialized training in leading
  therapy groups. Your group therapist should also have training in eating
  disorder treatment. Group therapists help group members help each
  other with their eating disorder problems. They also help members
  become aware of interaction patterns that develop within the group.
  This way, group participants gain insights from what happens among
  themselves to improve their relationship skills. These skills are an
  important part of recovery. (You can find out more about group therapy
  and other kinds of groups in Chapter 11.)

Sometimes the same person wears both the individual and the family therapy
hats. In one version of this, the family therapist sees everyone together for
family sessions and has separate sessions with the person with the eating
disorder. In another version, he sees the person with the eating disorder individually, but consults separately with parents instead of seeing everyone
together. Others mix and match these options.

The jury is still out on whether having one therapist wear multiple hats is a
good idea. Those who endorse the idea feel it's helpful to have one person
who can see the whole picture. All the better to coordinate what's happening
in different types of treatments. Opponents point out that young people with
eating disorders often tend to get lost in their families. They feel it's important for those with the eating disorder to have an entirely separate setting
where they can explore their feelings and develop their own points of view.

A therapist by any other name is still a therapist

What kinds of official credentials should you expect the therapists on your treatment team to have? Actually, people licensed in any of the following professions can be individual, family, couples, or group therapists:

- ✔ **Social work:** This person has a master's or doctorate of social work (MSW or DSW) degree. She may also have an LCSW (licensed clinical social worker) or similar designation to show state licensure.

- ✔ **Psychology:** This person's degree is a PhD or PsyD. (Make sure the person's degree is in psychology. A PhD in deep-sea fishing isn't likely to do you much good.)

- ✔ **Counseling:** A licensed professional counselor (LPC) has a master's or doctorate degree in counseling or a master's in psychology or some-times in education. Some LPCs focus on current problem intervention only; others provide a full range of psychotherapy treatment.

- ✔ **Pastoral counseling:** Recognized members of the clergy who have received any of the preceding degrees plus advanced training in psy-chotherapy may provide psychotherapy services.

- ✔ **Nursing:** A registered nurse with advanced training and a master's or doctorate degree may practice psychotherapy. The designation is advanced practice registered nurse (APRN).

- ✔ **Psychiatry:** This person's degree is an MD, so he can prescribe medications in addition to providing counseling.

People are often confused by the term *psychotherapist*. A psychotherapist is not necessarily someone who belongs to a licensed professional group. "Psychotherapist" is a general term for anyone who provides therapy by talk-ing with a patient to alleviate psychological symptoms. People in any of the professions listed above can choose to become psychotherapists. But, be on your toes! People without any kind of professional degree or training can legally use the term as well. You need to make sure you know the basis on which the person you're considering has set up shop.

Addressing physical health

Eating disorders get physical! They involve your body's fuel supply and its balance of a slew of hormones and other body chemicals that affect the way you function. The bottom line is that you may need some body experts on your team to help you achieve the right physical balance for your recovery.

Primary care provider (PCP)

Your primary care provider (PCP) can be an internist, pediatrician, or family doctor. He's the person who provides the initial medical evaluation sizing up the physical consequences of your disorder. He also provides ongoing treatment for any medical problems. If hospitalization is needed, he's the one who makes that call. If you need to restore your weight to get better, and can safely do so as an outpatient, your PCP may oversee this process. Or he may work together with your nutritionist until your weight is back in a healthy range.

Make sure your PCP specializes in working with eating disorders. He needs to be on top of the many medical risks specific to eating disorders. Also, if you have anorexia, he needs to understand and be prepared for the intensive work you two have ahead of you to get your weight and health back up to snuff.

PCPs frequently prescribe psychiatric medications. This arrangement has both plusses and minuses. On the plus side are

- **Familiarity:** You probably already know your PCP. You may appreciate a familiar face about now, and that's one fewer person you need to add to your team.

- **Cost:** Getting your medications prescribed by your PCP usually costs less money.

- **Case coordination:** Your PCP can easily coordinate any psychiatric medication you take with the rest of your physical picture.

On the minus side, PCPs usually

- **Have less expertise:** If your medication needs are in any way complicated, working with someone who specializes in psychological issues and psychiatric medications can be advantageous. Prescribing psychiatric medications is what this person does all day. She *should* be better at it than most PCPs.

- **Are less current:** A PCP is less likely than a psychopharmacologist to be up-to-date on what's new with medications like the ones you may be considering. He's got too many other fish to fry.

If your situation doesn't seem too complicated — you're not physically ill, your symptoms aren't severe, and your companion disorders don't include more than mild to moderate depression or anxiety — you may start with your PCP (assuming he's comfortable prescribing this kind of medication). If it all works out well, you're good to go. But if you're not getting the results you need in a reasonable amount of time (say, 6 to 8 weeks), consider consulting with a psychopharmacologist.

Nutritionist

A nutritionist — in some states a registered dietician (RD) — is the member of your team who gets into the trenches with you to help guide you back to healthy eating. She supplies you with accurate information and buries some eating disorder mythology along the way. She also provides you with tools, like food logs, to help you become more aware of your eating patterns and zero in on the trouble spots. Your nutritionist helps you set reasonable, reachable food goals and shows you how to problem-solve to reach them. Not all nutritionists specialize in working with eating disorders. Make sure yours does.

Psychopharmacologist

The psychopharmacologist on your team is the person who evaluates your need for psychiatric medication. (I discuss medications used for eating disorder treatment in Chapter 12.) A psychopharmacologist has a medical degree (MD) and is also board certified in psychiatry as a medical specialty.

If a psychopharmacologist recommends medication for you, and you agree to try it, she follows you for as long as you take the medication she prescribes. She monitors you for side effects, any changes in dosage, and the need to change medications or add new ones. You two have the most contact when you start a new medication or if you have problems with medications you're already on. When things are stable and you're getting the desired results from your medication, you and she may only be in contact every three to six months.

Some psychopharmacologists also do individual psychotherapy. If your individual psychotherapist is a psychiatrist, she can handle any medication needs you have. One-stop shopping.

Designating a team leader

With so many people thinking, evaluating, and making recommendations on your behalf, you're going to want someone coordinating all that energy. This doesn't mean your team leader is the boss of everybody. She just makes sure she knows what everybody on the team is thinking and planning so she can help bring everyone's ideas together into one overall plan.

If you're an adult or young adult, your individual therapist most likely is the central player on your team. She's usually the one you see the most — from one to several times per week when you begin treatment. So she may be the one who knows you best and has the bigger picture in her sights. (With younger people, emphasis is likely to shift to the family therapist.)

Leadership changes if you need to go into the hospital (see the next section). Your PCP usually leads this transition and coordinates your hospital stay.

Determining the Intervention You Need

Level of intervention refers to the intensity of your treatment. Two ingredients determine this factor:

- ✔ **Structure:** How much your time and choices are supervised, organized, and planned
- ✔ **Frequency:** How often you meet for treatment

Treatment in which you go to a special setting that focuses on your eating disorder around the clock is more intensive than treatment that allows you to stay home, go about your business, and see your experts a few times a week.

How do you decide what level of intervention you need? Is your situation an emergency? In this section I go over how to determine the answers to these questions and where you can turn for help.

If you're a minor child, your parents make most of these decisions in collaboration with your therapy team. If you're a teen, you're expected to share your opinions in the decision-making process. In some extreme instances, even if you're an adult, decision-making gets taken out of your hands. This only occurs when your life is in jeopardy (see the next section, "Do you need urgent hospitalization?"). The most clear-cut example of such a threat occurs when you present a suicide risk. Making decisions against your will when you're starving intentionally is much more controversial. The judgment call to hospitalize and feed you against your will depends on the treatment team you're working with.

Do you need urgent hospitalization?

You get the most intensive level of treatment on a hospital ward. It provides what's called a *controlled environment*, meaning you don't have much latitude for making bad choices. You're closely monitored, your food and weight choices are negotiated and contracted like international trade agreements, and you have no opportunity to make mistakes. Under what circumstances do you need such controlled conditions? In the following sections I outline the emergency and non-emergency situations that make hospitalization either necessary or desirable.

Urgent emergency hospitalization

Hospitalization comes up as an emergency measure when it's the only way to guarantee your life. Two circumstances require immediate hospitalization:

- ✔ **Suicidal impulses:** You have suicidal feelings *and* you can't be sure you won't act on them. (In Chapter 7 you can read more about determining your level of suicidal risk.) If you have any doubt about your current risk level or your ability to manage your impulses, call 911 or go straight to a hospital emergency room.

✓ **Severe weight loss in anorexia:** Your doctor will hospitalize you to keep you alive if all three of the following factors apply to you:

- Your weight has fallen below 25 percent of ideal weight (see Chapter 2) or is otherwise low enough to put your health at risk as determined by your doctor.

- Your key vital signs, like pulse and core body temperature, are in dangerous territory.

- You refuse to eat.

Warning signs for you or people around you to watch out for include

- Fainting

- Severe dizziness on standing (can also occur with bulimia)

- Collapsing

- Chest pain (can also occur with bulimia)

These symptoms mean you should head straight to your doctor or an emergency room. Ask questions later.

Urgent non-emergency hospitalization

Even if your situation isn't life-or-death, sometimes a hospital setting is still a good choice. For example:

✓ **Your level of starvation is making it difficult to concentrate or think clearly.** You can't participate well in your treatment if your brain isn't functioning on all cylinders. (I review the effects of starvation on the brain in Chapter 7.)

✓ **Your eating disorder symptom picture is highly unstable.** If you're bingeing and/or purging many times a day, it can be hard to focus on much else. If you're purging this often, you're at risk medically. Getting a handle on a pattern this entrenched is difficult outside a controlled environment.

✓ **You need to withdraw from severe abuse of laxatives, diuretics, or other means of purging.** Doing this under medical supervision is useful to avoid the risk of bowel obstruction.

✓ **You have other medical complications.** Your eating disorder may be causing other medical conditions, most commonly diabetes, to deteriorate. Hospitalization may be the most reliable way to get things back on track.

Though most of these situations focus on your medical condition, you're best off on a hospital unit that specializes in eating disorders. You want staff members who understand not only your physical condition, but also the psychological issues that are involved.

Is non-urgent intensive treatment a good option?

You don't have to be in a medical or psychological crisis for intensive treatment to be a good idea. While taking yourself out of your life for weeks or months is pretty disruptive, some circumstances may call for this kind of more drastic action:

- **Your disorder is chronic.** You've had your disorder for a very long time — years. This actually makes an eating disorder harder to treat. You may need bigger medicine.

- **You've tried outpatient options with inadequate results.** When you've given an outpatient plan your best effort but your symptoms remain pretty much as is, it's time to do something different. The same reasoning applies if you find you simply can't follow through with expectations in your outpatient treatment. Upping the level of treatment intensity is one thing to try in each case.

- **You have companion disorders.** The more companion disorders you have, the harder it is to get things stabilized on an outpatient basis. This is particularly true if the companion disorders include alcohol or drug addiction.

Letting things go too long without adequate treatment can be especially risky if you have anorexia. The mortality risk of your disorder increases over time.

Getting a Good Medical Work-Up

Getting a good medical work-up is one of the first things you need to do to get started with eating disorder treatment. It comes first because you need to know whether your health situation is an emergency. In an emergency, other components of your treatment must be put on hold until the emergency is taken care of. (See the section "Does your situation require urgent hospitalization?" earlier in this chapter.) Short of a medical emergency, what's the need for a medical evaluation? How do the results affect your treatment plans? How do you find the right person to do the evaluation? I answer these and related questions in this section.

How do I find a good doctor?

It's important to work with a doctor who knows what to look for and how to treat eating disorder–related medical problems. How do you find such a doctor? Start here:

- Check out the "Resource Guide" in the back of this book for Web sites with listings of doctors.
- Ask your therapist. He may know a doctor who specializes in eating disorders.
- Call the American Medical Association (AMA) or go to its Web site, `http://webapps.ama-assn.org/doctorfinder/home.html`.

Who needs a medical work-up?

Anyone who has an eating disorder needs to get a good medical work-up. The stakes are highest if you have anorexia. You're the most likely of anyone with an eating disorder to have a life-threatening condition. If you have bulimia, you are at the next-highest level of risk. Though your condition is less likely to be life-threatening, you may be doing some serious damage to your body with purging behavior. (You can read about the specific effects of starving and purging in Chapter 6.) Getting thoroughly checked out and treated for potential problems is critically important.

Even if your medical needs don't qualify as an emergency, being mindful about your physical health is part of your recovery. Taking care of business, self-care-wise, helps to build self-esteem.

What happens during a medical work-up?

Like almost any visit to the doctor, an eating disorder work-up has two parts. First, the doctor asks you questions about your symptoms, habits, and history, and then she conducts a physical exam.

Eating disorder symptom questions focus on dieting, starving, bingeing, purging, and exercise. Your doctor wants to know what you do, when you started doing it, how often you do it, and so on.

Eating disorder side-effect questions cover topics like your menstrual periods, energy level, unusual heart behavior (such as palpitations), digestive problems, and so on. Your doctor also takes a more general health history. She needs to know about any other medical conditions you may have, like diabetes, and whether your eating disorder affects them.

The thoroughness of the physical exam depends on your disorder and symptom picture. If you are starving and/or purging, your exam includes more than if your only eating disorder symptom is bingeing. Starving and purging do a lot more damage to your body with a lot more potentially deadly results. Your doctor may request the following tests:

- **Blood work:** The basics include testing for such things as anemia and determining your levels of electrolytes (minerals that keep your heart beating). More extensive blood testing may be needed to see if starvation has hurt the functioning of any of your organs.

- **Electrocardiogram:** This tests for possible damage to the way your heart functions.

- **Chest X-ray:** This shows whether starvation has made your heart shrink.

- **Bone density test:** This shows whether your bones have lost some of their substance to starvation.

Unless you're especially sensitive to needles (used for drawing samples for the blood work), all these tests are painless.

What gets decided?

What does your doctor do with the results of your medical evaluation? Your doctor uses them to make immediate decisions for your medical care, including

- Whether you need hospitalization to be safe

- Whether other health symptoms need to be treated and how

- Whether other medical specialists are needed

If you have anorexia, the medical evaluation is also useful in determining the following:

- What a healthy goal weight is for you and what the plan is for achieving it.

- Whether you need to gain weight before you'll be able to participate in other treatment. (Starvation affects your ability to think and make judgments.)

Making a Plan for Your Treatment

Eating disorders cover a lot of territory, so their treatment has to cover a lot of territory too. To cover a lot of territory *effectively*, you need a plan. Two major considerations go into the design of your treatment plan:

✔ What are your treatment priorities? If you have a number of things to work on, what comes first?

✔ Who's responsible for making the plan?

I discuss answers to both questions in this section.

First things first . . . but what comes first?

In Chapter 7, I point out that eating disorders seldom travel alone. They usually come with one or more companion disorders. Examples include alcohol and drug abuse, compulsive exercise, depression, OCD, and anxiety.

When a therapist or psychopharmacologist evaluates your situation, she looks for the presence of any of these companion disorders. They need to be treated, too. Recovery from your eating disorder may partly depend on improvement in companion disorders.

The problem is that you can't do everything at once! Some components of your treatment have to be addressed before others. But how do you decide what comes first? Though the answers depend on your particular situation, here are a few general guidelines:

✔ **Behaviors that are the most self-destructive come first.** If drug or alcohol addiction is threatening your job, your family, or your legal status, you need to focus on these conditions before you tackle the less destructive ones.

✔ **Behaviors and conditions that alter your brain come first.** Anything that interferes with participation in your recovery work has to be a priority in your treatment. This includes the starvation state as well as mind-altering substances. Severe states of depression and anxiety also fall in this category.

✔ **Out-of-control bingeing and/or purging usually demand an early, structured intervention.** Whether inpatient or outpatient, a more intensive symptom focus is usually necessary when symptoms are severe. With mild or moderate symptoms, you can afford to see if they get better in a less symptom-focused treatment.

✔ **Out-of-control eating disorder symptoms coexisting with out-of-control companion disorder behaviors usually require an inpatient setting for treatment.** With this combination, you have too much room for harm and too few resources for getting better. You need some outside containment until you can supply more of your own.

✔ **Treatment for underlying trauma usually comes later in your treatment, after you've created some external and internal stability.** Trauma treatment can be overwhelming. You need to be confident you've accumulated the resources you need to manage whatever comes up.

Often treatment for one disorder helps with another. For example, if you're medicated for depression, the same medication may help you with anxiety and obsessive-compulsive disorder symptoms. Similarly, meditation and self-soothing techniques you use to work on your addiction are also useful in recovering from your eating disorder.

Your therapist can recommend a plan

Your individual therapist is likely to take a position of team leadership in devising your treatment plan. He's the one who goes over with you the goals for your treatment and the overall plan for action, including what comes first. The blueprint for treatment he suggests needs to make sense to you because you're investing a lot of yourself in it.

At the same time, keep in mind that a lot can happen along the way that may call for changes in the original plan. So the key is for you and your therapist to hold the plan not only with some commitment, but also with some flexibility. Each of you should be prepared to speak up about how the plan is working out and whether some tinkering is called for.

Choosing Where to Get Treatment

Earlier in this chapter, in the section "Determining What Level of Intervention You Need," I discuss different levels of intervention, reflecting both how much structure you need in your treatment and how frequent intervention needs to be. The inpatient and outpatient options I go over in this section are listed from most intensive (highly structured and controlled) to least intensive (less structured and controlled).

Inpatient hospital care

If you need hospital care for an eating disorder, you're best off in a specialized unit which only treats eating disorders. Staff members are familiar with the medical and psychological issues you face and are trained to work with them.

Most eating disorder hospitalizations are for people with anorexia. Bulimia can usually be managed on an outpatient basis, although a small number of people with bulimia have symptoms severe enough to require hospitalization. Some of these hospitalizations are purely in order to stabilize medical effects of starvation (or purging, for bulimia) that have gotten out of hand. Your treatment on such a unit includes

- ✔ **Setting weight goals:** Your doctor or the hospital team determines what weight is medically safe for you.

- ✔ **Re-feeding:** This is the process of getting enough calories into your system for you to achieve your weight goals and become healthy again. It also involves getting your eating habits back to normal. Just how much of the re-feeding looks like normal food at the beginning depends on how much you need to gain. If your medical condition is dire, you may need nutritional supplements for awhile.

- ✔ **Limiting your physical activity:** If your weight is low enough, your medical safety may require bed rest or some other limit on your activity level until you gain enough weight.

- ✔ **Normalizing eating patterns and reducing purging behavior:** If you have a binge/purge pattern, you're supervised so you can't do either and you receive skills training to reduce your symptoms.

In the old days, *structure* on an inpatient unit meant *control*. Many inpatient programs are discovering that putting as much control in the hands of the patient as possible works better. How much you need to weigh to be discharged probably isn't going to be put up for a vote, but various options for getting there may be. One issue, however, continues to be upsetting and controversial: how much control to take with patients who can't seem to choose life over thinness.

Some hospital units focus only on treating the medical aspects of your eating disorder. Other eating disorder units focus on the psychological aspects as well. These units may include individual, group and/or family therapy.

Residential treatment

Residential treatment facilities, like hospital units, provide round-the-clock care for eating disorders. However, the environment in residential care is more informal and home-like. You're encouraged to shop for food, prepare meals, and eat with others. Residential facilities believe this more natural setting helps you apply the skills you acquire to your real life when you leave.

Residential facilities usually cost less than hospitals. People stay longer — on average, around three months. (Length of stay, of course, depends on factors like how severe your symptoms are and how fast you're getting better.) A longer stay means you have a better chance of achieving your treatment goals because new behaviors and thinking patterns have more time to take hold.

Programs vary considerably in what they offer to help you get better. Some are set up to work with people whose medical conditions are fragile; some aren't. Some focus on just a few treatment approaches, such as group therapy and family education. Others offer a pretty sophisticated menu of treatments, including alternative therapies and trauma treatment. Some have a particular spiritual or religious orientation. Almost all focus on whole-person recovery as opposed to just symptom reduction. Almost all rely on the power of a community of support to strengthen your healing process. You can get specifics on what treatments a particular program offers by taking a look at the program's Web site. (Check out the "Resource Guide" at the back of this book for Web sites that list residential facilities.)

Residential treatment may be a good first choice for you if your eating disorder symptoms have really dug in their heels, making them hard to disrupt on an outpatient basis. This is a good question to go over with your eating disorder specialist. For some people, trying outpatient therapy first is best. For others, the wisest course is to go straight to a residential program with greater structure. Here are a few indicators that you may need a more structured setting as a first step:

- Your symptoms are deeply entrenched.
- You have a history of relapse.
- You have a history of other treatments that didn't work out.
- You have companion disorders, especially substance or alcohol abuse or mood disorders, which have been hard to stabilize with medication.

Halfway houses

Halfway houses or *recovery houses* are often part of the aftercare programs provided by residential facilities. These are small, unstructured, live-in situations, usually with house parents as overseers. You attend some type of group program, and you also have an individual therapist, perhaps the same person you saw individually while in the residential program.

You must be medically stable and have the worst of your eating disorder symptoms behind you to stay in a halfway house. Participation in a halfway house

- Provides support for practicing the new skills and new ways of thinking about yourself that you acquired in residential care.
- Helps prevent relapse.
- Provides an immediate community of people who are also in recovery.
- Provides extended support for learning to live in the community again.

Day hospital (partial hospital)

Day hospital programs, also called *partial hospital* programs, are a step down from hospital or residential care in structure and frequency. Often a day hospital program is set up as an extension of a hospital program to meet the needs of patients who are being discharged from a full hospital program. A day hospital is also appropriate if you need an intensive program but don't need the level of medical monitoring a full hospital program provides. If you enter a day hospital program, you typically attend eight hours a day, four to seven days a week.

In a day hospital program, you work on reducing your eating disorder symptoms and building recovery skills (such as self-esteem and improved emotion management). You have individualized treatment goals and a plan for achieving them. The treatment team may recommend individual therapy, family therapy, and/or medication. You also have several supervised meals each day so you get the structure you need around food and eating.

Everyone participates in group treatment. Day hospital programs rely on the *therapeutic community* of mutual help and support as their main healing ingredient. If you're coming out of a residential or inpatient program, having this continued experience of reliable support for your recovery can be extremely important. Day hospital groups may be educational or problem-solving, focus on relationship skills within the group, or discuss eating disorder or recovery topics.

Intensive outpatient program (IOP)

An *intensive outpatient program (IOP)* is another transitional option if you're leaving inpatient hospitalization or residential treatment. If a day hospital program is one step down in structure and frequency from these intensive services, an IOP is two steps down. A typical IOP meets for several hours several evenings a week, allowing working people or students to resume jobs or school while still getting an intensive treatment experience.

An IOP can also be a valuable treatment choice if you're medically stable but your eating disorder symptoms are stuck, or you're experiencing a crisis that's making your symptoms significantly worse. In these cases, stepping up your level of treatment from ordinary outpatient care (see the next section) may be the way to get unstuck or to help you weather your crisis.

IOPs are generally group-based programs. Like residential facilities and day hospitals, they put their faith in the healing power of a therapeutic community guided by eating disorder professionals. In the group, you work on managing eating disorder symptoms and developing a strong recovery. An evening's activities are likely to include a supervised meal so you can discover ways to handle food and eating-related anxieties in a group setting.

Outpatient therapy

Outpatient therapy is treatment that you participate in while living at home and going about your life. You can engage in any of the forms of individual therapy, or family, couple, or group treatment on an outpatient basis. Though a particular form of treatment you choose may be more or less structured (you can read about these choices in Chapter 10), your time is pretty much unsupervised. So outpatient treatment is the least intensive level of treatment intervention.

You and your therapist may choose to increase or decrease the intensity level of your outpatient treatment by adding or subtracting sessions from your week. (Some people do the same thing by making sessions shorter or longer. A typical individual outpatient psychotherapy session is 45 to 50 minutes.) If you're just beginning treatment or going through a crisis period, you and your therapist may agree, for example, to meet two to three times per week. If your symptom picture is quite stable, you may do just fine with one session per week. These decisions are usually influenced by how many other treatments you're trying to juggle at the same time and by financial considerations as well.

Outpatient therapists are mainly found in one of two places: in *outpatient clinics* and in *private practice*. In the following sections, I discuss what each one involves and why you may choose one over the other.

Outpatient clinics

Outpatient clinics are often part of larger institutions, such as hospitals. In these cases, they may be set up partly to serve the community and partly to train new staff, who work under the supervision of more experienced clinicians. Other times, a clinic is government-sponsored to serve a particular neighborhood or population (for example, substance abusers or immigrants).

Outpatient clinics present several advantages. They can be a big advantage financially. They take most kinds of insurance, including Medicaid, and they usually operate on a sliding scale that's quite reasonable. What's more, if the clinic is affiliated with a larger institution that's interested in eating disorders, you're likely to get staff members who are up-to-date on the latest in eating disorder treatment.

To start your search, consider the following types of institutions, which may focus on eating disorders or have an eating disorder program. Any of them may also have an eating disorder outpatient clinic:

- Hospitals
- Universities

✔ Training institutes (programs set up to study eating disorders and train eating disorder professionals)

✔ Residential treatment facilities

You can also check for eating disorder specialists among the staff at other kinds of clinics. For example, if you need a family therapist who knows about eating disorders, you may check the clinic of a family therapy training institute or a family training program within a hospital department of psychiatry.

Private practice

Therapists who are in private practice either operate independently or in group practices with several other people for business purposes. Outpatient therapy with a private practitioner tends to be more costly than clinic services. Insurance covers less and less, though you need to check with your particular insurer. Many private therapists offer services on a sliding scale, so it's always worth checking, even if the original price quote sounds beyond your means.

The advantages of working with a private practitioner may include the following:

✔ **Privacy:** You usually meet in a more private setting than you would in a clinic. This may or may not matter to you.

✔ **Experience:** A private practitioner is usually someone who has been doing this work for awhile. But you can always check.

✔ **Choice:** You can choose who you want to see. In a clinic, you are assigned a therapist.

✔ **A known entity:** Chances are this therapist was recommended to you by someone who knows her work and thinks highly of it. Or you read about her and liked what you read.

Be sure to read the section "Finding the Right Therapist" at the beginning of this chapter for hints on picking a therapist who's a good fit for you. This applies even if you're going to a clinic and have been assigned a therapist. You have a right to speak up if the match just isn't working.

Exploring Experiential and Alternative Therapies

I emphasize throughout this chapter that eating disorders affect all aspects of being you. Unconventional treatment approaches often address the nooks and crannies of eating disorder experience that conventional therapies may miss. In this section I review the experiential and alternative therapies most widely used with eating disorders. Nobody's amassed much research on the effectiveness of any of the following out-of-the-mainstream approaches for eating disorders. Yet individual clients have found one or another of them to be invaluable additions to their core recovery work.

If any of the experiential or alternative therapies sound about right to you, talk with your primary therapist about it. The two of you can figure out whether it's an appropriate addition to your treatment plan. (Of course, when you start adding treatments, time and money can always become a consideration.) If you're getting ready to enter inpatient or residential care, you'll probably find at least some of these treatments are options in your program.

Experiential therapies

Experiential therapies aim at increasing your awareness of being in the present moment. Any technique, tool, or practice that increases present awareness puts you in stronger connection with yourself. That's because you have to be tuned in to yourself and your own sources of knowing — thoughts, feelings, sensations — in order to be aware. If you have an eating disorder, connecting to yourself probably hasn't felt all that rewarding. Experiential therapies may help you learn to tune in to yourself more comfortably and effectively. Possibilities include

- **Dance/movement therapy:** Helps you improve body image and boundaries, and to express feelings
- **Art therapy:** Provides safe ways to express feelings
- **Music therapy:** Provides ways to express yourself, relax, and participate safely with others

Chapter 10

Finding the Treatment Approach That's Right for You

*I*n this chapter you get to meet Julie, who is my fictitious therapy guinea pig. Julie tries out some of the treatment approaches I describe in this chapter to give you a feel for what to expect.

The treatment you choose becomes the centerpiece of your recovery efforts. Yet, unlike shopping for a car or a house, you usually sign on for therapy without getting to see the product first! By getting a "fly on the wall" view of Julie's experiences, you gain a better understanding of what to expect in individual therapy.

The "Resource Guide" at the end of this book provides more information on each of the therapies you meet in this chapter. The guide also tells you how to locate therapists who use each approach.

If you have anorexia, you won't be able to participate in therapy effectively in a state of starvation. A starved brain is in no shape to do the kind of work therapy requires. Getting the nourishment you need comes first. (Read more about this stage of treatment for anorexia in Chapter 9.)

Choosing Your Eating Disorder Treatment

When you choose a treatment approach, you want to select the one that best suits your individual needs. You may want to consider each prospective approach in light of the following questions:

- ✔ Is this approach good for my problem?
- ✔ Is this approach a good match for who I am?

You're not likely to find perfect answers to either of these questions. But in this section I get you started by providing some information that may help you choose your treatment approach more wisely.

Choosing the best approach

Is one approach to treating eating disorders more effective than another? That's a good question, but one for which, unfortunately, no great answer exists. Not a scientific one, anyway. Not enough research has been done to enable you to make useful comparisons. However, the discoveries that *have* been made through research so far regarding some of the most common therapies include the following:

- ✔ **Cognitive-Behavioral Therapy (CBT):** CBT shows better results for bulimia than for anorexia. For more information on CBT, see the section "Concentrating on Cognitive-Behavioral Therapy (CBT)," later in this chapter.

- ✔ **Interpersonal Therapy (IPT) and CBT:** In studies comparing CBT and IPT for the treatment of binge eating disorder (BED), the two treatments worked equally well to reduce binge eating as well as companion psychological symptoms (like depression). See the section "Investigating Interpersonal Therapy (IPT)," later in this chapter, to find out more about IPT.

- ✔ **Dialectical Behavioral Therapy (DBT):** Researchers have reported successful use of DBT for binge eating disorder. In one study, treatment lasted for 20 weeks. At a six month follow-up, seven of ten women reported no binge eating. The other three reported so few binges that they no longer qualified for the BED diagnosis.

Be cautious of widespread claims that CBT shows better results than *any other* treatment for eating disorders. When you read the fine print, you find that the only other psychological treatment to which CBT has been compared is IPT. And in those tests, IPT did just as well as CBT. No research has yet been done comparing CBT with the other treatments you read about in this chapter. CBT is a fine treatment and it may be the right treatment for you, but research proving that CBT is better than all other eating disorder treatments doesn't exist, no matter what anyone tells you.

Lack of research also plagues trauma treatment (see the section "Taking to the Trenches with Trauma Treatment" later in this chapter to find out more about the connection between eating disorders and trauma). CBT and EMDR are by far the best-studied. The American Psychological Association, reviewing the research to date, calls both approaches "effective" for treatment of Post-Traumatic Stress Disorder (PTSD).

Should you throw up your hands for lack of solid research to guide your decisions? Certainly not. Lack of research doesn't mean lack of *experience*. Lots of highly experienced, highly qualified eating disorder specialists out there have been fine-tuning their thinking about eating disorders for decades, even if their approaches are not well-researched. Other experienced therapists are pioneering the application of some of the newer therapies, like EMDR, to working with eating disorders.

Many, if not most, eating disorder therapists use a variety of treatment styles in their approach. If a therapist tells you his approach is *eclectic*, he means that he uses a combination of techniques to treat eating disorders. Don't be surprised, for example, to find that the EMDR therapist you're seeing talks to you about mindfulness with your bingeing or asks you to keep a food diary. Fortunately, most therapists understand that helping you to get better is what matters most. They don't mind stealing from each other's bag of tricks to help you do so.

Choosing an approach that fits who you are

A very important consideration when choosing a treatment approach is finding one that is not only effective but also suits your personal style. In other words, you want an approach with which you feel comfortable. As you chew over the various approaches discussed in this chapter, here are a few things for you to think about:

- ✔ If you're ready to make a special commitment, you may like CBT, IPT, or DBT, which require you to do homework assignments every week. The idea behind this is that the more work you put into therapy, the more you get out of it.

- ✔ If you feel best when you can get to the bottom of things, and you want to understand how things work and what makes you tick, you may do best in one of the therapies that explore issues in depth, like psychodynamic psychotherapy or feminist therapy.

- ✔ If you already meditate, do yoga, or use alternative (non-Western) health approaches, you may find yourself on familiar ground with the bottom-up therapies.

✔ If you tend to rely on logic, you may feel more at home with the purely logical approach of CBT or the problem-solving focus of IPT.

✔ If you haven't worked in your body before (see the section "Body-based therapies" later in this chapter), you may find that the opportunity opens up many new possibilities for healing and feeling whole.

✔ If you have a history of uncontrollable emotions and behavior, especially in ways that are dangerous to you, you may want to think seriously about DBT. Addressing such emotions and behavior is DBT's specialty!

Concentrating on Cognitive-Behavioral Therapy (CBT)

Cognitive-Behavioral Therapy (CBT) is best known for the effective treatment of depression and anxiety. CBT also has a track record for treating eating disorders that goes back several decades. CBT is a highly structured therapy, so every session is well-planned. The treatment time is limited, usually to 16 to 20 sessions. A CBT therapist believes that knowing this time limit makes both of you concentrate and work harder.

CBT is a here-and-now approach. Instead of focusing on historical causes for your problems, CBT practitioners look for conditions in the present that keep your eating disorder going and aim to disrupt those conditions. CBT practitioners believe that problems, including eating disorders, are usually maintained by distorted thinking. Distorted thinking, in turn, leads to troubling emotions and problematic behaviors.

In the case of eating disorders, CBT zooms in on the typical distorted thought that your worth is determined by your body size and shape (for example, "If I'm thin, I'll like myself better, and so will everyone else"). Related beliefs involve body image, an obsession with being thin, fat phobia, being in control, and being perfect. A cognitive-behavioral therapist aims to undermine these beliefs and help you replace them with more realistic, constructive ones. CBT assumes that when you undermine the core beliefs, you undermine the disorder itself. The behaviors aren't likely to continue without the beliefs that fuel them.

In CBT, you're expected to work from the beginning — with the support of the therapist and the techniques and information you discover — on gradually changing behaviors central to the disorder: bingeing, purging, dieting, food rituals, starving, and compulsive exercise. Overall, CBT for eating disorders aims at correcting symptomatic behavior and changing problem-causing attitudes about food, eating, and body image.

What you do in CBT

CBT is based on a few basic principles. The central ingredients of CBT that you encounter when you start your treatment are

- ✔ **Getting educated.** CBT takes a logical approach, wherein facts comprise the basis for your choices. You get a lot of up-front information about how dieting causes bingeing (and therefore purging). You also find out about the physical consequences of your disorder, the myths of purging as calorie-wasting, and so forth.

- ✔ **Discovering how to recognize and correct errors in your thinking and to replace distorted thoughts with rational ones.** CBT is not only logical but also scientific. Your therapist invites you to treat your beliefs as theories that can be put to the test. If you hold a distorted belief, she helps you use facts to look at different possible explanations. She may encourage you to experiment to decide whether your idea holds water or some other idea works better.

- ✔ **Finding out about techniques for handling bingeing and purging urges.** Your therapist may recommend relaxation and distraction techniques or help you substitute other activities for bingeing and purging.

- ✔ **Developing problem-solving skills.** You learn the same logical, fact-based approach as you use elsewhere in CBT to think about your problems and devise appropriate solutions for them.

- ✔ **Doing homework assignments.** Your therapist may have you keep a log or diary for challenging your erroneous thoughts, practice new behaviors, or take on previously avoided situations or activities between sessions.

Julie concentrates on CBT

On her first day in treatment, Julie gets a thorough education about the CBT approach. Education is important because knowledge supplies the reasoning for everything Julie's going to be asked to do. A lot of these new behaviors are scary, so they have to make sense to Julie or she won't follow through. She also gets her first homework assignment: She is to keep a thorough daily food log, including notes about the situation, thoughts, or feelings that accompany her eating.

Julie's therapist asks her to immediately begin a normal, predictable eating pattern: three square meals and two snacks, at regular intervals, every day. She explains to Julie how deprivation causes bingeing. Julie's own experiences back up this theory. Bingeing begins to fall off as Julie's eating normalizes.

Julie is surprised to see that her therapist reviews her log in great detail at the beginning of the next session. (She thinks, "Yikes! I'm really going to have to follow through. Some of this is embarrassing.") The careful review of the food log happens again at the beginning of every session, along with a review of other homework assignments. These reviews form the basis for much of the session work: challenging thoughts, finding binge triggers, and discovering new possibilities.

Julie's therapist asks her to expand her choices about eating even more. Julie challenges herself to join her friends for pizza — without vomiting afterward. Julie's therapist reminds her of some things she now knows:

- ✔ Vomiting encourages future bingeing.
- ✔ Eating in a more normal way hasn't caused her to gain weight so far.

Adding more fat is going to be a stretch. But the therapist also reminds Julie that forbidden foods become binge foods. Julie decides to experiment to see how the pizza affects her weight. She also makes a plan to use the restroom before the food arrives so she's not tempted to do so afterward, when she may purge.

The pizza experiment is a success, but Julie flops later when she tries to add a new "forbidden food." Julie's reaction is to think of herself as a loser, and she and her therapist go over this reaction in her next session. Julie's therapist acknowledges that Julie's reaction is one possible conclusion. She then suggests that Julie look at the facts of her life and her progress in treatment to see whether this conclusion holds up. Julie realizes that the facts don't support her conclusion. Finally, the therapist asks Julie to suggest some conclusions that fit the facts better. The one Julie lands on is that she doesn't have to do everything perfectly in order to make progress.

Before treatment ends, Julie's therapist tells her to expect her eating disorder symptoms to return in times of stress, but also to expect that she'll keep getting better. She gives her a detailed written outline of how to handle binge/purge episodes and urges to diet that sums up the work she and her therapist have already done together.

How CBT helps

CBT puts a lot of valuable experience under your belt. You begin to live without your symptoms and discover that you're okay. If you have bulimia or BED you find that your weight doesn't change significantly, even though you eat regularly, and you practice sitting through urges to purge without acting on them. You discover from experience that you can manage your urges and they will pass. If you have anorexia, you learn to manage urges to restrict and fears about adding additional foods and gaining weight.

You also get lots of practice with a method of recognizing and challenging the irrational thoughts that make you want to purge and diet. You know that urges will come up in the future, but you work out a process to turn to for help when they do. The same is true of bingeing: You determine what feelings and situations trigger you and what to do when binge impulses occur. And here's a big bonus: Your therapy successes provide you with some much-needed self-esteem and confidence.

Delving into Dialectical Behavioral Therapy (DBT)

Dialectical Behavioral Therapy (DBT), developed by University of Washington therapist Marsha Linehan, combines CBT (see the preceding section, "Concentrating on Cognitive-Behavioral Therapy") with Eastern mindfulness techniques. Linehan made a name for DBT by using it successfully with seriously impulsive and suicidal patients no one else had been able to help. DBT has since been adapted for work with substance abuse, eating disorders, and other problems.

DBT emphasizes a balance between acceptance and change. Acceptance doesn't mean throwing in the towel; rather, it means accepting who you are and what your circumstances are at the current moment (as opposed to concluding, "I'm disgusting" or "I hate myself"). In DBT, you discover ways to nurture this accepting stance while simultaneously working on making changes.

 DBT practitioners assume that your eating disorder symptoms — dieting, starving, binging, purging — are misguided attempts at emotion management. The focus of DBT work is on finding ways to handle emotions constructively through a balance of acceptance and change.

What you do in DBT

If you sign up for DBT, you may have an individual therapist, be part of a DBT group, or both. (Some people who are in other kinds of therapy for individual work also participate in DBT groups.) DBT is a short-term therapy, usually lasting for about 20 sessions.

In DBT you receive skills training for emotion management. You're expected to carry out homework assignments in which you apply these skills to your particular situation. You practice applying emotion management techniques when you feel the urge to engage in an eating disorder behavior, such as bingeing or purging. You also practice applying your new skills to situations that trigger your eating disorder behaviors, such as a fight with a friend or being criticized by your boss.

DBT teaches you four core sets of skills:

- **Mindfulness:** Drawn from meditation, these skills teach you to be aware — without judgment — of what is occurring in the present moment, both inside of you and on the outside.

- **Distress tolerance:** These skills involve accepting yourself and your life as they are right now and being able to observe without trying to control or change things. As a result, you gain a new tolerance of painful emotions.

- **Emotion regulation:** You find out how to use mindfulness skills to help you identify and be present with disturbing emotions. You also discover ways to cope with negative emotions, such as listening to music, talking with friends, writing in a journal, practicing slow breathing, and so on. You find out how to make better choices with regard to emotion-driven behavior.

- **Interpersonal effectiveness:** This set of skills teaches you how to get more of what you want from relationships — without hurting the relationship or your good image of yourself in the process. Skills include asking for what you want, being able to say no, and managing conflict.

Julie joins a DBT group

Julie joins a DBT group that's specifically for people with eating disorders. Five other women are in her group. One has bulimia, like Julie. The other four have binge eating disorder. Two also abuse substances. One self-injures by cutting herself.

Here is the usual drill for Julie's DBT group sessions. After any personal sharing at the beginning, each group member tells how she did with the week's homework. A particular week's assignment always involves one of the core mindfulness skills. Members talk about any problems they had with the homework. They also review diary cards on which they've recorded the DBT skills they practiced each day. Then they learn a new skill and practice it with each other. The next homework assignment is based on that skill. Before ending the session, the group does some kind of mindfulness or relaxation exercise together.

This week the group is going over an assignment to work on distress tolerance skills. The assignment was to pick a distressing situation and list the pros and cons of tolerating the distress versus bingeing (or engaging in another destructive behavior). Julie thought the assignment would be easy — until a fight on the phone with her mother ended with her mother hanging up on her and refusing to take her calls all week. Julie could think of no pros for tolerating what she was feeling. She binged and purged several times.

Julie is relieved to find that the group doesn't judge her, either for bingeing and purging or for having trouble completing the assignment. The group's tolerance serves as a reminder to her to practice being less judgmental and instead to become more curious about her behavior — "I wonder what was going on for me that led to that binge?" Julie laughs at a suggestion for her "pro" list (why to tolerate the situation): five full days of *not* having to hear her mom's criticisms! Group members also help Julie rehearse conflict resolution skills they've been working on, as well as distraction and self-soothing techniques in case she just can't make the situation with her mom right.

How DBT helps

DBT teaches you how to stay in awareness of the emotional states that trigger your eating disorder behaviors without acting on them. You also learn techniques for reducing intense negative emotions. Being less at the mercy of your emotions allows you to think more clearly and make good choices about the way you respond to situations and people — choices that don't involve eating or restricting. With time and practice, DBT training helps you improve your eating disorder symptoms and strengthens your approach to life in general.

Setting Your Sights on Psychodynamic Therapy

Get ready for a whole truckload of psychodynamic therapies. All of these therapies start with the belief that symptoms in the present represent emotional baggage from the past. Getting better in psychodynamic therapy involves unpacking the baggage and resolving old issues in a constructive way that doesn't include your symptoms. The relationship with your therapist is crucial because the assumption is that sooner or later all the key issues causing you trouble will come up in the ways you relate to her.

The following approaches constitute a small sampler of the different psychodynamic approaches in use (including a few that are more accurately called *psychoanalytic* approaches):

- ✓ **Freudian analysis — the original approach:** Freudian analysis encompasses everything you probably imagine therapy to be, including the couch and the therapist who doesn't say much. Freudian analysis supposes symptoms arise from unacceptable, unconscious sexual or aggressive impulses and that you can develop some pretty maladaptive patterns in life trying to keep these impulses out of awareness.

✔ **Object relations therapy:** This approach assumes you unconsciously take in the qualities of your early caregivers and the ways they relate to you, and that this, in turn, affects your future ability to trust, be intimate, be independent, and so on. You tend to repeat the patterns that you see in your early relationships in your adult relationships. In object relations therapy, you use the relationship with the therapist to become aware of what you took in and develop new patterns when the old ones aren't useful.

✔ **Self psychology:** Self psychologists think you are as entitled as the next guy to possess key abilities of a healthy adult personality, such as the ability to feel "together," to feel alive, to self-soothe, and to keep up your self-esteem. Normally these abilities develop in the relationship with a caregiver who is sensitive to a child's needs. Self psychological therapy offers a second chance at developing these abilities if you didn't get them in childhood.

✔ **Jungian therapy:** The idea behind Jungian therapy is to help you heal what hurts, to become more of who you are able to be, and to find personal meaning in your life. Jungians believe that in order to accomplish these goals you need to know what's going on in your unconscious and be able to read the symbolic messages, such as dreams, that it sends you.

Distinguishing between psychodynamic and psychoanalytic therapies

Psychodynamic and psychoanalytic approaches share the same theoretical beliefs about how psychological problems arise; that is, they are the result of unconscious conflicts. The main difference between the two approaches is in method. In psychoanalysis you are asked to commit to more frequent therapy (perhaps three to five times per week compared to one to two times per week in a psychodynamic therapy) and probably a longer time in treatment overall — several years or longer. Psychoanalytic treatment is more open-ended in the way it explores your feelings. This is best exemplified by the process of *free association* in which you talk about whatever comes to your mind. (Lying on the infamous couch is believed to help this process.) Psychoanalytic goals are also more general, aiming at personality transformation. In contrast, a psychodynamic therapist is likely to direct you to specific topics to explore (aspects of your childhood, your relationships, and so on) and to be focused on particular problems, such as anxiety or depression.

Psychodynamic psychotherapists have contributed most of what is known about the inner world of eating disorders. They've figured out how eating disorders subconsciously provide a way to work on problems that feel too threatening to work on directly or consciously. Food, weight, dieting, bingeing, and purging express issues like needing to be taken care of, needing others, needing more independence, being angry, feeling powerless, and so on. Therapy provides a safe environment for bringing these issues out into daylight. The idea is that you won't need your symptoms when you deal with the issues more openly.

What you do in psychodynamic therapy

Psychodynamic therapy is not a structured therapy like CBT (see the section "Concentrating on Cognitive-Based Therapy," earlier in this chapter). Sessions aren't planned, homework isn't assigned, and the therapy usually isn't time-limited. Treatment starts with your therapist finding out what you want from therapy and taking a thorough history. Your therapist then discusses her general ideas about your symptoms. Your part of the work of therapy is to bring your experiences — your current concerns, past memories, and impressions of what's happening in the therapy — to your sessions. Your therapist may direct you to certain parts of your history, ask for your ideas or feelings about significant issues, ask how you feel about the relationship between the two of you, or present her own ideas and impressions regarding your treatment.

Julie sets her sights on psychodynamic psychotherapy

Julie chooses a therapist whose combination method includes *object relations*, an approach that emphasizes the effects of early relationships. The therapist expresses interest not only in what Julie is doing — bingeing, purging, dieting, and so forth — but also in what Julie feels emotionally both when she engages in these behaviors and when she refrains from doing so. For example, Julie notices that when she tries not to binge, she experiences terrible emptiness. Her therapist asks her when she has felt that kind of emptiness before. Julie is right back in the great empty space between her and her chronically depressed mother. (Her dad abandoned them when she was born.)

A lot of Julie's therapy sessions are devoted to remembering how she coped as a little girl with such a distant, barely functioning mom. Julie realizes how early she had to grow up. Gradually she and her therapist piece together how her eating disorder symptoms came to the rescue when adolescence flooded her with issues of separation she was unprepared to handle. Dieting suggested to her that she was so strong she didn't really need other people. It also felt like she was taking the deprivation inside herself, where she could be in charge of it. Bingeing sometimes soothed her, but just as often it just made her numb. Purging restored some temporary order, but made her feel terrible.

Within the safety of the therapy relationship, Julie begins to understand how focusing on her symptoms seemed to keep her together during her teens when she so often felt she could fall apart. For the first time, she realizes just how terrifying it was to be expected to grow up when there was nobody there to rely on. Probably the hardest part of her therapy is feeling she needs her therapist. For awhile her symptoms get worse as her desire to finally have someone she can depend on increases. She finds unexpected relief in putting her needs into words and discovering that her neediness doesn't flood her or make her therapist run away!

Getting better for Julie in this therapy is a matter of shifting the trust she placed in food and dieting back into the world of other people. Julie had to skip many steps of normal development because of the unusual circumstances of her childhood, especially having a mom who always seemed to need more than she did. Now she can stop and take the steps she missed. She can become a fully functioning adult — she no longer has to fake it while turning to eating disorder symptoms for cover. In her psychodynamic therapy, Julie is able to discover who she is so she doesn't have to define herself with her symptoms anymore.

How psychodynamic psychotherapy helps

In psychodynamic therapy, you gradually build your strength from the inside out. Your therapist uses a careful read of the "hot spots" in your development to interact in ways that give you the growth experiences you need. A therapist who specializes in psychodynamic psychotherapy and has experience in treating eating disorders understands how eating disorder symptoms reflect missing or harmful developmental experiences. This understanding helps her offer you chances to heal and grow so that your symptoms are no longer necessary.

Focusing on Feminist Therapy

Many feminist therapies for eating disorders are based on psychodynamic principles. But feminist therapists also have some basic beliefs about gender and culture that make therapy with them different. Here are some of the differences you find with a feminist therapist:

> ✔ **A belief that men and women develop differently and view the world differently.** A man's world is one in which others are viewed in terms of power and competition. A woman's world is more about relationships and connections to others.

✔ **A therapy conversation that looks at the impact of the culture.** Depending on who you are and what you need, you're likely to cover issues like the following:

- Cultural pressures for women to be thin

- *Objectification* of women's bodies, meaning that they are treated by others as something separate from the person living inside — something that can be judged, criticized, ogled, or admired like an inanimate object

- Expectations that good women contain and control their needs and appetites rather than express them

- Expectations that feminine women are compliant and accommodating

- Cultural valuing of qualities in girls and women that aren't generally useful for developing personal identity or power

- Family power arrangements that often mirror the culture, to the disadvantage of girls and women

✔ **A collaborative therapy relationship that will be central to healing.** In a relationship of this type, the following ideas are considered important:

- **Connection and attachment are crucial for growth.** Traditional psychodynamic views of development have emphasized separation from the parents and autonomy as signs of maturity. Feminist approaches believe that the ability to form healthy connections to others, including intimate attachments, is just as important to growth and maturity. This includes qualities of support, understanding, and mutual respect in relationships we rely on.

- **The relationship is a partnership between equals.** Both you and the therapist have a share of the expertise instead of the therapist being viewed as having all the knowledge and expertise.

From a feminist point of view, a therapy that controls and contains symptoms under the therapist's direction runs the risk of repeating the errors of the culture and the family. Culture dictates that women are to be silenced and contained. The feminist therapist prefers to see your symptoms get better as part of a process in which you are encouraged to become a whole person with your own voice validated.

Like the traditional psychodynamic therapist, the feminist therapist sees eating disorder symptoms as an expression of a person who has lost faith in relationships with other people. If you have an eating disorder, you probably don't see relationships as a reliable place to get nurturing. You may not think you can get nurturing without losing yourself. And you probably don't believe you can be your own separate you without losing important relationships. Why even bother? Food isn't so picky about how you act. A feminist therapist understands where you're coming from. She knows that the journey to change is difficult and frightening, and that she will have to be in there with you in a real way for change to happen and for you to get better.

What you do in feminist therapy

In feminist therapy you and your therapist talk about your life and try to make sense of how your eating disorder became a part of it. The relationship between the two of you is part of the focus of your treatment and part of the healing process.

So far, I could be describing a psychodynamic therapy. Your feminist therapist may very well have a psychodynamic background. What she adds as a feminist therapist is an understanding of how being female (or male) in this culture contributes to your eating disorder symptoms as well as your more basic view of yourself. She is certain to ask you to challenge beliefs about yourself and your possibilities that are based on limiting gender stereotypes.

For example, saying no when you need to may be hard for you because you were taught that a good woman doesn't get into conflicts with others. Or you may binge and purge whenever you get angry because you were taught that nice girls don't get angry. You may find it hard to even think about who *you* are because you've been so well-trained to focus on others. Your eating disorder may have been filling in this identity gap. In feminist therapy, you see clearly how the culture has been rewarding you for being so selfless while at the same time making it hard for you to become the mature, self-directed adult you're expected to be.

Julie focuses on feminist therapy

Julie picks a feminist therapist. The emphasis on women's issues and on relationships feels important to her. But the relationship emphasis also scares her. She's been getting along in the world by being nice to everyone and avoiding conflicts. She's noticed that her actions never result in her feeling very connected to anyone, or even very alive. Is it possible to feel differently? Choosing a therapist who's asking the same question is an act of courage for Julie.

Feminist therapy isn't just for females

Can a man go to a feminist therapist? Sure! Feminist therapy isn't all about women being oppressed. A feminist therapist is interested in all the ways culturally dictated gender roles shape and limit your ability to define yourself, no matter what your gender. And the model of growth-in-attachment applies equally well to men. Men are often relieved to hear the messages of feminist therapy in contrast to the John Wayne, go-it-alone stuff the culture insists on for them.

Julie has to call on her courage many times in her therapy as she tries to be honest and open with her therapist. Her internal map of relationships tells her that openness is going to get her clobbered. She thinks her therapist will see her as one big needy monster and will be horrified, swamped, or disgusted.

One of the first times Julie's neediness comes up is when her therapist is away for the holidays. Julie taught herself a long time ago not to need people who aren't there for her, so she's upset with herself for needing her therapist now. She can't help but feel angry at her therapist for putting her in this position. It makes her feel weak and vulnerable. When she sees her therapist again, Julie tells her she thinks she should quit therapy because she's becoming too dependent.

In this session and others to follow, Julie and her therapist talk about the unique circumstances of her life that have made needing and separation feel so threatening. They also talk about the added problem of living in a culture that thinks of needing and connecting as weak. For the first time in her life, Julie begins to see her ability to need and connect as a strength. She can talk through the overwhelming parts — they don't get the better of her or her therapist. And in time, they don't feel so overwhelming.

Julie knew before she started feminist therapy how strongly the media influenced her desires to be thin. Her refrigerator was plastered with pictures of models and celebrities who were up there to inspire her to stay on her diet. She is surprised to find out how many other ways the culture affects her and how cultural stereotypes keep her eating disorder going. For example, she feels frightened any time she doesn't act the way the feminine "good girl" is supposed to, and this feeling triggers urges to binge and purge. She experiences this scenario when she contradicts a guy she works with. Her therapy reminds her that she's entitled to have a voice and to begin to create her own definition of what makes a good woman.

How feminist therapy helps

When you're able to see clearly what the culture is prescribing and the effect its prescriptions are having on you, you have a better chance to weed out the parts that aren't good for you. A feminist therapy will offer you the perspective and support for thinking through the culture's impact on your eating disorder symptoms and on your life more generally. A feminist therapist helps you develop personal strength and a sense of identity so you have less need for your symptoms.

Feminists believe you are most likely to develop a strong individual self when attachment and connection are also part of the picture. You don't have to worry that you can have one only at the expense of the other. Feminist therapy is a place to test this theory and experiment with new possibilities with someone who understands what's at stake. In the process, you leave the need to rely on your eating disorder symptoms behind.

Investigating Interpersonal Therapy (IPT)

Interpersonal therapy (IPT) is another short-term treatment for eating disorders. Like feminist and some psychodynamic models (see the preceding sections, "Focusing on Feminist Therapy" and "Setting Your Sights on Psychodynamic Therapy"), IPT places its main emphasis on relationships. Unlike these two approaches, however, IPT doesn't try to find reasons for the development of your disorder in your history. In fact, IPT doesn't try to explain the development of your eating disorder at all. Instead, like CBT (see the section "Concentrating on Cognitive-Based Therapy," earlier in this chapter), IPT looks for current factors that are keeping your symptoms going and tries to help you change them.

IPT therapists believe that psychological problems occur when people's needs for attachment and connection aren't being met. Therefore, they put all their eggs in that basket for your 12–20 sessions of therapy. Your IPT therapist will pay little-to-no attention to your eating disorder symptoms, at least not as a focus for work. The aim of the therapy is to figure out how you can change what you're doing in your relationships so you get more of what you need from them. The assumption is that as you improve your relationships, your symptoms get better accordingly.

What you do in IPT

In the first few sessions, you and your IPT therapist draw up a list of your most important relationships. You then go over these relationships, checking them against four categories of potential interpersonal problems. These categories are

- **Interpersonal disputes:** Conflicts you may be having that don't seem to get resolved are interpersonal disputes.

- **Role transitions:** Changes in relationships which may be due to development, aging, job loss, breakups, and the like constitute role transitions.

- **Grief:** From the IPT therapist's point of view, grief refers only to loss through death.

- **Interpersonal deficits:** These deficits occur when you have too few relationships and/or the ones you have aren't very fulfilling.

Your therapist helps you use this review to size up what you need to work on. He also uses his observations of interactions between the two of you to help identify relationship snags. The two of you then spend most of your remaining sessions working on ways for you to improve things.

In general, your IPT therapist tries to help you improve your ability to communicate in relationships, express emotions, adjust your expectations where appropriate, problem-solve, and increase your overall set of relationship skills and options. He helps you come up with your own solutions in specific situations and put them into practice.

Julie investigates IPT

Julie decides the IPT combination of a relationship focus with a short-term model is just right for her. She and her therapist identify the following areas Julie needs to work on:

- ✔ **Julie experiences her friendships as one-sided**. Everyone seems to lean on her and confide in her, but nobody expresses interest in Julie or her problems.

- ✔ **Julie's relationship with her mother is a little formal and stiff.** Julie is afraid to "rock the boat," even though her mother's depression has been stabilized through medication for some years.

- ✔ **Julie never got to grieve the relationship with her grandfather** who died when she was eight. Though living in the next town, he was a reliable source of affection and the one person who let Julie be a little girl.

- ✔ **Julie can't figure out what went wrong with her last boyfriend.** Despite the fact that she always tried to be supportive and there for him, he broke things off because he said she was too needy. The breakup left Julie feeling confused, betrayed, and afraid to try again.

Julie's therapist helps her become aware of a pattern that threads through all her relationships: She is behaving selflessly in the hope that others will notice and repay her in kind. That way, she won't have to ask for what she wants and needs, something she finds excruciating. Julie admits this arrangement hasn't exactly been working out so well for her. She agrees with her therapist that the strategy leaves her needs to the imagination of others and is disempowering.

Julie begins practicing speaking up with her friends, first about minor issues — where to have dinner, what movie to see — and later about meatier issues — hurt feelings, her desire to spend time talking about her problems, and so on. Julie and her therapist role-play these situations so Julie can try out her approaches ahead of time and anticipate possible problems.

The situation with her mom is more complicated (surprise!) because it involves finding out if her mom can or will behave any differently toward her. Julie also has to confront how *angry* she's been at her mother (how can you be angry at a poor depressed woman?). Julie realizes she's been afraid her anger will come out if she starts asking that the relationship include her needs as well as her mom's. Through some well-rehearsed efforts to speak up more and talk about how their current pattern is affecting her, Julie discovers that, within limits, her mom can be more responsive.

Julie spends several sessions allowing herself to mourn the loss of her grandfather. Though she may not be able to put all her feelings into words, having another person (the therapist) witness and accept her profound emotions gives Julie a new sense of the possibilities for human connection.

In the last few sessions, Julie and her therapist go over what she's accomplished. They try to anticipate how these issues may come up in the future and how Julie may deal with such circumstances.

How IPT helps

The truth is that nobody exactly knows why IPT helps with eating disorder symptoms. Practitioners believe that helping people experience some success in identifying their relationship needs and getting them met a little more often has a big impact on eating disorder symptoms.

Getting to the Bottom of "Bottom-Up" Therapies

If the name of this category makes you picture yourself turning cartwheels, think of that as what you'll be doing in recovery when you're better. In the meantime, the name *bottom-up* contrasts the approaches of some newer therapies with more traditional therapies which are considered to be *top-down* in their approach. In a top-down therapy, you use your logical mind to impose some law and order on disorderly internal processes and behaviors. When you learn and practice skills, apply insights, or make logical choices, you are working from the top — your logical mind — down.

When you work from the bottom up, you go straight to where feelings, impulses, and urges live — right in the gut — to change how you feel from the inside. Clients who experience bottom-up therapy claim the changes feel more solid and believable and seem more long-lasting.

How a bottom-up therapy helps

Bottom-up therapies can be especially useful for working on eating disorders. Several reasons exist for this, including the following:

- ✔ **Breaking through despair:** By the time you reach treatment you are probably pretty worn down from battling your symptoms. You've exhausted your own efforts and find it hard to believe that anything will make things better. A treatment that works from a different angle or produces a little "magic" may be just the right prescription for injecting some hope.

- ✔ **Working in the body makes particular sense:** If you have an eating disorder, you've already chosen your body as the arena for working out what's wrong. Becoming more comfortable from the inside out seems like just the right recipe!

- ✔ **Making up for what's been missing:** If you have an eating disorder, "what's wrong" probably includes a lot of missing pieces in your relationships with caregivers. In several of the bottom-up therapies you work on developing resources in yourself related to these missing pieces.

- ✔ **Healing what's been hurting:** When you heal old injuries, you no longer need your eating disorder symptoms to pull you out of awareness.

Many developing therapies may fit the bottom-up description, but only a few have gained any broad-based acceptance and/or have been adapted for eating disorders. These include body-based therapies, EMDR, and the energy therapies.

Body-based therapies

Perhaps you're thinking, "Body-based therapy. Hmm. She must mean something like massage or acupuncture." Nope. Not that I think these body treatments can't be terrific. They can. But here I use the term to refer to a group of therapies that take into account the continuous loop of influence between your mind and your body. A body-based therapy taps into this back-and-forth connection between mind and body to help facilitate healing.

You already know something about this mind-body connection. You caught a cold because you were under so much stress. The fight with your friend gave you that headache. Your stomach has been in knots ever since your teacher announced the exam on Friday. Each of these examples demonstrates a common way emotion can translate to body symptoms.

Emotions don't always turn into physical symptoms, but they do always register someplace inside you as a body sensation. Perhaps you feel a slight pressure in your chest when you're nervous. Or maybe your mouth and throat feel like you just ate your gym socks. Maybe when you know you've aced something, you feel your spine lengthening or your body temperature warming up a little.

Generally speaking, your body knows how you feel before your conscious mind does! Tuning in to this channel of information can be a great addition to self-awareness. Not only that, once you've tuned in, you can learn to influence how your body feels in the present — which in turn influences how you feel emotionally.

The best-known and developed of the body-based therapies are Somatic Experiencing (SE) and Sensorimotor Psychotherapy (SP). In each approach you find out how to track your body's responses to experiences in the moment and to events from the past that continue to upset you. Using skills your therapist helps you develop, you're able to quiet down nervous system arousal (see the sidebar "Addressing your autonomic nervous system") and experience once-upsetting events in a calmer and more confident way. You may also discover how to develop body states that aren't so familiar to you but can be useful, such as assertiveness or relaxation.

Somatic Experiencing is based on the fact that when your physical or psychological survival is threatened, an instinctive part of your brain throws you into survival mode and chooses one of three paths to safety: "fight" (stand and defend yourself), "flight" (run away!) or "freeze" (play dead). In childhood, neither fight nor flight is a realistic option if an adult, especially a parent, is the one threatening you. What's left? Freeze. Though it's a state of numbness and immobility, the freeze state is still super-charged with HUGE survival energy. When survival energy hangs around in your body, it's constantly warning your brain that something bad is about to happen, so your brain is constantly telling your body to brace and get ready. The aim of SE is to help your body safely discharge all that stored-up survival energy and restore you to a normal energy balance. This reduces your symptoms and helps you connect more fully to a world that until now has felt too dangerous.

What do body-based therapies have to do with your eating disorder? That depends partly on the approach you choose and the outlook of your therapist. Following are some important ways a body-based therapy can help you with eating disorder symptoms:

- ✔ **Emotion regulation:** Body-based therapies teach you skills for managing your emotions from the bottom up. When you change what's happening in your nervous system, your feelings follow.

- ✔ **Management of binge or restriction urges:** When you're able to quiet the nervous system arousal that's underlying an urge, the urge tends to fizzle.

- ✔ **Processing early experiences that are "feeding" your eating disorder in the present:** When you're able to quiet the nervous system arousal that goes with early wounding, you're able to transform the way you hold that experience inside and the way it affects you. Childhood experiences that had an impact on your self-esteem, body image, sense of security with other people, acceptance of making mistakes, and so on may all be relevant to your eating disorder in the present.

EMDR therapy

EMDR stands for *Eye Movement Desensitization and Reprocessing*. Don't let the name scare you. The approach puts things in information processing terms, much like your computer does when you work with it. The *processor* is your brain and the *information* your brain processes is stuff that happens to you in life that you gain new knowledge from. Some of what you discover is useful — you want to keep calling on it to guide you in the future. For example, you may feel confident meeting people because you've found from experience that people really like to be your friend.

EMDR therapists believe that your brain has a mechanism that can process experience effectively. But this mechanism can get jammed up when experience overwhelms it — like the way your paper shredder gets jammed when you put too many sheets in it at once. EMDR specialists think this is what happens when you experience trauma or even smaller events that are just too much to handle at the time they occur.

TECHNICAL STUFF

Addressing your autonomic nervous system

Body-based therapies work by affecting your *autonomic nervous system* (ANS). Your ANS controls automatic functions in your body — things like heartbeat, breathing, and digestion that you don't have to think about every day. The ANS is also in charge of the flow of body energy, meaning it can speed us up or slow us down.

One ANS branch, the *sympathetic branch,* is an arousing or energy-spending branch. Among other things, your sympathetic nervous system controls your reaction to threat. It sends adrenaline and other hormones into your system when you feel threatened. (Feeling threatened can refer to big things like getting mugged or day-to-day things like having somebody look at you the wrong way.) You may know this reaction

as the "fight or flight response." You may also know it as sweaty palms; rapid, shallow breathing; and your heart speeding up a little or a lot. A second ANS branch, the *parasympathetic* nervous system, quiets arousal. Unlike the energy-inducing sympathetic branch, the parasympathetic branch is the "rest and digest" branch. You experience parasympathetic activity as calm and relaxation.

You may be guessing right now that it would be a good thing to be able to control the switches of your nervous system's ability to rev you up or slow you down. Controlling these switches is not only a good thing, but also something you can actually discover how to do. Body-based therapists teach you how.

EMDR therapists believe that their approach un-jams this jammed-up system so that your brain's own natural ability to process experiences can take over again. In the process, the old stuff gets linked up with newer, more helpful information. When experiences that have been badly stored are reprocessed with the help of EMDR, symptoms are relieved and you gain a perspective of yourself that's based on more grown-up information.

An unusual aspect of EMDR is the use of eye movements to un-jam the processing system and jumpstart the linking-up of different networks of information in your brain. *Eye movements* (yours) are what happen when the therapist holds up a couple of fingers in front of your face and then moves them from left to right and back again repeatedly while you follow with your eyes. (Actually other techniques are also used to create the same effect, for example, using sound instead of sight.) Nobody knows precisely what this focus is contributing, apart from allowing you to keep one foot safely in the present when working with disturbing memories. What EMDR therapists do know is that when they put all these pieces together — with appropriate precautions for emotional safety — those badly stored memories tend to fade in intensity while the person undergoing treatment relates more and more strongly to more current, useful information about herself.

The basic outline of how EMDR can be applied to work on your eating disorder is quite similar to that for a body-based therapy. You are likely to do a lot of work up-front on developing emotion management skills. These skills do double-duty: They help you cope in the present in ways that don't involve your eating disorder symptoms, and they help prepare you for reprocessing difficult memories later in the therapy.

Anything that stirs up powerful negative emotions (and sometimes even positive emotions) can trigger your eating disorder symptoms. Your therapy can be such a trigger! You and your therapist need to be mindful of this possibility and take it into account in the way you work. You may decide to do this by

✔ Simply acknowledging and talking about what's happening

✔ Slowing the pace of work temporarily

✔ Remembering and practicing emotion management or self-care skills that you've found helpful

The important thing to remember is that now you have options. You don't have to be stuck just feeling worse and worse the way you did earlier in your life.

Energy therapies

Energy therapies combine Western ideas of psychology with Eastern beliefs about body energy fields to create a rapid method of healing. An energy therapist tells you that symptoms — negative thoughts and emotions — represent patterns of imbalance in the energy *meridians* or channels that run through the body. These are the same meridians an acupuncturist taps into when he uses needles to treat you. In an energy therapy, you learn a quick method of tapping at various meridian points with your fingers. That's right; this is a do-it-yourself treatment method. The tapping is said to rebalance body energy, which in turn alters the way the brain processes information in relation to the problem you're working on, helping to resolve and heal the problem.

The first of the energy therapies to become well-known is Thought Field Therapy (TFT). A TFT practitioner uses information about the *thought field* connected to your symptom — that is, the thoughts, emotions, and body sensations you associate with it — to make a diagnosis and decide on the pattern of tapping that you need to do to get relief. Sometimes symptoms, like long-time phobias, disappear with breathtaking speed. Other times you have to do a *lot* of tapping to get results.

A TFT therapist treats anorexia as a phobia. A phobia is a morbid fear of something. In the case of anorexia, the fear is of eating and thus gaining weight. He applies a phobia protocol. He thinks of bulimia and BED as addictions. He assumes the addiction is fed by anxiety. He believes the person with bulimia or BED is actually addicted to the anxiety-calming effects of eating.

The problems with TFT are that it's expensive to learn and complicated to do. Emotional Freedom Techniques (EFT) is a streamlined alternative. As in TFT, the EFT practitioner believes you need to restore your body energy fields to balance in relation to a problem that has unbalanced them. Also like TFT, you tap on meridian points in a certain way while thinking about your problem to create the rebalancing. Unlike TFT, you don't need a specific diagnosis of each problem to determine the correct pattern of tapping. There's just one pattern, and it's much less complicated than the TFT patterns. The EFT approach addresses eating disorders in the short term by calming urges to perform eating disorder behaviors (eating too little, bingeing, purging) and in the long term by quieting underlying emotional disturbances (such as anxiety, self-doubt, anger, and so on) — all with the same repeated pattern of tapping.

Taking to the Trenches with Trauma Treatment

Trauma refers to any experience that overwhelms your ability to cope at the time it occurs. A traumatic experience threatens your very survival, terrifies you, and leaves you feeling helpless. Trauma ruptures your sense of a safe boundary between yourself and the world.

If you have an eating disorder, particularly if you are bulimic, chances are good that you've experienced trauma in your history. You can read more about trauma's effects on the development of eating disorders in Chapter 5. If trauma is part of your history, your recovery may be significantly strengthened by undertaking specific treatment to heal lingering trauma effects in your life. The individual therapist you choose may or may not be equipped to do that work with you. You may wish to take this into account when choosing an individual therapist. At the end of this section I list some approaches for treating trauma.

When you are unable to bounce back from the effects of trauma with the help of family, friends, community, and time, you suffer from what's called Post-Traumatic Stress Disorder (PTSD). If you have PTSD, it severely disrupts your life. Its symptoms can include nightmares, flashbacks, panic attacks, numbing, depression, irritability, body aches and pains, a sense of loss of meaning in life, and more. *PTSD requires treatment.* (You can read more about PTSD and its treatment in *PTSD For Dummies* by Mark Goulston [Wiley].)

All trauma is strikingly similar in some respects. However, experiencing a one-time traumatic event as a stable adult (for example, being the victim of a crime or a car accident, or losing someone unexpectedly) is very different from experiencing chronic trauma as a child. The most important difference is that an adult has many more resources to call on than a child. Adults have more internal psychological resources, such as judgment, perspective, and the ability to self-soothe, as well as external resources, such as family, friends, a stable work environment, and so forth.

Children have not developed these buffering resources. What's more, in childhood, the caregiver who is supposed to provide the buffering is often the source of the trauma. The chronically traumatized child feels very deeply that she is a powerless person in an unsafe world where overwhelming experiences can and do happen on a regular basis.

If you experienced chronic trauma in your childhood, you are likely to have a symptom picture that includes the following:

- **PTSD:** A pattern of symptoms that include both memories or sensations of the trauma and various kinds of shutting down to distance yourself from it.

- **Dissociation:** An effect of trauma that leaves you less connected to yourself and to life. You can read more about dissociation in Chapter 5.

- **A persistent pattern of interacting with yourself and the world:** This pattern may include impulsive behavior, difficulty tolerating emotions, problems getting along with or trusting others, and low self-esteem.

If you have a trauma history, your eating disorder probably represents your attempt to cope with it. Too much is coming at you and you've been unable to develop the resources you need to manage. Your treatment needs to take into account not only your eating disorder but also the trauma that fuels it.

What is trauma treatment?

Treatment for a single-event adult trauma aims at *restoration*. You want to get back, or restore, your sense of safety, and the reassurance of having solid boundaries and meaning in the world that you had before the traumatic event occurred. (Of course, if triumphing over the trauma leaves you feeling even *stronger* than before, that's okay too!)

If you've been traumatized, the most natural instinct is to avoid thinking about what happened. Yet getting better usually requires confronting the traumatic experience head-on. The trick is to face the trauma in a way that doesn't overwhelm you all over again. The idea is for you to be able to "digest" an experience that was too much when it happened. That way the trauma can take its place among other things that have happened in your life — and you can move on.

 In contrast to the restorative, getting-back-to-where-you-were-before work of single-event adult trauma, treatment for chronic childhood trauma usually means building in what was never there to start with. Before you can even think of taking on the overwhelming events of the trauma itself, you need the life skills trauma robbed you of. You need to be able to

- ✔ Manage your emotions in a constructive way
- ✔ Use the therapy relationship for support and stability
- ✔ Maintain other supportive relationships
- ✔ Contain impulsive behavior, including self-injury
- ✔ Minimize your use of dissociation
- ✔ Show good judgment, especially concerning personal safety

Developing these abilities may actually be the biggest part of your trauma treatment. It's certainly the part that comes first. When both you and your therapist agree that you've gained enough stability inside and outside from working on these skills, you may be ready to work on your trauma directly.

 You may want to jump right into direct work on your trauma experiences with both feet, skipping the part about stabilizing your life and finding ways to manage your emotions. A lot of traumatized people fiercely believe or hope that some kind of cathartic encounter with their trauma experiences will relieve them of their suffering. Nothing could be farther from the truth.

When you take on the powerful emotions associated with your trauma history without adequate preparation, one of two things happens:

✔ Your system, in its wisdom, shuts down (dissociates) before you can get flooded.

✔ You are once again overwhelmed by the feelings and memories and, in the process, become traumatized all over again. Reliving trauma in this way may very well lead to a relapse of your eating disorder symptoms.

Most treatments for chronic childhood trauma occur in stages, beginning with a stage for building personal stability. Depending on your needs, this stage of treatment can last anywhere from several months to several years. Much of what you work on to make your life more stable — like emotion management or building a social support network — is also very relevant to your eating disorder.

Several major approaches to therapy can treat trauma as well as eating disorders. These include the following, each of which is discussed earlier in this chapter in the section indicated:

✔ **Cognitive-Behavioral Therapy (CBT):** See "Concentrating on Cognitive-Behavioral Therapy (CBT)."

✔ **Psychodynamic psychotherapy:** See "Setting Your Sights on Psychodynamic Therapy."

✔ **Somatic Experiencing (SE):** See "Body-based therapies."

✔ **EMDR:** See "EMDR therapy."

✔ **Thought Field Therapy (TFT):** See "Energy therapies."

How do trauma treatments help?

What can you expect to happen when you make it through the trials and tribulations of trauma treatment? Your symptom picture certainly improves: You experience less dissociation, fewer intrusive experiences (like nightmares or flashbacks), and better relationships with others. You also have a new version of what happened to you, one from which distortions about yourself have been deleted. This new version includes the feeling that the trauma is now in the past, not part of your present. Your view of yourself is more positive. The world seems safer. Your future looks brighter and filled with possibilities.

Chapter 11

Including Other People in Your Treatment

*N*o matter how you slice it, your relationships are pretty central to your eating disorder. Your family, with only the best of intentions, may have passed on ideas that turned out to be too rigid or limited. Or they may have lacked the nurturing themselves to give you experiences vital to a sense of security in the world. Peers may play a big role in causing you to believe that your eating disorder is necessary in order for you to be accepted. They may have even introduced you to eating disorder behaviors. Romantic rejections or mistreatment can convince you that people are just as untrustworthy as you feared. Food and thinness are reliable when people fail you.

Just as people are part of the problem, people can also be part of the solution. This chapter describes the major treatment approaches that include other people in your therapy. These approaches may involve going back to get things right with your family, making sure you get off on the right foot with your current partner, or depending on the kindness of strangers in groups. The curative ingredient in all of them is that they take advantage of the safety of the therapy environment to try out new, healthy ways to connect with others — ways that help make your eating disorder obsolete.

For the most part, these therapies are not substitutes for individual, one-on-one treatment. However, children and young teens in family therapy and people with Type A therapists who seem to be able to cover all the bases may do fine without one-on-one time. (See Chapter 10 for more information on choosing the best treatment approach for you.)

You can find out how to locate therapists or groups for each of the approaches I outline in this chapter in the "Resource Guide" at the end of this book.

Family Therapy: Everybody Gets into the Act

Family therapy is one of several ways you and your family can come together to talk about your eating disorder. (You can read about other options in Chapter 24.) Family therapy can take many forms, but one thing they all have in common is that you are no longer the *client* (the one seeking help from a therapist) by yourself. Your family — as a unit or entity — becomes the client.

The fact that your family may be involved in your therapy doesn't mean that your family is to blame for your eating disorder. Family therapists understand that eating disorder behaviors — like any repeated behavior in a family — naturally become linked into a pattern with your family members' responses. For example, maybe whenever you cut back on your eating your mother begs you to eat and your father threatens you — and you respond to both of them by digging in your heels and restricting even more. Then your mother begs you to eat again, and so the cycle repeats.

Eating disorders can fit into many family patterns. Maybe you noticed that when your parents became involved with your eating disorder, they put aside their bickering to focus on solving your problems. Perhaps your big sister, who had drifted away from the family, has been pulled back in to help with your crisis. Or maybe your father's preoccupation with his business failings faded as his attention turned to you when your symptoms became evident. In these types of patterns, the worse your eating disorder symptoms become, the more some other problem appears to get better.

None of these family events caused your eating disorder, but they've all become interlocking pieces with it, like a giant jigsaw puzzle. The interlocking pieces have to change in order for you to get better. Family therapy helps widen the view so everyone can see how all the pieces connect. Having this broader view begins to make clear how everyone can help.

But, you may think, "My little sister has nothing to do with this. Why should she have to come?" The reality is that everyone in the family is affected and everyone can potentially help. A common scenario is to involve everyone in your immediate family and even others, if your particular situation calls for it. For instance, maybe your Aunt Louise has been very close to you and your family and has your mother's ear about your eating disorder. Inviting Aunt Louise is probably a good idea.

When to choose family therapy

Anyone who deals with an eating disorder and who lives with a family can benefit from family therapy. In some cases, choosing family therapy is an option rather than an absolute requirement. In other situations, however, family therapy is a must. Family therapy is a necessity if

- ✔ **You're a child or teenager.** If you're a dependent child, your parents are still responsible for issues related to your development and well-being. You still need their help and support. If your eating disorder reflects other problems in the family, you can't fix them by yourself. The whole family needs to be included in making things better.

- ✔ **You live at home.** No matter how old you are, if you live under the same roof as other family members, your eating disorder behaviors inevitably are influenced by your family's responses to your symptoms.

- ✔ **Your eating disorder is intertwined with other family issues.** Perhaps another family problem — such as a conflict or the emotional or physical issues of another family member — appears to get better or fades into the background as your eating disorder becomes worse. Maybe a parent or other relative expresses concern that you're growing up too soon, but these worries fade as your eating disorder settles in. Or perhaps one parent seems to always understand you, while the other parent is always fighting with you.

- ✔ **Your eating disorder is having a negative affect on family life.** If your eating disorder causes your family to fight or worry more than usual, or if everything revolves around you and your symptoms, both you and your family need help.

Sometimes including the whole family may not seem so critical, but it still may be a good strategy. Family therapy may be a good idea if

- ✔ **You're an adult child who hasn't "launched."** If you're a young adult struggling to achieve independence, you may benefit from your family's help. Family therapy is a good place to figure out what actually helps at this stage versus what gets in the way.

- ✔ **You're reluctant to become involved in treatment.** Even though you may have issues with your family, you may still feel a sense of safety in numbers. The support of your family may help you overcome any fears you have about entering treatment alone. Plus, the thought of your entire family going off to talk about you to a stranger may motivate you to be there too, if only to defend yourself!

If your parents or other family members are hostile toward you and your eating disorder, and are unable to move into a more supportive position, family therapy is probably a bad idea. Likewise, family therapy is impossible if you or your parents consistently come to therapy sessions under the influence of alcohol or drugs. If family therapy is a no-go in your situation, you still have plenty of individual therapy options to choose from. I cover these treatment approaches in Chapter 10.

What you do in family therapy

When you and your family go into therapy together, your family therapist helps you figure out what's linking family behavior to your eating disorder, and then helps you disentangle these issues. The following linking patterns need to be unlinked:

- ✔ **Family responses are meant to help you, but instead they keep the eating disorder going.** Families may get stuck in responses that don't help because they simply don't know what else to do. Family therapy can be a great place to explore better options. For example, your mother may find out that setting firm weight recovery expectations, with clear consequences, is more helpful than begging and pleading with you.

- ✔ **Family problems seem to be solved by your eating disorder.** Maybe you believe another family member relies on your symptoms, and you aren't ready to take chances on what would happen without your eating disorder. Maybe you fear Mom will become depressed if she no longer has the closeness you two have achieved by working together to overcome your problems. Or maybe you don't trust that Mom and Dad will have anything to talk about if you get better. In family therapy, worries like these come to light. Family members have the chance to reassure you that you're wrong or, if you're right, to find their own ways to work on the issues that worry you.

Three patterns of family organization show up frequently in families where a child has an eating disorder: overorganization, underorganization, and a shame focus. Each of these family patterns is a piece of the eating disorder puzzle and, as such, contributes to keeping the eating disorder going. If your family fits one of these patterns, a family therapist can help you determine how to move outside of that pattern. I describe these family patterns in greater detail in Chapter 5, but the following summarizes the characteristics of each pattern:

- ✔ **An overorganized pattern:** Families that fit this pattern are all about togetherness and unity, sticking to the rules, and conforming. You may have a great sense of belonging, but this family pattern may make it hard for you to know yourself as an individual. An eating disorder, particularly anorexia, may pop up to help you gain some individual control. If you're facing the prospect of separating from your family, for example, to go to college, your eating disorder may be an expression of your family's anxieties about how your leaving will rupture the family's togetherness. Depending on your needs, your family therapist may help you with some or all of the following:

- Encouraging each person to have their own say

- Finding ways to deal with conflict and resolve it

- Flexing up family rules to deal with growing children

- Tolerating the inevitable loss of togetherness as children grow

✔ **An underorganized pattern:** Underorganized families have too little structure. Parents frequently suffer from what was missing in their own upbringing. The eating disorder, usually bulimia, frequently expresses missing nurturing, going back for generations. Family therapy for an underorganized family aims at

- Helping parents establish structure and rules for family life

- Helping members connect with each other in supportive ways

- Teaching members how to cope with anger and express it safely

- Helping the family to manage crises in constructive ways

✔ **A shame focus:** The family with a shame focus forever fears loss of face and feeling worthless. Family members emphasize public appearance and being perfect to avoid worthless feelings. An eating disorder is just an exaggerated version of what the rest of the family feels. If you live in a shame-based family, family therapy can be a place for everyone to work on:

- Being imperfect

- Discovering inner qualities and feelings that have been overlooked while focusing on appearance and achievement

- Connecting to each other and the world in less competitive ways

A special form of family therapy, known as the Maudsley approach, is proving to be very promising for teens with anorexia. In the Maudsley approach, parents are viewed as their child's best resource for recovery, and accordingly, they're essentially put in charge of the process. You can read more about this approach in Chapter 12.

How family therapy helps recovery

A family whose rules are clear but flexible, who can respond to the emotional needs of its members, who can tolerate and resolve conflict, and who can change as the kids grow is in much better shape to respond to the crisis of an eating disorder. Developing a stable, supportive family environment allows you to focus on recovering from your eating disorder, secure in the knowledge that other members of your family can take care of their own needs.

Couples Therapy: Just the Two of Us

Just as the family becomes the "client" in family therapy, your relationship with your partner becomes the client in couples therapy. The focus shifts from the individual to the relationship. If you live with a partner, your eating disorder

✔ Affects your partner and your relationship

✔ Draws responses from your partner, which, repeated over time, become part of the pattern of your disorder

✔ Draws responses from each of you that reflect how you handle issues as a couple

If you and your partner are engaged in constant struggles about your eating disorder, whether openly or secretly, it will prolong your eating disorder and make you both feel bad about your relationship. In this section I review the warning signals and tell you about what couples therapy involves.

When to consider couples therapy

If you wonder whether you and your partner would benefit from couples therapy, you may find it helpful to review the items in the following list, and consider whether they apply to your relationship with your partner. Warning signs that indicate couples therapy is a good idea include the following:

✔ **Your partner threatens to leave because of your eating disorder.**

✔ **You and your partner constantly fight about how to handle your eating disorder.**

✔ **Your eating disorder symptoms started or got worse when you entered the relationship.** *Note:* This doesn't necessarily mean that your relationship is bad — in fact, sometimes the opposite is true. The problem may be that you're not accustomed to your partner's kindness or reliability and are having trouble trusting them.

✔ **You and your partner can't agree about your parents' involvement in your eating disorder.**

✔ **You and your partner have other problems in the relationship.** Such problems may include physical or emotional abuse, addictive behaviors, affairs, or keeping secrets that damage your relationship.

What you do in couples therapy

Your couples therapist not only wants to know how you're doing with your eating disorder, but also how you and your partner are doing as a couple. Most of the time, the way the two of you are managing with the eating disorder is a good indicator of what your strengths are as a couple and where you may need to do some work.

Creating healthy boundaries

In Chapter 8 I talk about healthy *individual* boundaries. But relationships have boundaries, too. They distinguish who's included in and who's excluded from various aspects of your life. Boundaries show up in your determination of who gets information, who's included in activities, who's in on planning and decision-making, who you share emotional and sexual intimacy with, and who's responsible for what.

Healthy boundaries in a couple accomplish a lot. They draw a line around the two of you so you can develop couple strengths and intimacy without outside interference. But the lines are flexible enough to allow for social resources (family, friends, and community) and outside help when you need them. Boundaries also exist between the two of you. Healthy boundaries allow each of you to feel your individuality and separateness, while also allowing you to step inside each other's individual boundaries for the practical stuff, like planning, and for emotional sharing. Some boundary problems that couples commonly face when one of the individuals in the relationship has an eating disorder include:

- ✔ **Family-of-origin:** If involvement with your *family-of-origin* (that's the family you grew up in) regularly takes priority over your current partnership in terms of time, activities, or emotional energy, you may find it hard to form a strong boundary around you and your partner as your own unit. Your eating disorder may provide an ongoing line of connection with your family-of-origin. You may feel that without this connection, your family would be overly upset by the prospect of losing you to your new relationship.

- ✔ **Personal responsibility:** Although you are expected to manage your own eating disorder behaviors, you may feel that your partner expects you to hand this management over to him. Or maybe you worry that he'll feel left out if you insist on handling your disorder yourself. These concerns may effect how you handle your disorder.

- ✔ **Closeness and distance:** Individuals vary a lot in the amount of intimacy and closeness they're comfortable with. For example, sometimes talking about eating disorder symptoms can offer closeness, but living with those same symptoms can create distance. If you feel like an accordion with your partner around your symptoms — constantly moving in and out — trying to achieve a balance between closeness and distance is likely to be a theme for the two of you in other areas of your relationship as well.

Your couples therapist will help you negotiate with your partner to develop stronger boundary-related choices and behaviors. If your boundary issues include your family-of-origin, you may be asked to include them in some of the work. The idea is not to exclude your family from your life but to find the right balance between your relationship with them and your relationship with your partner.

Dealing with control issues

Whether you're aware of it or not, you and your partner face the issue of control — who influences whom and how — from the moment you become a couple. Management of your eating disorder can be an arena for expressing control issues. Does your partner get to tell you what to eat? When you're allowed in the kitchen or bathroom? What you're supposed to weigh? Do you openly go along with the arrangement, yet manage to hold onto your symptoms anyway?

Control issues are no small matters. You may struggle over whether your relationship is a partnership of equals or one in which one of you gets to be "more equal." The fact that the struggle has gotten tangled up with your eating disorder just makes the stakes that much higher. If you and your partner are in a control struggle over your eating disorder, your couples therapy is a place where you can stop, take a breath, and see this clearly. You can then work on dividing up responsibility in a way that helps you not only in the management of your eating disorder, but when it comes to other jobs and decisions you face as a couple as well.

You may have come to your adult partnership with a lot of wounds from your family-of-origin. Or you may have gotten lots of good stuff but found that you now want to change some not-so-good stuff that also came with the package, like an emphasis on appearance or squishy boundaries. In couples therapy you create a relationship in which you get to modify the bad stuff. This makes couples therapy a great opportunity for healing.

How couples therapy helps recovery

Your couples therapy has the immediate job of helping you and your partner stop behaving in any ways that may unintentionally feed your eating disorder. In the long term, couples therapy should help your relationship become a place where each of you can grow, thrive, and safely connect as equals. Working with your partner on relationship problems that you tried to cover with your eating disorder in your childhood is a major plus for your recovery. Working with your partner on needs that your eating disorder was meeting allows you to let go of the eating disorder and embrace the relationship.

Group Therapy: Safety in Numbers

Like family and couples therapy (see the preceding sections, "Family Therapy: Everybody Gets into the Act" and "Couples Therapy: Just the Two of Us" for more on these), group therapy includes other people in your eating disorder treatment. But unlike family and couples therapy, group therapy involves total strangers, people you may never have connected with in life. Why would you possibly want to do that? In this section, I lay out the reasons — along with a snapshot of the process — and let you decide.

Group therapy is different from support groups, which I discuss in the next section, "Self-Help Groups: Grass Roots Support." In group therapy, you have a professional therapist as the group's leader. You may focus on patterns of relating among members during group sessions as part of treatment. You're expected to attend each meeting. Support groups, on the other hand, rely mainly on mutual support and often draw leadership from their members. You attend only when you want to. Support groups are usually free, whereas you're expected to pay a fee for group therapy.

Group therapy may be short-term, say 10 to 12 sessions, or open-ended, meaning they continue indefinitely. Open-ended groups usually meet weekly. In these groups, you're able to get into a wider range of topics related to your eating disorder and your recovery, such as family, relationships, school/ career, and so on. In most cases, you also get to know other people in the group better.

Your group may have as few as 3 or 4 members or as many as 12, but 6 to 8 people is an average group size. Some groups only have members with one kind of eating disorder, but the trend is to mix it up. If you're in a mixed group, you should expect at least one other person in the group to have the same eating disorder that you do.

Why you may consider group therapy

Some people specifically seek out group therapy because they feel they don't have a good support system. At the beginning, the group itself fills this void. In time, the hope is that the social skills you gain in your group will result in improvements in your support system outside of the group. Other benefits you're likely to get from group therapy include

 ✔ **Feeling accepted:** Almost all groups emphasize a nonjudgmental environment. This is a big part of what makes a group feel safe.

 ✔ **Getting support:** Getting encouragement from other members to make changes and take on tough issues is like having your own cheering section.

✔ **Feeling connected:** Many people come to group therapy feeling very isolated because of their eating disorder. You may find it a big relief to feel understood and not so alone.

✔ **Practicing new skills:** Group therapy serves as a great place to practice new skills. For example, you may practice expressing your feelings (including anger), stating your opinions, giving and receiving honest feedback, or disagreeing.

✔ **Trusting others:** Group therapy provides an opportunity to discover that others can be trustworthy, reliable, and supportive.

✔ **Being yourself:** Group therapy provides a safe environment for exploring who you are with other people who will be accepting.

Some of the benefits in the preceding list may actually sound more scary than beneficial. You should know that most groups spend a lot of time giving members a chance to get to know each other and to feel safe and comfortable as a group before delving into the hard stuff. Members take on only small, manageable challenges with each other as they develop skills and confidence in the group setting.

What happens in group therapy

Just what happens in group therapy? Group formats vary, but two common sources of group discussion are leader-suggested topics and group members' own issues. Often a particular group session will include time for both. Your leader might suggest topics like

✔ What does it mean to say you "feel fat"?

✔ What helps you most when you feel like purging?

✔ Who in your family is having the most difficulty with you getting better?

Your own issues may be anything from handling the fight you just had with your sister to your shame about how competent everyone in your workplace thinks you are — if they only knew! As your participation in the group goes on, you're likely to get better and better at knowing the specific kind of help you want from other members when you bring up a particular subject.

Your group therapist guides you as a group in using *group processes* — that is, being able to notice things that happen among you as group members and finding ways to grow and gain insight from them.

How group therapy helps recovery

A lot of your eating disorder reflects your feelings of discomfort and inadequacy in relation to other human beings. Some of this is due to shame. Some comes from lack of trust. Some is because you don't feel entitled to have others respect your needs or listen to your point of view or feelings. And some is about lacking the skills and experience for expressing yourself. Group therapy provides an environment in which you can heal and grow in all these areas. When you do, your need to turn to food lessens.

Self-Help Groups: Grass Roots Support

Self-help or *mutual support* groups are made up of people with eating disorders, much like the group therapy I discuss in the previous section, "Group Therapy: Safety in Numbers." However, unlike therapy groups, self-help groups are free-of-charge, they usually aren't led by professionals, and you aren't expected to make a commitment to regular attendance. (I discuss similar groups for families of people with eating disorders in Chapter 24.)

While self-help groups are free, don't think of them as doing treatment on the cheap or not providing real value. Self-help groups do offer value and are good sources of support. The freebie aspect is useful to people who can't otherwise afford treatment, but self-help groups aren't really intended to be a substitute for professional treatment. In this section I discuss the contributions self-help groups make as an *addition* to your primary treatment. I zero in on Overeaters Anonymous (OA) as a special case.

Overeaters Anonymous

Overeaters Anonymous (OA) is a self-help group modeled on Alcoholics Anonymous (AA), a program for people addicted to alcohol. OA started as a group for people who overeat, but now it's common for people with anorexia, bulimia, and binge eating disorder to attend OA as well. (In some places you can find Eating Disorders Anonymous [EDA].)

Like AA, OA is called a *twelve–step* program because being a member includes working on principles of recovery organized into twelve separate steps. Unfortunately, some of what OA has borrowed from AA can spell trouble for eating disorder recovery. At the same time, other parts of the program can be healing and helpful to people with eating disorders — so much so, that many have been willing to work around the problems.

You can find OA meetings in your area by going online to www.oa.org. If you live in a large city, you'll have a choice of groups. Be sure to visit several to find the meeting where the membership feels like a good fit for you.

Knowing the pitfalls of OA for eating disorders

Because OA is based on the principles developed by AA, it adheres to many of the same standards. Many of the guidelines that were established with alcoholics in mind may also be applicable to overeaters, but they can translate into trouble for those with eating disorders. The following AA/OA ways of thinking can cause problems for those recovering from an eating disorder:

- **Compulsive overeating as a disease:** Alcoholism is considered a lifelong disease, and few alcoholic people seem to be able to take up normal drinking. The same story doesn't apply to eating disorders. You can reasonably expect complete recovery if you follow through with your treatment. Predicting a lifelong disease could make it come true.

- **Admitting powerlessness:** The first of the twelve steps, admitting powerlessness, seems pretty useful as a way to break through alcoholic denial. However, if you have an eating disorder, you probably struggle all the time with feelings of powerlessness. The breakthrough for you is discovering your power!

- **Abstinence:** With alcohol, complete abstinence makes sense. With food, not so much. What else can you abstain from? In OA, the answer is up to you, but it has to be something. Some say bingeing. Others say certain "forbidden" foods, like sugar. Still others say snacking. Trying to hold onto the AA principle of abstinence in OA can lead to a lot of all-or-nothing thinking — just when you need to be working on moderation.

Using OA effectively

The people with eating disorders who use OA most effectively are those who adapt OA's way of thinking to better suit their specific needs. Some successful ways to do this are to

- **Focus on the community, spirituality, and emotional support OA offers.**

- **Keep flexible about ideology.** This includes defining OA expectations in personally meaningful ways. For example, your "abstinence" might be following your own healthy way of eating.

- **Find a sponsor (OA mentor) who supports flexible use of the program.**

People who figure out a good way to use OA find that it benefits their recovery. Participation in OA can aid your eating disorder recovery plan by

- **Reducing shame:** Everybody's been there and done that.

- **Reducing isolation:** In the OA community, you're not alone.

- **Encouraging you to deal with your feelings:** OA is a place where talking about feelings is welcomed.

- **Promoting healthy relationship behaviors:** Part of the 12 steps involves examination of how your behaviors affect others.

- **Supporting your efforts to change:** Other members understand the significance of even baby steps toward change and are a cheering section for your success.

- **Providing hope:** You meet people who've been where you are — and gotten better

Chapter 12

Exploring Medication and Other Approaches

An eating disorder affects every part of you — your body, mind, and spirit — so the process of getting better is composed of many treatment elements. For this reason, in Chapters 9, 10, and 11, I discuss a team approach to your recovery, as well as taking advantage of more than just one approach. This chapter focuses on some additional treatment options for you to consider.

Additional options include using medication, trying an innovative family approach to treating eating disorders, and using online therapy. These treatment approaches aren't appropriate for everyone with an eating disorder. If you're in individual therapy, you'll want to discuss any additions to your treatment with your therapist.

Designating a "coach" for your recovery team — someone who helps you coordinate your recovery team and its efforts to get you well — gives you a big advantage. For many people, that coach is their individual psychotherapist.

Getting Your Biology on Board with Medication

If you have an eating disorder, or any psychological disorder, part of the problem may be that your brain chemistry is out of whack. The brain requires certain hormones to be present in just the right places and just the right amounts for the body's systems to run smoothly. In Chapter 5 I discuss how brain chemistry that's off-kilter can both contribute to developing an eating disorder as well as be the result of an eating disorder. Either way, medication may help get things back in order. (Surprisingly, so can psychotherapy!)

When people think about taking medication to treat psychological disorders, two reactions representing opposite extremes are common. At the one extreme is the desire for a pill that simply fixes everything (since food and restricting don't). At the other extreme is the fear that medication may control you or turn you into a zombie. Each extreme gives medication more power than it actually has. In this section I go over what medication can realistically do for your eating disorder.

Actually, if you have an eating disorder, you probably have to think about more than your eating disorder symptoms with regard to medication. In Chapter 7, I cover the major psychological disorders that commonly go hand-in-hand with eating disorders. These companion disorders include mood and anxiety disorders as well as substance abuse. Depending on your personal needs, medication can play a role in the treatment of any of them. (Fortunately, they probably don't all require separate medications!) I discuss medication for these companion disorders in this section as well.

The part of your treatment that involves medication is guided by your psychopharmacologist. *Psychopharmacologist* is the designation for an M.D. who specializes in medication for psychological conditions. Your psychopharmacologist will review your health and psychological history, make recommendations about medication for you, and follow your progress on any medication you take.

Seeking the cure for your eating disorder in medication

You may think, "I've tried so many things and I'm tired. Can't I just take medication and be done with it?" Unfortunately, the answer is no. Medication alone is not the answer for any eating disorder. Think of your treatment package as a mosaic. Medication may or may not be one of the pieces, but it never comprises the entire mosaic by itself. Key reasons for this include the following:

- ✔ **Many eating disorder symptoms are not treatable at all with existing medications.** In the next section, "Rebalancing the brain chemistry behind your eating disorder," I go over which eating disorder symptoms psychopharmacologists find they can treat with medication.

- ✔ **Lots of people don't get the desired effects or only get partial effects.** Reactions to medications vary widely from person to person. Somebody else may get a great benefit from a drug that fizzles for you.

✔ **Medication's effects on eating disorder symptoms are generally short-term (usually six months or so).** Medicine may offer some short-term relief, but you need to approach your symptoms in ways that have more lasting effects (I discuss ways to do this in Chapters 10–14).

Several of the researched psychotherapies have a better track record than does medication with regard to both cure and relapse. The best approach is usually to try psychotherapy first and consider adding medication later if your symptoms prove to be stubborn. You and your pharmacologist may decide not to wait if your symptoms are especially severe or if you are being treated for depression in addition to your eating disorder. (See the section "Treating companion disorders," later in this chapter, for more information on treating depression.)

Rebalancing the brain chemistry behind your eating disorder

Medication can't cure everything, and it can't cure anything permanently, but it does seem to help in some situations. Medication's helpfulness varies depending upon the eating disorder. In this section, I go over what you can expect from medication for each of the major eating disorders.

Medicating anorexia

A basic rule about medication applies to you if you are anorexic: *gain weight first!* In Chapters 6 and 7 I review the physical and psychological symptoms you're likely to experience just because your body and brain are starving. Give your body the nourishment and substance it needs to take care of itself. At that point, you and your doctor can see what symptoms are still hanging around that may need medicating.

The picture for treating anorexia with medication isn't very rosy. So far, not much has proven especially useful for helping sufferers with their acute symptoms, such as the urge to restrict or the distorted thinking and body image that go with it. Ditto for preventing relapse. However, some hopeful possibilities are under study, including

✔ **Zyprexa (olanzapine):** Zyprexa is a drug originally used for the symptoms of psychosis, but newer uses include treatment of the acute symptoms of anorexia. Zyprexa is a find because, unlike some other drugs, your brain doesn't need to be well-fed in order for the medication to do its job. So far, Zyprexa seems most helpful in decreasing the obsessive thoughts and fears about weight that keep you starving yourself. Zyprexa also promotes weight gain. But not to worry — you stop taking the drug when you reach your target weight.

✔ **Naltrexone:** Naltrexone is an *opiate antagonist*. Opiate antagonists block the activity of opiates in your brain. Opiates are brain chemicals associated with pleasure. Naltrexone blocks the pleasure sensations an alcoholic gets from alcohol. Researchers are experimenting with naltrexone as a way to similarly block an addiction to dieting in people with anorexia.

Medicating bulimia and binge eating disorder

Medication works better for bulimia and binge eating disorder than for anorexia, though results aren't guaranteed. Antidepressants are your best bet. And among the antidepressants, the SSRIs (selective serotonin reuptake inhibitors) have the safest side-effect profile, so they're most often pre-scribed. (See the sidebar "How do SSRIs do what they do?" to discover how the SSRIs work.) Though Prozac (fluoxetine) is the SSRI that's been most studied, experts believe other SSRIs are likely to be equally effective. These include

✔ Celexa (citalopram)

✔ Lexapro (escitalopram oxalate)

✔ Luvox (fluvoxamine)

✔ Paxil (paroxetine)

✔ Zoloft (sertraline)

A significant number of people with bulimia who try antidepressant drugs experience a reduction in their bingeing and purging behavior and in their preoccupation with weight. People with binge eating disorder respond to antidepressants with reduced bingeing. Researchers used to think these effects were indirect benefits of being less depressed. But now researchers are finding that even people who aren't depressed show improvement in their bulimic or binge eating disorder symptoms when they take antidepressants.

A few other medications are under investigation for treating bulimia and/or binge eating disorder. These drugs include

✔ **Topimax (topiramate):** Topimax, a brand name for the generic drug topi-ramate, is an anti-seizure drug which reduces bingeing and purging. The problem with Topimax is that it may make your brain go goofy — many people can't concentrate or think straight on Topimax. Researchers are looking into Zonegran, a cousin of Topimax that has fewer side effects, for similar results.

✔ **ReVia (naltrexone):** ReVia, a brand name for the generic drug naltrex-one, seems to reduce bingeing and purging behavior. See the previous section "Medicating anorexia" to find out about naltrexone's effects in blocking the brain's pleasurable experience of addictive behaviors.

How do SSRIs do what they do?

SSRI stands for *selective serotonin reuptake inhibitor.* That mouthful actually describes a process that helps you use your on-hand supply of an important natural brain chemical, *serotonin*, more effectively. Serotonin is responsible for a multitude of tasks throughout the brain and body. Among these tasks is the regulation of moods and appetite. When a supply of serotonin has just been out on its job and is ready to be absorbed back into its neural storehouse, an SSRI acts to block the exits ("reuptake"), sending the serotonin back for another shift. This supply joins the serotonin already headed out for work. That way you end up with more serotonin in your circulation at any particular time.

✔ **Zofran (ondansetron):** Zofran, a brand-name form of the generic ondansetron, is an *antiemetic*. Antiemetics help control vomiting caused by chemotherapy. They may also stop you from bingeing and purging. (Zofran hasn't been researched for binge eating disorder.)

Ironically, if you suffer from bulimia, medication may not be an option until your symptoms are under control. No medication can be helpful to your bulimic symptoms if you purge it out of your system!

Treating companion disorders

Using medication to treat your mood and anxiety symptoms doesn't usually help your eating disorder symptoms. However, treating depression and anxiety does provide a better platform for recovery. Plus, you deserve to feel as good as you can.

Three companion disorders common to eating disorders — depression, anxiety, and obsessive compulsive disorder (OCD) — are routinely treated with a class of antidepressant medications called selective serotonin reuptake inhibitors (SSRIs). (See the sidebar "How do SSRIs do what they do?" for more information on how SSRIs work.)

More than one type of medication is available to treat each of these disorders, but SSRIs are often the first choice of medical professionals. (I mention the SSRIs in the preceding section for treatment of bulimic and BED symptoms.) SSRIs have a high rate of effectiveness and a low side-effect profile compared to other drugs. Prozac is probably the best known of the SSRIs, but newer models of SSRIs coming on the market have fewer and fewer of Prozac's side effects, such as drowsiness and loss of libido.

Bipolar disorder is another frequent companion of the eating disorders. Bipolar disorder almost always needs to be medicated and is almost bound to get worse over time if medication isn't prescribed. A class of drugs called *mood stabilizers* is usually used to treat bipolar disorder. Lithium is probably the best known. Some mood stabilizers, like lithium, cause weight gain. Others, like Zonegran, not so much. You need to discuss your options carefully with your psychopharmacologist if you are diagnosed with bipolar disorder.

You may want to turn to the following sources for more information on medicating these disorders: *Depression For Dummies, Overcoming Anxiety For Dummies,* and *Seasonal Affective Disorder For Dummies,* all by Laura L. Smith, Ph.D., and Charles H. Elliot, Ph.D., plus *Bipolar Disorder for Dummies* by Candida Fink, M.D., and Joe Kraynak (all available from Wiley).

If you're the parent of a child or adolescent who needs psychiatric medication, beware of being overcautious or under-cautious. On the overcautious side, don't be so alarmed by the thought of medicating your child that you are closed off to its possibilities for relieving some serious symptoms and suffering. This is especially difficult these days with some of the stories that have been in the news about potential dangerous effects of the SSRI antidepressant drugs. Just how these drugs may affect children differently than they do adults is still under investigation. For this reason, try not to be under-cautious either. Because so many unanswered questions still exist, if your child is placed on an SSRI antidepressant for depression, anxiety, OCD, or eating disorder symptoms, you need to be on the lookout for mood changes at the beginning of treatment or at any time dosages are changed. At these times, a small minority of kids show an increase in depression or suicidal thoughts and feelings.

Exploring New Frontiers in Eating Disorder Treatment

Progress isn't found only in the test tube. In this section I describe two innovations in eating disorder treatment that have developed outside the lab. The first is a new way of working with the families of teenagers who have anorexia. (You can read about the more traditional approaches in Chapter 11.) The second — it had to happen — is the use of the Internet as a way to deliver treatment to people with eating disorders who may not otherwise have access to services.

Putting parents in charge with the Maudsley model

A very promising treatment for teens with anorexia has come out of the Maudsley Hospital in London, an institution already well-respected for its work with eating disorders. The treatment is a special form of family therapy. It engages parents as the most important resources for treatment — the ones who can save their daughter's life.

In a handful of studies, the Maudsley model has already proven to be superior to individual therapy for adolescents with anorexia. In the original study, two-thirds of kids avoided hospitalization and showed reduced preoccupation with dieting and body shape. At a five year follow-up, they were still doing better than a comparison group of kids who'd had individual treatment at the same time. Teens who'd had anorexia for a short time — three years or less — did best.

Maudsley may be too much for a single parent or families with special needs members to manage. If, for legitimate reasons, parents can't commit the time needed to take this treatment approach, the other therapy options discussed in this book are all viable and good choices that have proven track records of yielding successful results.

What the program involves

The major plus, as well as the primary challenge, of Maudsley is that parents have to really, really be committed for it to be successful. They have to get everybody in the family to sessions and often have to take time off work. (Your therapist may remind your parents that they'd do it if you had cancer.) Your parents also have to get you to eat. In the Maudsley model, your parents are viewed as your best shot at staying alive. Why? Your parents know you best. Your parents are asked to become your hospital unit and to supervise what you eat until you gain the weight you need in order to be healthy again.

During the first phase of treatment, the entire family puts all other family issues aside to focus on your life-threatening condition. Your parents are asked to think of you as a much younger child — an effect of the anorexia — who has to be fed to get well. Early on in treatment, you have a family meal in the therapist's presence. He coaches your parents on how best to get you to eat. He also suggests other changes they may need to make for you to get better.

Once you achieve a healthy weight, the family enters another phase of treatment. During this phase, your parents help you with normal tasks of adolescence, including being a little more independent. They can also start bringing up other family issues — beefs with you, disagreements with siblings, or other family business.

How Maudsley helps

The Maudsley model appears to help by putting families back in order when anorexia has thrown them into serious disorder. Where parents (understandably) feel helpless and unable to protect their children, Maudsley provides a way for them to feel effective and in charge again. Anorexia is dethroned and you get to experience your parents as competent and able to take care of you when you need them most. You are also encouraged to become competent, in a teenage sort of way, and to find better sources of control in your life than being thin.

Family researchers are now looking at ways to adapt the Maudsley model beyond individual teens and young adults with anorexia to adults with eating disorders, people with bulimia, and chronic eating disorder sufferers. Studies with bulimic teens are showing good results, while other areas of study have yet to be undertaken.

You can find a listing of therapists and programs that use the Maudsley approach at the Something Fishy Web site at www.something-fishy.org/ treatmentfinder/.

Looking to the Internet for therapy

So many online resources are available for eating disorders, looking at them all could make your eyes cross. (You can find a pretty good sampling of what's available in the "Resource Guide" at the back of this book.) Web sites are available to give you eating disorder information, recommend books, help you locate eating disorder specialists, supply you with chat rooms or support groups, offer general advice, and so on.

But can actually getting *treatment* online even work? Surprisingly, in specific limited circumstances for those with bulimia or binge eating disorder, the answer seems to be "yes." And the amount of research to support this is increasing.

Online therapy is absolutely *not* a good choice in the following circumstances:

- ✔ **You have anorexia:** The health risks are just too great and your disorder prevents you from seeing this clearly. You need a team that includes real people, including medical professionals.

- ✔ **Your eating disorder is severe:** If you aren't sure whether yours is severe, assume it is and get a good, in-person evaluation.

- ✔ **You're suicidal:** You must have real people on your team if you struggle with wanting to stay alive.

Considering an online treatment program

The bottom line is that you are always on safest ground when you work with another human being, one who has gotten to know you well and can help you flag risky situations. That said, the following conditions may make working with an online program anything from better-than-nothing to actually-pretty-good:

- ✔ **Shame:** You may feel so ashamed about your symptoms that you simply can't bring yourself to tell someone what's going on face-to-face.

- ✔ **Fear:** You may be nervous about entering treatment and need a way to get your feet wet before you go public.

- ✔ **Lack of financial resources:** Online treatment isn't free, but it's generally less expensive than in-person treatment.

- ✔ **Lack of access:** In many locations, no one who knows how to treat eating disorders is available.

- ✔ **An intention to supplement your in-person therapy:** Many eating disorder sufferers who work with a therapist find additional ways to work on their treatment on their own. Talk about this possibility with your therapist to make sure what you do online doesn't clash with what you're doing with him. Some online programs have a specialized focus which may fit in well with your primary therapy, such as nutritional counseling or body image work.

Finding help with online therapy

Mouse-clickers beware! Being online is like being in the Wild West. People make up the rules as they go along, and no regulations exist to govern what anyone may offer you. Be sure to check the credentials of the Web sponsor. Finding your Web-based program through a reputable eating disorder network, such as those listed in the "Resource Guide" at the back of this book, is one good way to check a potential provider's credibility.

The following models represent the types of online treatment that are available:

- ✔ Online workbooks with questions and exercises that you complete at your own pace

- ✔ Programs timed with other participants in which you read, journal, and "meet" in chat rooms with a facilitator

- ✔ Educational programs divided into sessions that offer advice and strategies for symptom management and dealing with relapse

Depending on the site and program sponsor, you may find a lot of mixing-and-matching within these models. For example, some programs may only involve you and your computer screen. Other programs may require you to have phone sessions with a sponsoring therapist. Or you may have to start out with an in-person evaluation.

Internet sites may be hazardous to your physical and emotional health!

Just as the Web is used to promote and support eating disorder recovery, some people use the Internet to undermine recovery. Though not exactly the plan, undermining recovery is often the effect of a group of underground Web sites known as pro-ana (pro-anorexia), pro-mia (pro-bulimia) and pro-ed (pro-eating disorder).

These sites are generally described as glorifying eating disorders as a lifestyle. If you read the sites' content, you can easily see how they've earned this reputation. However, the truth is a little more complicated and a lot sadder than what you see on the surface. In some communities members might recognize their disorder, but have given up on recovery. In "lifestyle" communities, whether members embrace or deny their own disorder, they aim to emulate anorexic qualities of grit, determination, and endurance in the pursuit of thinness. Pro-ana groups share *thinspiration*, that is, inspiration in the form of photos of emaciated heroines and weight loss slogans and tips. Pro-mia groups add tips for bulimic activities such as purging and keeping it a secret. ("Pro-ed" seems to be a moving target for definition, often used to refer to all such communities.)

The heart of these groups is individuals reaching out of isolation for community and understanding — just what you'd want an eating disordered person to do, right? The tragedy and risk of the community they form is that its members have given up on the possibility that things could ever be different for them. So they support each other in this belief and make a virtue of defeat. Who can be thinnest? Who can endure most? (People who die from starvation are considered martyrs.) A participant believes her eating disorder — the pursuit of perfection, the possibility of reaching her goal weight, of being "good" — is all she has to protect her from the oncoming tide of her own unworthiness.

Because despair is never far from anyone who has struggled with an eating disorder, a vulnerable person who wanders onto one of these sites out of curiosity or with the hope of finding connection and understanding (a common theme) may be at risk of being drawn into the vortex. Feeling understood and not judged feels good, especially if you're feeling like a failure. These sites, like secret clubs, have their own language, vows, rituals, and — above all — loyalty to one another, or at least to one another's suffering.

The allure of the pro-ana, pro-mia, and pro-ed Internet underground is dangerous because the basic instincts that draw people to these sites are understandable human needs (like acceptance and community) in the face of disabling, demoralizing disorders. These sites seem to fulfill these human needs, but they do so in a destructive way. If you have an eating disorder and find yourself tempted by pro-ana–type sites, consider the following alternatives:

- If face-to-face support feels too overwhelming, consider online support in the form of groups or chat rooms (see the "Resource Guide" at the end of this book).

- If you've tried a recovery-based group (online or real time) and were disappointed, maybe you need to give it another chance. Unlike pro-ana, support groups are made up of real people who are bound to disappoint at times as well as help.

- If you feel judged or pushed to do more than you feel you can at this moment in a support group, you need to speak up. That's part of recovery too!

- If you feel like giving up on recovery, remember that — unlike your eating disorder — your treatment team doesn't require or expect you to be perfect.

Chapter 13

Making Good Use of the Approach You Choose

Say you've lined up the best treatment team you can find to help with your recovery. Your team includes an individual therapist whose approach and personality you like, a reputable nutritionist, and maybe a psychopharmacologist and a support group. Everything's in place — almost.

You still have one more team member to focus on to make sure you get the results you deserve: *you*! Recovering from an eating disorder is one of the hardest challenges you'll ever face. You want to bring your "A" game.

You may be wondering, "What does this even mean? I'm the one with the problem. Didn't I hire the experts to figure this out for me and make me better?" Well, you're half right. You *are* in treatment to work on your problem — your eating disorder. And you *did* hire your team members because they're eating disorder experts. But successful treatment requires you to partner up *with* your team members; they can show you the way, but *you* have to walk the path.

In this chapter I go over four areas where your way of partnering up can make a big difference: your expectations of treatment, your view of recovery goals, your relationship with your therapist, and your participation in group treatment.

Letting Go of Magic for Reality

Unrealistic expectations for treatment can undermine the process before you even set foot in the door. If your ideas about how the treatment should go or what your part in it should be don't match what actually needs to happen for you to get better, you aren't headed for a good treatment outcome. Two unrealistic treatment expectations are particularly common among people with eating disorders:

✔ The longing for a quick fix from therapy, one that will involve a minimum of time and discomfort.

✔ The expectation that someone else can fix things for you.

What makes you bring unrealistic expectations to your treatment? Sometimes you simply don't know what's supposed to happen. A frank discussion with your therapist at the beginning of treatment is a good way to clarify what you can realistically expect from each other and from the process. (Read more on establishing a successful working relationship with your therapist in the section "Partnering with Your Therapist in a Treatment-Boosting Way," later in this chapter.)

People who find that longings for magic hang around in spite of such a conversation usually have very little confidence in what they can bring to the team effort. In this section I describe more about how expectations for magical treatments develop, how they affect treatment, and why surrendering them is more likely to get you the results you want.

Giving up the longing for a quick fix

Living right alongside fears of giving up your eating disorder is a small volcano of urgency that says you must get over your symptoms *now*! You're especially likely to feel this way if bingeing is one of your symptoms. Even if you reduce your symptoms fairly quickly in treatment, that same volcano fires away for you to be over all your other discomforts yesterday. You don't want to feel frustrated about your future or friends. It's hard to experience loneliness, disappointment, or anger.

The urgency to get rid of uncomfortable feelings is part of what causes the development of an eating disorder in the first place. Tolerating discomfort is a recovery skill that takes time to develop.

Longing for a quick fix also reflects your feelings of hopelessness. You've been struggling for a long time, always ending up in the same demoralizing place. Some of the urgency you feel may be your desire for immediate reassurance that you actually *can* get better.

Your feelings completely make sense, given where you've been. Yet, if you're going to dig in for the long-haul work of recovery, someplace along the line you need to let go of the expectation that you'll get better fast. Holding on to your longing for a quick fix impacts your treatment negatively by leading you to conclusions like the following:

- ✔ You believe your treatment is failing because you think it's not working fast enough.

- ✔ You believe *you* are failing because you think you'd be getting better faster if you were doing everything right.

- ✔ You don't dig in for the work that takes longer because it doesn't match your idea that recovery is supposed to happen right away.

- ✔ You're highly vulnerable to relapse because you want to turn to something that makes you feel better *now* (such as food or dieting).

If you have questions about your progress, talk them over with your therapist. To address the issue of how well things are going, you may ask:

- ✔ How does your therapist think you're doing, considering how long you've been in treatment?

- ✔ Does she see signs of progress you may be missing?

- ✔ Can she think of anything you can do differently to benefit your treatment?

- ✔ Does she think adding any other kinds of treatment or practices may improve your progress? (See Chapter 9 for a discussion of some possibilities.)

Just because *everything* isn't better now, that doesn't mean *nothing* is better. Recovery is about progress, not perfection. Some of the joys of recovery are the unexpected nuggets of progress that develop along the way: You find you're able to do something you never imagined doing before; you understand something in your situation with a new compassion you didn't believe possible; or you become aware of a positive trait or a resource in yourself that you didn't see before. These jewels often provide just the injections of hope and confidence you need to keep you going.

Losing the longing for an outside fix

Not only may you feel powerless and unable to do anything about your eating disorder, but you may also feel powerless and ineffective in managing your life as a whole. These feelings steered you into your eating disorder in the first place. Longing for someone or something outside of you to fix not only the eating disorder but also your life in general reflects your vote of no-confidence in your own worth and abilities.

You may have devoted a lot of energy to finding the outside fix. Besides food and thinness, you may have tried drugs, alcohol, sex, or shopping. If you haven't turned off from relationships, you may have hoped another person could supply what feels missing. Hoping your therapist or the therapy process can be the outside fix is just another in a line of efforts doomed to failure. The good news is that once you've committed to developing your own inside fix — the real road to recovery — your therapist can be a great source of guidance and support.

Beyond symptom management, the heart of your recovery is the process of building yourself up from the inside out. Self-esteem and self-confidence can only come from an *inside* fix. You achieve this by developing skills that help you feel empowered and effective as a person.

How can you tell whether you're bringing a desire for an outside fix to your therapy? Be on the alert for the following telltale signs:

- ✔ You regularly wait for your therapist to say or suggest something to make you feel better.

- ✔ You resist your therapist's efforts to engage you in self-soothing or other emotion management techniques. (Isn't that your therapist's job?)

- ✔ You frequently try to convince your therapist that expecting you to try to make the kinds of changes in your life that the two of you are discussing isn't reasonable or fair.

Surrendering the longing for someone or something outside of you to fix you is necessary in order to face the challenges of working on an inside fix. Giving up this longing is one of the bravest and most meaningful leaps of your recovery. It signals the beginning of your understanding that

- ✔ You are the only one who can rescue you.

- ✔ You have or can develop the resources and skills you need for self-rescue.

- ✔ You'll never find a better fix than this one.

Your therapist can't do the work for you, any more than a personal trainer can exercise for you. But your therapist can certainly offer you support, recognize your courage and efforts, help you see where you're tripping over your own feet, point the direction to recovery, commiserate with your setbacks, and applaud your big and little victories. You have a lot to gain by having your therapist in your corner.

Substituting Recovery Goals for Eating Disorder Goals

Many changes in thinking mark your shift from eating disorder into recovery (see Chapter 8 for more on evaluating your recovery). One of the most important changes in your thinking is that you surrender "thin" as your measure of success. This change may feel like one of the scariest. If you don't measure your success by your thinness, how *do* you measure it? You need a lot of courage to invest hope or energy in a future "you" that you can barely imagine, let alone believe in. But the more you invest in that future you, the more buffering you create between yourself and your eating disorder. The choices you make can have either boosting or busting effects on your treatment. I discuss your choices and their effects in this section.

Surrendering "thin" as your measure of success

With your eating disorder, "thin" is your measure of success and you think being thin is what will make you happy in life. These beliefs are part-and-parcel of your eating disorder. Keeping "thin" as your goal, with the belief that it can make you happy, has a treatment-busting effect.

How does this stance undermine your treatment? Here are some examples:

✔ If you're mostly talking about getting thin in your therapy sessions, you're not working on the issues that caused your eating disorder or developing the skills that can free you of it.

✔ If you're still putting your energies into getting thin, you're probably not investing in recovery skills outside of treatment.

✔ The more focused you are on getting and staying thin, the more at risk you are for relapse, even when you've reduced your eating disorder symptoms.

If you have a particularly hard time shifting away from thin as your goal, you may be having difficulty imagining that other things about you matter or that you can be accepted if you're less than perfect. These issues are fundamentally important. Aim to resolve these issues in your therapy sessions rather than trying to resolve them by being thin. In the meantime, you may want to check out Chapter 8 for ways to work on building a positive self-image unrelated to weight.

Does surrendering "thin" as your goal mean your sensitivities about your body size and shape will disappear? Not likely, if only because of the constant cultural and media drumbeat to be thin. Shifting your focus away from thin may be purely a leap of faith for you at the beginning — an acknowledgment that your way hasn't worked, so maybe the time is right to try something different. And that's enough to start with. Putting your energies into other goals proves to be a worthy approach when you begin to see results from your efforts.

Knowing you need to do more than stop bingeing

One of the most common mistakes people with eating disorders make is to drop out of treatment as soon as their acute symptoms are gone, before doing any recovery work. If you're thinking about dropping out, *don't do it*! Failing to get a good toehold in recovery sharply increases your risk of relapse.

On the other hand, the more recovery work you get under your belt, the less your chances of relapse. Think of the recovery process as building up a reserve bank account. The reserves you store supply you with a buffer from eating disorder behaviors. When challenges come up, you have more and more skills and an improved self-image to draw on.

Looking beyond your focus on food and weight

Peeking around the corner from the monster issues of food and weight to see whether anything else is out there for you is a great act of courage in recovery. Could you have a life with better relationships, more education, or a career you care about? Sometimes hanging around in the familiar territory of your eating disorder feels a lot safer than trying something new, even though your eating disorder makes you miserable. You may feel like you're being asked to choose between the devil you know and the devil you don't know.

Thinking about the outer aspects of your life may not feel as scary as facing what may be *inside*. You may be afraid of finding feelings that jolt your image of yourself. The "nice girl" in you doesn't want to discover that you're angry at someone. Perhaps you're fearful of tapping into emotions that may overwhelm you. Or maybe your worst fear is finding no feelings at all.

If facing big life questions or inner truths makes you tiptoe or stop and start, don't worry. Treatment isn't a sprint to the finish line. Only when you retreat to your eating disorder as a safer focus and *stay there* are you in a treatment-busting situation. If you think this is where you may be headed, talk with your therapist about it. How can the two of you work together to better recognize your fears? Does just talking openly about them help? A conversation like this is likely to be treatment-boosting by opening the door to topics that help your therapy progress.

Recognizing signs of recovery unrelated to weight

Part of your eating disorder recovery involves recognizing results that are unrelated to weight. If you count only what you see on the scales, you put yourself at great risk for relapse. On the other hand, when you begin to recognize and enjoy results that have nothing to do with getting thin, you plant at least one foot and several toes in recovery. And you reduce your relapse risk.

Discovering how to recognize signs of recovery unrelated to weight offers a great opportunity for you to partner up with your therapy in a treatment-boosting way. You can't will yourself to stop having thoughts and fears about weight, but you can choose what to do when such thoughts and fears pop up. The treatment-busting choice is to hang out with your fears and give them lots of air space. The treatment-boosting choice is to shift your thinking to some aspect of your recovery instead.

In Chapter 8 you find charts for tracking your progress with common markers of recovery, such as emotion management and healthy relationships. Working with these progress charts may give you just the change of focus you need. Or you and your therapist may identify progress markers that apply specifically to you, such as leaving the job with the abusive boss, telling your girlfriend you don't like being called "Shrimp," or noticing that you're more likely to restrict when your mom and dad aren't talking to each other.

Therapists and therapy group members often notice small signs of recovery before you do, or see the significance of a new behavior in a way that you don't yet see. Here are some examples of ways recovery progress may show up:

  ✔ *Sheri* has always been afraid of her anger. She's annoyed at her mom for walking into her room without knocking, but she's afraid to say so. Simply acknowledging these feelings is progress.

> ✔ *Anna,* who can never assert her own needs, asks if it would be okay to turn up the air conditioning in her therapist's office.
>
> ✔ *Mike's* group notices his posture has changed and he's been looking people right in the eye when he speaks.

If the feedback or recognition you get doesn't match your image of yourself or involves a direction that feels scary (like getting angry or being assertive), one response is to shrug off the comment. This is a treatment-busting response. A treatment-boosting response is to stay curious and interested — ask yourself what may happen if you take the feedback seriously. When feedback involves a direction that feels scary, remember that you can take all the time you need to build the skills and confidence required to get to the next step in your recovery. Acknowledging your improvement doesn't obligate you to jump off the high dive!

Partnering with Your Therapist in a Treatment-Boosting Way

No matter what form of treatment you choose, the outcome depends on the quality of the work you and your therapist do together. I assume you've picked the best therapist you can, so your team is strong on that side. But what are the ingredients *you* need to bring to the mix to round out your team and make sure you and your therapist do the best possible work on your behalf? In this section, I go over therapy-boosting ways to partner with your therapist.

Working collaboratively

Working collaboratively is an ongoing treatment-boosting approach. *Collaboration* means you and your therapist each jump in and do your share of the work to solve your problems and help you get better. The opposite of this approach would be if somehow your therapist could "do treatment" to you without much input from you, like getting a massage or a haircut. Holding out for this fantasy treatment is a treatment-busting approach and can seriously interfere with getting the results you want and deserve.

In a collaborative therapy partnership, you bring your therapist on board for her expertise about eating disorders and the treatment process in general. But you are also an expert. What your expertise covers is *you*: how you feel about things, how you feel in the moment, how you view things, what works for you, what doesn't, and so forth. You and your therapist can both contribute ideas about what makes you tick and what may be a good direction for you in a particular situation.

Believing you have as much to contribute to the outcome of your treatment as your therapist is a treatment-boosting approach. It shows up in all the remaining ways I outline for participating in your therapy.

Showing up

Showing up sounds like a silly thing to mention. But actually showing up for your sessions is a minimum way to express collaboration. When you're there, something helpful can happen. This is true even on the days you're full of despair and feel that your body in the chair is the maximum contribution you can make. Allowing your therapist to support you in moments when you need to catch your breath contributes to your recovery!

It can also be important to show up for appointments even when you've had a good week or day. Sometimes you may not be aware of important actions you took or ways you looked at events to make things go well. You'll want to know about your "secrets to success" so you can repeat them. And it doesn't hurt to get your therapist's affirmation!

Another part of showing up is being fully present. You're not fully present if you go to sessions under the influence of drugs or alcohol. Even if you "get away with it" and your therapist can't tell, you still aren't able to do your best collaborating under these conditions. Definitely a treatment-buster.

Following through

What's expected of you between sessions depends on your therapist and the kind of therapy you're in. In certain kinds of therapy, such as cognitive-behavioral therapy, interpersonal therapy, and dialectical behavioral therapy, formal homework assignments are a built-in part of the approach. (You can read more about these approaches in Chapter 10.) Other therapists make up homework assignments regularly or once-in-awhile to reflect something you've just worked on in session.

The obvious follow-through for therapy homework is to just do it. But that doesn't mean you have to succeed at what you try in order for your treatment collaboration to be a success. Kelly supplies an example:

> In Kelly's last therapy session, she and her therapist talked about the fact that Kelly has no long-range goals for herself and is sort of drifting from one dead-end job to another. Her therapist describes a goal-setting exercise for Kelly to do at home that starts with visualizing her ideal life five years down the line.

Kelly sits down to do her assignment. Staring at the blank sheet, she starts to feel panicky. She wisely puts the paper away and does something else to quiet herself down. In her next session, Kelly is able to report that she's never thought of her life five years ahead, and that she feels flooded with fear and a sense of inadequacy when she tries to do so. This opens up an important conversation with her therapist about the crisis-to-crisis way her family lives and how scary it is to imagine being different from them.

Even if your therapist rarely or never suggests homework, you can find treatment-boosting ways to follow through on your own after a session. You can continue to think about what you were working on. Maybe you have more ideas about it or see the issue in a new light. Maybe something that felt true in your session feels wrong now — or the other way around. Maybe just having the ideas percolating in your mind impacts your feelings or behavior during the week. Or maybe keeping track of what you've done since your session helps you know where you want to pick up the thread when you return. All these forms of follow-through are definitely treatment-boosting. They help you get maximum mileage out of your therapy.

Taking risks

In the movie *The Accidental Tourist,* the main character explains his view of foreign travel: You bring as many familiar items with you as you can and expose yourself to as little as possible of that which feels strange in the foreign culture. Approaching your treatment in a similar way is good for keeping things familiar, but bad for helping you change and get better. Nothing changes if nothing changes!

How much risk you take in therapy depends on your individual circumstances, what you're working on at a particular time, and how much trust you've developed in your therapist and the therapy process. Part of good collaboration with your therapist includes figuring out the amount of risk you can reasonably take, given your current circumstances. Taking on some risk is important; otherwise, your symptoms stay just as they are and you feel frustrated and disappointed with your treatment.

You can take some really valuable risks right in your therapy sessions. Depending on your individual circumstances, any of the following may feel risky:

- Revealing things about yourself
- Feeling emotions you're not used to feeling
- Finding out new things about yourself
- Exploring hopes and dreams that seem out of reach

Trying new behaviors outside of therapy — otherwise known as *life* — is the other big arena for risk-taking. The list of risks you can take outside therapy is as long as the list of goals you may have for treatment. Here are some examples related to recovery:

- **Eating:** Trying new foods, eating socially without purging afterward, eating breakfast

- **Relationships:** Telling people "no," weeding abusive people out of your network, telling your friend about your eating disorder

- **Emotions:** Tolerating awareness of grief a little longer before distracting yourself, trying out a meditation class

- **Self-image:** Trying to imagine other things about yourself that are worthwhile besides your weight, focusing on body parts other than the ones you think are fat

Your risk-taking efforts don't all have to hit the mark to be successful. As long as you gain new insights from what happens, the effort is a success. However, some risks feel particularly — well, risky. While you can never control all possible outcomes (if you could, you wouldn't be risking anything!), you and your therapist probably want to collaborate especially carefully to make the risky risks manageable.

Being truthful

Being truthful means telling your therapist exactly what's going on with you — things he needs to know in order to help you but can only know if you tell him.

Your therapist needs to know what you're doing outside the therapy sessions. Be sure to tell him about things like

- **Self-injuring behaviors:** For example, cutting or burning yourself, tearing out your hair, or similar behaviors

- **Reckless or dangerous behaviors:** For example, drinking and driving, driving way over the speed limit, or any other behavior that risks your life or safety

- **Relapse behaviors:** Dieting, restricting, bingeing, purging, or compulsive exercise

- **Illegal behaviors:** For example, shoplifting or petty stealing to pay for drugs, laxatives, and so on

- **Dropping out of school or failing most of your classes:** Class work or educational goals have taken a back seat to your eating disorder.

 ✔ **Losing a job you need:** You failed to show up or your job performance suffered due to your eating disorder

 ✔ **Relationship breakups:** Ending a romance or a friendship has big emotional repercussions. You may be tempted to use eating disorder behaviors to cope.

You may keep information like this to yourself because you're ashamed or afraid that your therapist may be disappointed or angry. Or perhaps you're not used to having people take you seriously when bad things happen to you. This is an excellent time for some treatment-boosting risk taking. When you bring your therapist on board with problems, especially things you may not be so proud of, you give the collaborative relationship a chance to get stronger. You discover that the two of you can take on the tough stuff.

Another time you need to be truthful with your therapist is when you're thinking or feeling things that may hurt you or hurt your treatment. He especially needs to know if you are having any of the following kinds of thoughts or feelings:

 ✔ Suicidal feelings

 ✔ Hopelessness or feelings of despair

 ✔ Thoughts about dropping out of treatment

Your instinct when you're feeling any of these things may be to withdraw. For your treatment to be helpful, you need to counteract this instinct. Thinking of people as a source of help when you're feeling your worst may be new to you. Finding that you can bring your most difficult thoughts and feelings to therapy is definitely a treatment-booster.

Speaking up

If you're close to someone, you know that at times that person makes you mad, hurts you, or disagrees with you, right? The same is true of your relationship with your therapist. Any or all of the following reactions to your therapist are to be expected at some point:

 ✔ You don't like something your therapist is saying or doing.

 ✔ You don't find something she's doing or saying helpful.

 ✔ Something she says hurts your feelings.

 ✔ You disagree with her opinion or suggestion about something.

Telling your therapist when you're not happy with her or the two of you are out of sync is a form of risk-taking. It may feel especially risky if you think having negative feelings toward someone you like is unsafe or not nice.

You pay a high price for not speaking up when you have negative reactions. The relationship with your therapist may begin to feel fake. Therapy may end up feeling like one more place where you just have to go along, where your feelings and needs don't matter. And the worst of it is, you're missing out on a great opportunity! Therapy can be the perfect two-person lab for experimenting with relationship behaviors you need to work on for your recovery. After all, you're with someone who knows that what you're doing feels risky and who supports your efforts.

Every time you risk speaking up with your therapist when you're unhappy or disagree with her, you engage in therapy-boosting behavior. You become stronger. The relationship becomes stronger and you trust it more. And — the bonus — you're a little more likely to try these valuable behaviors out in the "real world."

Participating in repair

Sometimes things that feel really bad happen with your therapist. The misunderstanding may be a really big one. The hurt cuts to the bone. You feel abandoned. Or humiliated. Furious. Frightened. Any of these unwanted experiences can feel like they've shredded the relationship with your therapist and your trust in him.

You may consider pulling up stakes and getting out of there. Maybe that's what you typically do when something happens to hurt a relationship you're in. Or maybe you just don't know how people make things better at a point like this. Or you can't picture how this particular rupture can be mended. Of course, the possibility exists that it can't. But you have a world to gain from hanging in a little longer and trying to repair the relationship.

When you and your therapist roll up your sleeves and go to work to repair a rupture between you, you are both saying your feelings matter and the relationship matters. This sends a healing message. More healing may be had by figuring out what went wrong, acknowledging your hurt, and looking together for a way to resolve things. You also feel effective when you're able to do this kind of repair work. You gain the confidence of knowing that you and your therapist can handle the situation if things go wrong again. What's more, the experience shows you how to do this in other relationships.

Making the Most of Groups

Group situations call on you to bring parts of yourself to therapy that you can leave at home in one-on-one situations. If you decide to include group therapy or a support group in your treatment plan, you need to determine what qualities you need to bring in order to get the most from the experience. In this section I go over the treatment-boosters for each kind of group.

Group therapy is different from a support group. A therapy group is led by a professional group therapist. You're expected to attend each time the group meets. Though support groups may sometimes be facilitated by professionals, they are often led by group members. You can go to meetings when you want to.

Group therapy

In group therapy, you talk about your eating disorder and how you're doing with recovery-related behaviors. You develop relationship skills by experiencing what happens among group members and practicing new relationship behaviors. (You can read more about group therapy in Chapter 11.)

Most of the treatment-boosting approaches I advocate earlier in this chapter for getting the most from individual therapy also help you maximize a group therapy experience. Treatment-boosting approaches include

- Having realistic goals for treatment results
- Focusing on recovery goals instead of eating disorder goals
- Showing up
- Following through
- Taking risks
- Being truthful
- Speaking up
- Participating in repair

But hold on! You can bring a few more qualities, specific to group therapy, to help you get the most from the situation, such as

- **Willingness to get involved with other people:** You can't get much from group therapy by keeping your thoughts to yourself (although many people start group therapy this way and gradually expand).

- **Willingness and ability to commit to the group process on a regular basis:** For a group to work, you have to know people are going to show up. For you to get something out of it, you have to feel you're a real part of the group. This can only happen if you're a reliable, regular part of what goes on there.

- **Openness to new things:** This quality is especially useful if your group is finding out about specific, new skills (like a dialectical-behavioral skills training group).

✔ **Open-mindedness:** You listen to other points of view, and think about what they may have to offer you. You take in what others have to say about you and think about it, whether you end up agreeing or not.

✔ **Ability to tolerate having the focus on someone else's needs:** Not everybody is up for sharing their therapy time with other people.

✔ **Ability to tolerate having the focus on your own needs:** You may find this surprisingly hard in a group situation, especially when you're aware of others who may want the spotlight at the same time.

Besides these therapy boosting approaches, a few practical considerations affect your ability to benefit from group therapy. The main ones to keep in mind are

✔ **Acute crisis:** If you or someone in your family is going through some kind of crisis situation — illness, job loss, relationship breakup, death, severe suicidal feelings — you probably need to put maximum energy into resolving or weathering the crisis. This probably isn't a good time to try to share your energies with others.

✔ **Life demands that make regular attendance impossible:** For example, you travel regularly for your business; you've promised to be at all your kids' soccer and basketball games; you have to take freelance jobs whenever you get called.

Support groups

Support groups really differ from one another. The qualities that do you the most good in one type of group aren't necessarily the ones you need to benefit from another type of group. For instance, are you in a large group with an invited speaker? You need the ability to listen, to get something out of educational material, and to assert yourself if you have questions. Are you in an intimate group of three or four people sharing your personal stories? There you want to bring a lot of the qualities you'd bring to group therapy, such as being prepared to focus on recovery skills rather than weight and food, the ability to express yourself and be truthful, the ability to let others have the group's attention, and openness to other points of view.

You tend to get more from any group situation when you participate. But you can benefit just by listening, too. Overeaters Anonymous (OA) is a good example of this. You can go to OA meeting after OA meeting and never say a word. And if that's the only way you can participate, by all means, do it! Just keep in mind that the people who become actively involved in the practices and community of the group seem to have the strongest sense of being able to lean on the group for their recovery.

Chapter 14

Managing Early Stage Recovery and the Reality of Relapse

In This Chapter

▶ Understanding the recovery process

▶ Identifying key recovery skills

▶ Getting a grip on resistance

▶ Finding out how to handle relapse

Choosing to begin letting go of your eating disorder and pursue recovery can feel like stepping off a cliff into an abyss; your eating disorder is familiar ground, while recovery is unknown territory. The prospect of venturing into the unknown is understandably scary. But as you begin your adventure down the recovery path, keep in mind that the challenges you encounter in the early stage can serve to make you even stronger, paving the way to a fuller recovery.

At this point, the worst of your eating disorder symptoms are receding, providing you some breathing room to focus on other areas of development. In this chapter, I discuss how you can use this valuable time to build a stronger recovery and make yourself more resilient.

The recovery process takes a lot of grit and courage because you are facing all the things about yourself and your life that, up until now, you thought you couldn't face without an eating disorder. Throughout this chapter, I advise you on how to make use of your treatment team and other resources to develop the skills you need to stay the course and waylay the obstacles of fear and resistance.

Without doubt, there will be times when your symptoms will resurface. In the section on relapse, I discuss how to weather and make use of these expected events as part of a normal recovery process. Recovery is a challenging time, for sure, but one in which you may surprise yourself with what you can do if you arm yourself with the right resources and give yourself a chance.

Stepping into the Unknown: A Recovery Overview

Recovery is the process of leaving your eating disorder behind and building your life around a healthier center. You want to make this healthy center as strong as possible. Doing so not only makes the return of your eating disorder less likely, but also makes your life richer and more fulfilling — the ultimate win-win situation.

Determining how long recovery will take

Understandably, you want to know how long your treatment will take. Unfortunately, no one-size-fits-all answer to this question exists. Treatment will probably take longer than you'd like, but it won't last forever. If you catch the problem early and don't have too many complicating wrinkles, you may be able to count the length of your treatment in months.

Generally, a full recovery for an eating disorder is far more likely to be counted in years. Anorexia Nervosa and Related Eating Disorders (ANRED), Inc., an eating disorder information source (www.anred.com), cites an average treatment time of three to seven years. Making a full recovery means not only addressing your disordered eating patterns, but also committing to resolve the underlying issues that led you to them in the first place. See the section "Building the Habits and Skills of Recovery" to discover some skills you can arm yourself with to expedite the recovery process.

- **A traumatic history:** Trauma can include such experiences as physical or sexual abuse, neglect or catastrophic loss. (I discuss trauma effects in more detail in Chapter 5.)

- **Very difficult family problems:** These can include chronic, unresolved conflict between parents, high–conflict divorce, addictions, inability of parents to provide for basic material or emotional needs of children and so on.

- **One or more companion disorders:** These can include drug abuse or bipolar disorder (you can read more about companion disorders in Chapter 7).

Making a commitment to recovery

Your recovery process will be as individual as you are. Recovery partly depends on how big a hold your eating disorder has on you, how extensive the root system is of internal issues holding it in place, and the kinds of personal resources you bring to working on it. Your recovery starts when you

1. **Make the decision to give up the disorder.** This is the commitment you make to yourself. It's the moment when you admit your eating disorder is making things worse, not better. Or when you decide it's better to let people know you're in trouble than to keep going in the same self–harming direction.

2. **Take a step to commit to this decision.** You may choose to do this by admitting to someone that you have an eating disorder, asking your family for help, or making an appointment with a professional. The important thing is to *do* something to make good on your resolve to change things.

Recovery includes your treatment process and all the members of your treatment team. But these helpers are really there just to guide, facilitate, and cheerlead a process that happens inside you. In recovery you are doing more than surrendering your eating disorder. You are reshaping your feelings about yourself and the way you go about living your life.

Reducing your symptoms

Reducing eating disorder symptoms — dieting, starving, bingeing, purging — is a typical starting point for many treatment plans, such as those begun in a hospital or residential center and some behavioral treatments. (See Chapter 10 for more on behavioral therapies.) To keep things simple, I approach recovery as if you begin it by focusing on reducing your symptoms, such as

- ✔ **Becoming aware of what triggers your symptom:** For example, emotional distress, feelings of loss of control, or problems in a relationship.

- ✔ **Managing urges to binge or purge:** For example, learning to delay the behavior, distract yourself, comfort yourself in a constructive way, and so forth.

- ✔ **Managing anxiety around increasing food intake**: For example, making the increases in small, manageable "doses," giving more positive meanings to the food (for instance, food, not starving, allows you to be strong) and so on.

You will not be able to participate in any aspects of recovery other than weight regain if you are in a state of starvation. Your brain and body won't be up to the demands. If you are starving, your recovery will have to start with weight gain.

Depending on the circumstances of your situation, your treatment plan may take another tack. For instance, you may reduce your symptoms on the installment plan — a little bit at a time over a long treatment period. Or you may do a lot of work on the underlying emotional factors before seeing much change in your symptoms.

Discovering the real person within

Many people with eating disorders are surprised to discover in recovery that an actual person exists within them! Finding a "you" with real opinions, feelings, and needs that have nothing to do with being thin may be a benefit of recovery you never expected. Much of recovery is about giving this "you" what she needs to develop and flourish.

You may find that discovering a "you" inside includes finding your own personal "start" button — the personal energy you possess to make things happen. This energy is what's at play when you dream a dream — big or small — and see it through to reality. Some people call this *initiative* or a sense of *personal agency*. You may have been turning to your eating disorder to supply a sense of purpose and direction you don't otherwise feel in your life. Imagine focusing all the drive and energy you've used for thinness on some goal outside yourself. As scary as that may be to think of now, a sense of direction and the power to take yourself where you want to go can be some of your most valued recovery side effects. You can begin the discovery process by

- Noticing how the things you like differ from the preferences of your siblings and friends.

- Noticing your daydreams. Even if you're tempted to dismiss them as foolish, they're your own unique creations. They tell you a little more about who you are.

- Writing in a diary or journal. You can begin to hear your own particular voice.

- Drawing or taking photographs. You can begin to notice your own special "take" on things.

Four secrets of a successful recovery

A few components are common to all treatment plans and are essential to a successful recovery. To make the most of your journey, commit to the following secrets of success:

- Stay in treatment, even if your eating disorder symptoms have subsided.

- Seek support — family, friends, a group.

- Develop coping skills that allow you to feel effective in your life.

- Be prepared for relapse to happen, and use the experience to gain new insights.

Building Recovery Habits and Skills

Surrendering your eating disorder symptoms is not recovery, but it makes recovery possible. Recovery is a *building* process as much as a healing one. In this section, I focus on developing the skills, abilities, and underused resources within yourself that allow you to feel personally powerful and confident. You can become someone you can safely rely on for advice about caring for your body, managing your emotions, navigating relationships, and challenging cultural body prescriptions that aren't right for you.

Consolidating healthy eating habits

In the symptom-focused phase of your treatment, the emphasis is on a few eating facts of life: You have to eat at least three square meals a day at regular intervals and get the kind of nourishment you can only get from a wide variety of foods. Eating this way not only takes care of your body's physical needs, but also reverses or reduces eating disorder symptoms of restricting and bingeing. So is that all there is? Thankfully, no! In recovery you work on developing an inside guide for eating, whereby making healthy eating choices becomes an automatic part of the way you think and act. You also regain a sense of pleasure in food and eating (no kidding!). The following sections can help you to formulate that inside guide.

Finding eating patterns that work best for you

If you're still struggling with eating disorder symptoms or you're at the beginning of your post-symptom recovery process, the focus for your eating will be on installing a basic template for health that has been missing. As your recovery continues and this basic commitment to meeting your body's needs becomes part of you, you begin to shift your focus to designing your own way of eating.

Customizing your eating plan doesn't mean that you can skip breakfast if you don't like eating it or go back to cutting out all fats. These forms of freelancing (making up your own rules) bypass that basic template for health. You can no longer sacrifice your health to meet emotional needs or cultural prescriptions. But after you take your health as a given, you can start to experiment with what works best for you. Maybe you don't like traditional breakfast foods but you're okay with a sandwich. Or maybe you're one of those people who does better with six smaller meals a day rather than three bigger ones. These types of alterations are perfectly acceptable.

Eating mindfully

Mindfulness is another word for awareness. When you eat mindfully, you're fully in the present moment, noticing everything you can about what you're experiencing. The following exercise, frequently suggested by teachers of mindful eating, can help you get the hang of it:

1. Put a bite of food, such as some fruit, on your tongue. Let it sit there for a moment, without chewing.

2. Notice how the bite feels on your tongue. Focus on its texture, taste, and temperature.

3. Notice how you know when it's time to chew, what the chewing feels like, and how it changes the quality of the bite.

4. Notice how you know when it's time to swallow, and focus on all the sensations that go with swallowing.

This is not, of course, how you would eat a meal. But it can help you discover how to eat with awareness. Eating with awareness helps you

✔ Tune in to when you are satisfied so you know when to start and when to stop.

✔ Determine the distinction between emotional triggers for eating and genuine hunger.

✔ Discover what gives you pleasure in food and eating.

You're now developing internal guides for eating. As you gain confidence in your ability to combine them with that template for health, you'll find that they take much better care of you than the grapefruit diet or any other outside rules and regulations. In time you'll be able to use body signals of hunger and fullness, along with current eating urges as reliable guidelines for when and what to eat.

Adding physical activity safely

In Chapter 8 I discuss healthy exercise as a marker of recovery. Your doctor is the person on your recovery team most likely to help you with decisions about safely adding exercise, but when you hit that point in your recovery, you want to focus on making exercise *healthy*.

Healthy exercise includes using awareness of how exercise is affecting you to help guide your exercise choices. This awareness is similar to being guided from the inside for eating choices, which is what you are doing when you eat mindfully (see the preceding section). Following are ways you can use this exercise awareness to your advantage:

✔ Your body will reliably tell you when enough is enough. This will protect you from fatigue and injury.

✔ You can learn which types of exercise you enjoy when you're tuned into your body and not focused on losing weight.

✔ When you exercise mindfully, you and your body become a collaborative team, working together for your heath and well-being. Your body is no longer the enemy.

As you tune in to what exercise makes your body feel best, be on the alert for two big warning flags:

1. Are you already exercising compulsively?

2. Are you tempted to add compulsive exercise to substitute for the eating disorder symptoms you are surrendering? You can read more about compulsive exercise, including how to recognize it, in Chapter 7.

If you still need to gain weight, exercise is not going to be on your menu until you reach your weight goals. In recovery, the new standard is this: What makes you healthy?

Staying tuned in to your feelings

One of the big reasons giving up your eating disorder is so hard is because you've relied on it so much to help you manage your emotions. Your eating disorder is a pretty blunt instrument, and you've paid a big price for using it. But it's been your life raft when you've had no idea how else to cope. Your recovery is a great time to discover other ways to handle your emotional life.

All coping skills have the opposite effect of your eating disorder in one crucial way. Your eating disorder takes you out of awareness of what's upsetting you, at least temporarily. Any emotion coping skills you discover will involve finding out how to stay in awareness, at least long enough to figure out what's bothering you and what you want to do about it. In this section I go over some skills of emotion management plus the special skills of calming or soothing yourself.

Expanding your ability to tolerate your emotions

To paraphrase Woody Allen, 90 percent of emotion management is showing up, or being aware of your emotions. Knowing what you feel requires tolerating a certain amount of discomfort. So far in life, you've been telling yourself that you can't tolerate any discomfort, at least not the emotional kind. In recovery, part of your job is to discover, a little bit at a time, that you can. You'll probably do a lot of this work in individual or group therapy. But here's an exercise you can try right now to start expanding your tolerance level:

1. Think of something that may be upsetting you. Nothing too intense — this is practice — but enough that your reflex is to get away from the feeling.

2. Now ask yourself to stay with the feeling just 30 seconds longer. If 30 seconds is too long, make it 15 seconds.

3. Notice how it feels to tolerate just a small dose of the upset. Is it manageable? Excellent! You've expanded!

If you have experienced physical abuse, medical problems, or other trauma to your body, being in your body may not feel safe. Your body may have taken itself out of the loop of emotional information. This is an example of a self-protective process called *dissociation*. (You can read more about dissociation and eating disorders in Chapter 5.) If you sense that you have closed down the connection to your body in this way, you need to respect this critical body wisdom about what feels manageable. Make sure your eating disorder therapist understands trauma and dissociation so he can help you take these experiences into account as you are becoming more aware of your emotions.

Using body-based therapies for emotion management

Body-based therapists (you can read about them in Chapter 10) spend a lot of time helping people become aware of signals of emotional distress as they show up in the body (rapid breathing, tight chest, butterflies in the tummy, and so on). Awareness of these signals is central to the therapy. Somatic Experiencing, Body-Mind Psychotherapy, and other therapies offer body-based approaches to help you expand your awareness of distressing emotions. Following are a few of their techniques:

✔ **Naming the physical sensation(s):** Locating your upset in a body sensation immediately makes the upset smaller because it's surrounded by the rest of you, which is bigger!

For example, Linda is feeling very hurt by her friend Joyce who broke their shopping date to go to a movie with a different friend. As she thinks about how she feels, Linda senses the tension in her stomach. But all around her stomach is the rest of her body, which isn't experiencing the tension. Linda begins to feel the strength and calm of the rest of her body. These feelings quiet the tension just a little.

✔ **Titrating:** Titrating is experiencing a big upset a bite at a time (think baby steps). The numbered exercise at the beginning of this section is a form of titration. You can visualize the concept by thinking of an I.V. drip or a thermostat that moves just a degree at a time.

✔ **Looping:** You can almost always find a part of your body that isn't feeling the upset. Settle into that part, and then make trips back and forth between the quiet part and the upset part, importing the quieted part into the upset one. Try it, and notice what happens.

✔ **Breathing:** This involves simply directing your breathing to the spots in the body that are feeling the upset.

You can find books that describe these approaches and other emotion management tools in the Resource Guide at the back of this book.

Strengthening skills of self-soothing

You've been trying to comfort and soothe yourself with food when you're upset. Because you're not turning to your eating disorder in recovery, you have a chance to discover effective alternatives. In recovery you want to develop a whole cupboard full of these alternatives. And practice them! The more you practice other ways to soothe, quiet, and comfort yourself, the more likely you are to turn to them the next time you're upset instead of bingeing or restricting.

The answer to what is soothing and comforting lies within you and within a particular moment or problem. Some situations may call for a combination of problem-solving and self-soothing in order for you to feel better. Sometimes you problem-solve better if you do a little self-soothing first. (You think more clearly when you're less overwhelmed.) Other times it works best the other way around.

Resources are healthy ways of comforting and soothing yourself. (Resources can do other things, too, like give you courage or confidence.) You have to try possible resources on for size to find out what works for you. The following list of suggestions is a way to get you started. Your own list should grow over time — you can never have too many resources! It should include a balance of resources that are outside yourself and ones that come from inside yourself (you want to be sure you have resources available at 3 a.m. or if you get stranded on a deserted island!).

Outside resources (includes actual people, objects or activities outside yourself):

- Talk to someone
- Take a walk
- Do something you enjoy, like gardening, listening to music, reading, or painting
- Write in a journal, diary, or blog

Inside resources (involves processes that occur inside you without outside props, meaning you'll have them available anytime, anyplace; thoughts, images and imagination are especially important):

- Breathe slowly and deeply
- Speak to yourself in a reassuring way (*You'll be okay. You're alright. It'll be fine.*)
- Picture a scene that you find peaceful or soothing
- Imagine the presence of someone you find comforting, whether real or made-up
- Pray, chant, or engage in some other spiritual practice

Nothing on this list will provide the instant sense of relief that you get from giving in to your eating disorder or using alcohol or drugs. But, on the other hand, you don't pay an emotional or physical price for anything on this list either. Instead, you become stronger and better able to take care of yourself as you practice using healthy, self-soothing methods.

Trying meditation, tai chi, or yoga

Many people in recovery find that practicing meditation, tai chi, or yoga can contribute to emotion management and overall emotional quieting. Following is a brief overview:

- **Meditation, especially mindfulness meditation:** *Meditation* is the name for a variety of practices for focusing the mind, any of which can be useful for becoming more calm and centered. *Mindfulness meditation* helps you stay grounded and connected to the calm and safety of the present moment, no matter how distressing the content of your thoughts may be. These practices help you to observe your emotions rather than be caught up in them or carried away by them. You can read more about the use of mindfulness meditation in the treatment of eating disorders in Chapter 9.

- **Tai chi:** Tai chi, a martial arts practice, is often called "meditation in motion." Tai chi consists of a series of gentle movements using the whole body. Practice of tai chi has been shown to reduce stress and improve symptoms of anxiety and depression.

- **Yoga:** Yoga is a set of practices using body postures, meditation, and breathing which create a sense of calm and well-being. You can read more about the use of yoga in the treatment of eating disorders in Chapter 9.

Staying tuned in to your needs

A strong recovery includes being able to identify your needs. When your desire to be thin isn't screaming at you with quite so much urgency anymore, you can begin to hear your own thoughts that inform you of what you want in life or from a particular situation. These thoughts, which were formerly being drowned out by your eating disorder, may be related to life goals, job or career situations, relationships, or other areas of your life. For example, maybe you begin to hear yourself thinking things such as

- My life won't be complete if I don't sing the lead in *Tosca* once on stage.

- Getting my degree will really make a difference in whether I can get the kind of job I want.

- I have to get my boss to quit interrupting me every time I open my mouth at this meeting.

✔ I've worked so hard, I have to have some down time or my brain will be fried.

✔ I need to be included in the decision-making in order for this relationship to feel fair.

Of course, you will only be listening if you have begun to trust that what you want or need matters. This belief might not come to you automatically. However, it's so important to your recovery that it's worth working on in therapy if you're not there yet. Individual, family, or group therapy can all be great places to take risks with treating your needs like they matter.

Knowing your needs and desires is important to your recovery. This knowledge will benefit you individually and will improve your relationships. I describe these benefits in the sections that follow.

Building in a personal navigator

Many people begin to experience their own initiative — a sense of being able to make things happen in their lives — for the first time in recovery. But how do you know which direction to go when you have the will and the energy? The game plan comes from knowing what you care about in life, what your values are, what moves you, and what your passions are. The energy that sparks an urge to do something in life often comes from your feeling that that something is important. When you were in the throes of your eating disorder, you directed all that energy to the pursuit of weight loss because being thin was of utmost importance. Now you have the space to discover other options and dreams that you feel that strongly about.

Though it's probably too early to be figuring these things out now, you may want to just stick a toe in the water. You might find clues to future passions by thinking about any of the following:

✔ **Book or movie themes you keep coming back to**: Wild life, foreign travel, women who run their own businesses, helping kids.

✔ **Adults you admire or who have inspired you**: Teachers, coaches, politicians, poets.

✔ **Life experiences that made you feel good about yourself or excited in some way**: Charitable work, discovering an artist whose work moves you, being at the beach.

✔ **Images — no matter how fleeting — of future activities you might enjoy**: Working in fashion, using your writing skills, using your people skills, doing something that allows you to see different parts of the country.

Building in a relationship navigator

Making your needs part of any relationship completely changes the way it feels to be part of that relationship. This is true whether it involves your family, friends, neighbors, romantic partner, teachers, work colleagues, or boss. Of course, the amount of space you have to negotiate your needs differs, depending on which of these relationships you're talking about. But when you have an eating disorder, you tend to think that no space exists for your needs in *any* relationship. This is particularly true if you're female. You've likely determined that thinking of your needs at all is selfish. You imagine that nobody will like you if you sometimes want your way. You envision feeling devastated and rejected if you speak up and your needs aren't honored. These risks feel impossible to take.

Consider, however, the risks of *not* making your needs known in a relationship. Here are just a few of them:

✔ You start to feel like the relationship is more for the other person than you.

✔ You feel like the other person agrees with you that his or her needs are more important than yours.

✔ You end up resenting the other person.

✔ You end up not trusting the other person.

✔ The other person doesn't really get to know who you are, so no real closeness can develop.

✔ You feel you could lose yourself in the relationship.

If you're having a lot of difficulty getting to know your needs, individual therapy can often be a safe place to think them through. The more reflective therapies such as psychodynamic or feminist therapy can be particularly good for this. You can read more about how to express yourself effectively in relationships in Chapter 8.

Expressing yourself!

You may be surprised to find that speaking what's on your mind can help your recovery. It's likely that neither your personal history nor your self-image have made such self-expression easy for you. But as you get better at it, you'll find *two recovery–related benefits:*

✔ **A stronger self-image:** A stronger self-image replaces the sense of worthlessness that makes you desperate to be thin and places you at high risk for an eating disorder.

✔ **Stronger relationships:** Stronger relationships give you a place of real support and connection so you no longer have to rely on food and dieting.

Strengthening your sense of self

Many people who work toward recovery in a group setting — be it family, couple, or group therapy; 12-step groups; or other support groups — are shocked to find that they have their own opinions and points of view about so many subjects. Or even *any* subjects!

Sometimes not knowing your views is due to coming from a family environment where differing opinions weren't valued — so you learned not to have them. Or sometimes it's a reflection of your low sense of worth — how could your opinions matter to others? Safer not to know you have them in the first place. That way you won't risk embarrassing yourself.

Making sure you have a place where you can regularly take risks expressing yourself and your newly discovered opinions can be very valuable to your personal recovery, even if the risks feel very tiny at first. Self-expression in a safe setting is frequently one of the first places for discovering that "you" inside who's going to become more — way more — than your eating disorder.

Strengthening yourself in your relationships

When you know what you need in relation to others and speak up about it, relationships get less scary. That may seem counterintuitive since speaking up can feel scary! But the truth is that you don't need to turn to food in order to avoid being swamped by relationship demands or a relationship's emptiness. Instead, you can state what you need in a relationship. In fact, the good news is that you will trust your relationships more as they do a better job of meeting your needs. Then you'll be more likely to turn to them for the support you previously sought in food.

All of your recovery skills involve some kind of self-awareness and a degree of self-acceptance for what you discover. Knowing and accepting yourself may be the greatest gift of recovery. The more you know and accept who you are and what you need, the more you can make decisions from the inside, based on what's right for you. This self-awareness makes you strong and sturdy to negotiate in relationships with others who also know what they need.

Dealing with Fear and Resistance

Nobody enters a change process without fears and doubts about how the change will affect them. Worries typically come up at the beginning of eating disorder recovery, and make it harder to go forward. Here is just a sampling of the kinds of worries you may experience:

- Will I be able to manage life without my symptoms?
- Will I seem boring or ordinary without my disorder?

✔ Will anyone pay attention to me without my symptoms?

✔ Will I be able to function like a normal person?

✔ If people get to see the real me beneath my eating disorder, will they abandon me?

✔ If I see the real me beneath my eating disorder, will I see things I can't stand?

You get to start over with a new round of doubts and fears with each new stage and each new step of your treatment. But the good news is, it's okay! Having doubts and fears is perfectly normal when you are venturing into new territory, whether it's going into recovery, starting a new job, moving to a new town, or any of dozens of new life directions. Even better, as you discover in this section, you can make these fears and doubts work to your advantage.

Accepting fear as part of recovery

Moments of doubt are to be expected as part of the recovery process. It's like putting on the brakes when you reach a curve and don't know what lies on the road ahead. It's a normal response. Therapists call this braking response *resistance*. Unfortunately, the term implies stubbornness, and for a few people, that may be a fair comparison. More often, though, resistance signals a need to slow down and regroup, perhaps getting some reassurances before moving ahead. Resistance comes from a part of you that is worried that things will get worse, not better, if you continue in the direction someone on your treatment team is suggesting for you.

A lot of confusion happens with resistance because people often put on the brakes without realizing that that's what they've done or why. Their fears and doubts simply haven't made it into conscious awareness yet, but some internal wisdom says: "Stop!" Here are some common forms resistance can take:

✔ Missing appointments; being late

✔ Not doing homework assignments

✔ Shutting down, responding to every question with "I don't know"

✔ Using the majority of treatment time to report on other people or events rather than to talk about yourself

✔ Picking petty arguments with your therapist to avoid focusing on yourself

Like so many other situations in recovery, awareness is your first friend when it comes to dealing with moments of resistance. When you know your behavior is coming from resistance, this awareness allows you to make other choices that might be more to the point. Here arc two things you can do to increase awareness of your own resistance moments:

1. **Be on the lookout for telltale signs of your heels digging in.** For example, you may feel a physical sensation or hear a small voice inside you saying "no."

2. **Be willing to question any of your behavior that interferes with forward movement in treatment or recovery in general.** Ask yourself: Am I afraid or doubtful in any way about where things are headed? Am I feeling mistrustful of my therapist's ability to guide me there?

Making constructive use of resistance

Resistance is not futile — when questioned! A good way to respond to resistance and turn it to your advantage is to be curious as to what's going on and why. Ask questions and explore possible answers about what could be making you put on the brakes. This exploration works best if you and your treatment provider work together. When you stop and use your curiosity, some very good things can happen:

✔ You quit sparring with your therapist's agenda and come back into collaboration (which *doesn't* necessarily mean doing things her way!).

✔ You have a chance to find out about some meaningful concern that simply hasn't made it into your awareness before now.

✔ After you know what's really bothering you about the road ahead, you can make course corrections to take your worries into account. For example:

   • You just need to move a little more slowly to be able to digest what's happening.

   • You need to know that if you're losing something by getting better, you can compensate for that loss in some other way. For example, you've used restricting to say "no" to people. You need to know that you'll be able to say "no" directly.

   • You can change without becoming someone you no longer recognize. What do you want to keep unchanged in yourself?

   • If you tell your friend you're angry at her, as your therapist suggests, won't she just drop you? Maybe you need to experiment with smaller challenges of speaking up first to gain confidence in yourself and the friendship.

✔ Exploring moments of resistance allows you to know yourself better. When you understand what's making you tick, you can respond to yourself more effectively.

Rebounding from Relapse

Being successful in recovery doesn't mean never relapsing, that is, going back to eating disordered behaviors. Successful recovery means finding ways to manage relapses when they occur. In this section I tell you more about relapse and take you through the steps of managing relapse episodes.

The risk of relapse is sharply increased for people who leave treatment before dealing with the underlying issues that make up a full recovery process. For information on how to address these issues and avoid this pitfall, see the earlier section, "Building the Habits and Skills of Recovery."

Distinguishing big ones from little ones

Not all relapses are created equal. Some people binge once or restrict a little, and then get right back on their recovery track, and that's that. Addiction experts don't even call this a relapse. They call these minor episodes from which you rebound quickly *slips*. It is also typical for people in recovery to spend days, weeks, or months revisiting old eating disorder behavior. In the worst case, the *partial relapse* of these visits can put you back where you started. This is called *total relapse*.

Total relapse, as you might guess, is a lot harder to return from than partial relapses or slips. Researchers at the University of Toronto found that rebound time makes a big difference when it comes to partial relapse turning into total relapse. In a study reported in *Eating Disorders: The Journal of Treatment and Prevention*, people who got back on track from relapse within six to eight weeks were likely to pick up their recovery again successfully. On the other hand, people whose partial relapses lasted three months or more were very likely to deteriorate into total relapses from which they did not rebound. Thus, the sooner you get back on track, the better your chances of success.

Seeing relapse as part of getting better

It's really, really important for you to understand that relapses are something to expect in your recovery. Why? Because you, like the rest of us, are human and will make mistakes. (Read more on this later in this chapter in the section "Practicing imperfection; discovering middle ground.") Why am I making such a big deal of this? Because your mindset about relapse has everything to do with how you handle it and how likely you are to rebound.

Two basic mindsets make the most difference when it comes to relapse. The first is your attitude about the relapse: What does it mean about you and about your possibilities for getting better? The second important mindset is your willingness and determination to gain new insights from the experience of relapse. I go over these two mindsets in the next sections.

Getting your head straight

A black-and-white, all-or-nothing way of thinking makes you more vulnerable to developing an eating disorder (see Chapter 5). The same thinking pattern, where things are all one way or another, can also make trouble if you're trying to cope with a relapse episode. People who have a hard time bouncing back from relapse tend to tell themselves things like

- ✔ I've blown it now; I might as well keep going with my eating disorder.

- ✔ This proves it; I'll never get better. Why even bother?

- ✔ I had 38 days (or 4 months) (or 2 years) of not bingeing or purging. This ruins it.

When you know relapse episodes will be part of recovery, you can prepare yourself to approach them differently. Here are some possibilities to get you started developing positive responses to relapse:

- ✔ One mistake doesn't blot out all the successes. I've got lots to take credit for.

- ✔ What I'll remember about this episode is how I responded to it effectively.

- ✔ I can gain new insights from this experience.

- ✔ I don't have to be perfect to be okay.

- ✔ I don't have to be perfect to be acceptable.

In thinking of positive ways to respond to relapse, you may find it helpful to think of what you'd say to a friend in a similar situation. Chances are you wouldn't be nearly as harsh with someone else as you are with yourself.

Using relapse to gain new insights

When you experience a relapse of any size, the best way to avoid doing it again is to seek to understand what triggered this one. With the help of your therapist and/or support group, examine what was going on: Why did it happen now? Why not last week or next month? What was going on that made you more vulnerable at that particular moment?

Think of relapse as a chance to find out more about your relapse triggers. If you know what's likely to trigger relapse behavior, you can work on improving your prevention and rebound skills.

By far the most common trigger for relapse is some kind of emotional experience. Let's say you figure out that your relapse episode started when you were either very depressed or very angry. That tells you two important things:

✔ You need to step up your work for managing the depression or anger.

✔ You need to be on the lookout when those emotions are triggered in you.

If you know you're more at risk for relapse behavior when, for example, you're depressed or angry, you can take pre-planned steps to help yourself manage without relapse. Such steps might include

✔ Seeking support from friends, family, or fellow group members

✔ Talking to your sponsor if you are in a 12-step program

✔ Asking for additional treatment sessions with your therapist

✔ Working with emotion management tools you've already discovered

✔ Increasing self-soothing practices

Relapse can also be a signal about some aspect of your recovery process, providing you with some useful direction. A relapse may highlight some area of recovery you haven't been ready to take on until now. But now you may need to focus on that area for your recovery to move forward. Following are some examples of what your relapse may be telling you:

✔ It may be time to work on expressing yourself instead of swallowing your feelings.

✔ Perhaps the time has come to start setting better limits with family boundary intrusions.

✔ Your treatment process may be moving too fast, in which case you need to slow down.

The big message here is that the only way relapse can be a failure is if you refuse to explore the reasons for it and rebound from it. Some of your biggest growth spurts can follow a relapse.

Knowing steps to take when relapse occurs

So you've had a relapse episode. You feel horrible and you probably aren't thinking all that clearly. Only one thing matters right now: Do whatever you can to get back on track with your recovery as soon as possible. The following do's and don'ts can steer you in the right direction:

✔ *Don't* do any of your old eating disordered behavior to compensate. It will only dig you in deeper and extend the relapse.

- *Don't* fast.

- *Don't* diet.

- *Don't* purge.

✔ *Don't* isolate yourself.

✔ *Don't* berate yourself.

✔ *Don't* ignore the episode, believing that's the best way to move past it.

✔ *Do* take any step you can to normalize your eating as soon as possible. Most importantly, eat the next meal you would normally eat.

✔ *Do* talk to people on your treatment team and those who are supportive of your efforts immediately. It will help you contain the episode and begin to put it into perspective.

✔ *Do* start your thinking process about what happened. Understanding what happened will also help you get perspective. Do this work with your individual or group therapist if your blame gremlins are too likely to take over when you work alone.

✔ *Do* remember you actually *can* pick up wherever you left off with your recovery, weaving in whatever knowledge you gain from the relapse.

Practicing imperfection

Working on recovery is working on living. When you work on coming back from a relapse, you're working on something you share with all your fellow humans: how to live with being imperfect. Fighting the facts of human imperfection, as you tried to do with your eating disorder, didn't go so well. Relapse, with the support of your recovery team, can be a great opportunity to try a new approach: embracing, or at least accepting, imperfection.

If you've instilled a very harsh internal critic, she's going to have trouble with newfangled ideas involving less than all-or-nothing standards regarding performance and mistake-making. Part of your recovery work is to help your internal critic develop a more mature and human outlook. But what do you do in the meantime while your critic is growing up? This is a great time to be drawing on the resources of friends, group members, therapists — anyone whose approach to mistake-making you admire or find helpful. For example, you can think, "What would Emily say if she were here? What would she do if she were in my shoes? What would my group say if I told them about this?" Do this enough and the approach will become almost automatic!

When you've lived most of your life in the land of black-and-white and all-or-nothing, discovering that territory in the middle actually exists can be a real eye-opener. You won't trust it at first because it may seem like swampland that disappears under your feet when you try to put your weight on it. You'll probably want to experiment a little rather than jumping in from the high dive! Exploring the part of middle ground that's about making mistakes and being imperfect is a good-enough place to stick your toe in.

Imagine that instead of flying on a plane from Completely Perfect to Complete Failure, you get on a bike to ride from one place to the other, so you can see every stop along the way. Take a minute now to picture the trip. Make sure not to miss those special attractions along the way, such as

> ✔ *Great Effort, Needs Some Fine-Tuning*
>
> ✔ *Parts of That Went Really Well, Others Not So Well*
>
> ✔ *Wow! That Was a Courageous Try. What a Great Risk-Taker!*

All of these valuable stops are accessible when you decide to inhabit middle ground. As you continue to experiment with landing there instead of at the extreme ends, you'll find that the ground is, in fact, a lot more solid than in all-or-nothing land. And you'll feel a lot more secure when you aren't trying to live somewhere humans were never meant to live.

Part III
Eating Disorders in Special Populations

The 5th Wave   By Rich Tennant

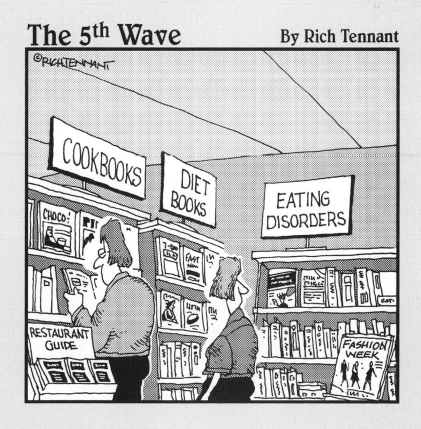

In this part . . .

1 delve into the special issues and concerns of six "minority" groups within the world of people with eating disorders: men, athletes, people in fashion and entertainment, children, the middle-aged and elderly, and people who are obese. I tell you what increases eating disorder risk for people in each group and what's needed to reduce risk. For instance, you find that athletes are greatly affected by certain qualities in the sports they choose and by their coaches. I also report on some surprising trends. For example, little boys and older men develop anorexia at much higher rates than young men do. And middle-aged women are developing eating disorders at increasing rates as they struggle to stay thin to look young.

For each group, I discuss special considerations for eating disorder treatment. This may include specific issues for treatment, difficulties in diagnosis, or choosing the best form of therapy.

Chapter 15

Eating Disorders in Males

A male with an eating disorder is thought to be a rarity. Sudden weight loss in a man is usually assumed to be due to something like depression, drug abuse, or AIDS. If a male tanks up on the buffet line or downs an entire pizza alone, he's not binge eating, he's just following the popular adage that boys will be boys.

These misconceptions are just a few of the many that abound regarding males and eating disorders. In this chapter I set the record straight with current information. I also review the major risk factors that make a male vulnerable to developing an eating disorder. And finally, I consider some issues specific to males when it comes to treatment.

Recognizing That Guys Suffer from Eating Disorders, Too!

A lot more men have eating disorders than you may guess. As many as a million men in the United States are said to have an eating disorder. The latest research from Harvard University Medical School suggests that up to 25 percent of American adults with eating disorders are men.

Women still have the edge when it comes to anorexia and bulimia. Only about 5 to 10 percent of people with these disorders are male. But estimates indicate that as many as 40 percent of people with binge eating disorder (BED) are men. Some put the percentages for men even higher.

Eating disorders in men are on the upswing

More than ever, men are being diagnosed with eating disorders and requesting treatment. The increase has been particularly noticeable in the last decade. During the same time period, men have also been reporting greater and greater dissatisfaction with their bodies — an important risk factor for developing an eating disorder. Body dissatisfaction used to be women's turf, but men are encroaching on that territory.

Cultural observers believe the gap between men and women is closing because social pressures on men to achieve an ideal body type have increased. Women have long been encouraged to think that they can endlessly perfect their bodies with diet, exercise, surgery, and other remedies. Advertising, magazine articles, and model images now tell men the same thing.

Seeing how men and women differ in terms of eating disorders

Generally speaking, eating disorders in men look a lot like eating disorders in women. The symptom pictures are quite similar; for example, fear of fat, distorted body image, a narrowing of life focus to body/weight goals, and so on are present in both genders. So are the underlying psychological dynamics fueling the disorder — for example, worth that is based on weight and shape, perfectionism, obsessive-compulsive features, and so forth.

Men and women part ways when it comes to the body changes they're aiming at and what these changes mean to them. Whereas women focus on becoming thin, men focus on becoming buff. The perfect male body has zero fat and its V-shaped, bigger-is-better muscular distribution is marked by huge biceps and "six-pack" abs. Women fear fat because it makes them unattractive. Men fear fat because it makes them appear flabby and weak.

Half of men who are dissatisfied with their bodies want to lose weight while the other half want to gain. What these two camps have in common is that, for the most part, both are aiming at the bulked-up cultural ideal. Steroid use to help achieve this muscular perfection is an essentially male addition to the scary things people can do when driven by eating-disordered thinking. (You can read more about how a fixation on bulking up affects men in the sidebar, "Getting into gear on reverse anorexia.")

Other differences exist in the ways that men and women experience each of the three major eating disorders: anorexia, bulimia, and BED. These differences (by disorder) include

- ✔ **Anorexia:** In men, starvation lowers levels of testosterone. This appears to have the immediate effect of killing libido. In some men, it may have lasting effects on their fertility even when their weight is restored.

- ✔ **Bulimia:** Men are less likely to purge and more likely to rely on compensatory behavior, like cutting calories or compulsive exercising.

- ✔ **BED:** Men who binge are generally less upset about their behavior than women who binge. Women feel shame in the act of bingeing, while men save their shameful feelings for the effect bingeing has on their bodies; males eat without shame, yet are embarrassed by the fat that results.

Uncovering Risk Factors for Eating Disorders in Males

What makes one man more at risk than another for developing an eating disorder? In some instances, the risk factors are the same as for women. Other risk factors have a particularly male stamp. In this section I review what's currently known about what puts men at risk for eating disorders. Keep in mind that men with eating disorders are still an understudied group, so some of this information is based on the best guesses of experts rather than definitive studies.

Psychological factors

Internal vulnerabilities — personal characteristics that make you more susceptible to developing an eating disorder — are pretty much the same for men as they are for women. Internal vulnerabilities include personality traits like the following:

- ✔ Low self-esteem
- ✔ Perfectionism
- ✔ Problems managing emotions
- ✔ Need for external approval

Getting into gear on reverse anorexia

Reverse anorexia, also called *muscle dysmorphia or bigorexia,* is a condition in which a man, regardless of his muscle mass, imagines himself weak and under-muscled. This body image distortion is very similar to the person with anorexia who imagines herself fat, no matter what her weight. The person with reverse anorexia becomes obsessed with bulking up. He takes any and every measure to build more muscle. This probably includes extremes in his exercise routine, where he favors weight training over aerobics. He's also likely to be using dietary supplements touted by an unregulated — and therefore risky — market.

Increasingly, bulking up involves the use of anabolic steroids. Steroids increase muscle mass and physical strength and reduce body fat, but the downside far outweighs these benefits. Using steroids too much or for too long can damage your liver and lead to liver cancer. Steroids also increase your risk for heart disease, heart attack, or stroke, and they appear to produce irritability and other negative mood effects (not to mention acne and enlarged breasts).

Reverse anorexia has a lot in common with compulsive exercise, which I explore in Chapter 7. The person with reverse anorexia is driven to his weight training with the same obsessional energy as the compulsive exerciser. Bulking up, like losing weight or keeping up an aerobic routine, comes before well-being or responsibilities to others. If you suspect you may have reverse anorexia, ask yourself if any of the following are true of your weight training:

- I've risked my health with unproven supplements and steroids to enhance my strength.

- I've risked injury with overtraining.

- I've risked my social life, school performance, or job by repeatedly putting my workouts first.

- I can't feel good about myself unless I like the shape my body is in.

- I never think I'm in good enough shape, no matter what anyone says.

Men with eating disorders also show companion psychological disorders at rates similar to those displayed by women. Psychological disorders that commonly accompany eating disorders in men include the following:

- Anxiety
- Depression
- Obsessive-compulsive disorder (OCD)
- Substance abuse

Whether these disorders predispose a man to an eating disorder or whether something else causes both of them is hard to tell. (You can read more about vulnerability traits in Chapter 5 and companion disorders in Chapter 7.)

Biographical factors

Your background may have an impact on your likelihood of developing an eating disorder. Two factors that stand out as eating disorder risks in women's backgrounds also stand out in the backgrounds of men. These risk factors are

- ✔ **Family history:** Certain family styles appear to pose a greater risk for eating disorder development than others. Overly rule-bound or *over-organized* families appear more often in the histories of people with anorexia. *Underorganized* families lack the structure needed to support and protect family members sufficiently. Many people with bulimia describe underorganized family histories.

- ✔ **Trauma history:** People with eating disorders have more than their fair share of trauma in their histories. This is apparently true of men as well as women. Trauma includes physical and sexual abuse, neglect, and catastrophic loss. It also includes a caregiver's chronic failure to respond sensitively to a child's emotional needs.

For more information regarding these risk factors, turn to Chapter 5. I describe the effects of various family styles and trauma history on eating disorders in greater detail there.

A third biographical risk factor appears to be exclusive to men. Unlike their female counterparts, many men with eating disorders report being overweight or obese in childhood. A number of these men remember being teased, made a scapegoat, or left out because of their weight. Not surprisingly, these men may develop a lot of shame related to their body image, although this kind of body shame is still more typical of women than men in our culture.

Body dissatisfaction

Dissatisfaction with body size or shape can be a powerful motivator to diet or take other corrective action. In men who have low self-esteem and believe they need to be perfect to be acceptable, body dissatisfaction can be a lethal weapon, leading vulnerable men to eating disordered behaviors to "fix" themselves.

Men engage in exactly the same dangerous ED behaviors as women. The only thing that's different — and it's not exclusively male — is bulking up. I discuss it in the sidebar on reverse anorexia.

Men are being subjected to increasing media pressure to look like an ideal body shape and size. As the pressure increases, so does male body dissatisfaction. Body mass index (BMI) is a far more reliable (and achievable) indicator of health than are the images projected by the media.

Dieting habits

Dieting is a well-known risk factor for developing an eating disorder. (See Chapter 5 for more about this.) Both men and women are more likely to diet when they are unhappy about their body shape or size. The biggest social pressures are still on women when it comes to being thin. But the heat is increasingly on men. Certain subgroups of men — for example, athletes or the overweight — feel the heat even more. As these groups jump on board the dieting bandwagon, their risk levels go up.

Thinning down for sports

Sports in which thinness helps you excel are famous gateways to eating disorders (see Chapter 16, "Athletes and Eating Disorders"). Sports that extol being thin include wrestling, running, swimming, gymnastics, being a jockey, and so on. In an all-too-common story, a guy who's never had an eating disorder on his mind fasts a few days to "make weight." It works. To ensure ongoing success, the fast becomes a necessary ritual. However, fasting requires more and more effort over time. It also takes a greater effort to get to the next level. The result is a guy who's regularly fasting, obsessing over what he eats, and engaging in dangerous exercise practices (such as excessive exercise, exercising while fasting, or exercising to the point of injury) to keep his weight under control.

Being gay

It's estimated that as many as 20 percent of the males with eating disorders are gay. Nobody knows enough to say whether specific characteristics of being a gay male actually increase your risk for an eating disorder. Many guess that a greater emphasis on appearance in the gay community plays an important role. In fact, surveys find that pressure to achieve an ideal body type among gay men is second only to that experienced by heterosexual women in Western cultures.

Gaining Awareness of Special Issues for Treatment

All studies so far suggest that men respond as well as women to sound eating disorder treatment, and that they need the same kinds of treatment programs to recover. Men have a good chance of recovery if they follow through with treatment. Specifically, men need to

- ✔ Regain a healthy weight if they've been starving

- ✔ Establish normal eating habits

- ✔ Reduce bingeing and purging

- ✔ Receive treatment for companion disorders

- ✔ Stay in treatment to build a strong recovery repertoire

While many elements are the same between males and females with eating disorders, a couple of factors compound the problem for men. Men are less likely to be diagnosed than women, and when they are, they're faced with the challenge of trying to fit into treatment programs designed for women. I discuss both these issues in this section.

Escaping diagnosis

Men often suffer with their eating disorders for years before anyone catches on. This matters because the longer an eating disorder has been around, the harder it is to treat. Delayed treatment is especially serious for anorexia sufferers because the risk of death steadily increases with anorexia over time.

Why are men able to fly under the radar when it comes to eating disorders? Simply because many people don't know that men can get eating disorders, including the men who become entrapped by them. The affected men and those around them aren't on the alert for symptoms and warning signs. This is true at every level at which someone might identify the disorder, starting with the man himself. These levels include

- ✔ **The individual man with the eating disorder:** Men haven't been exposed to the prevention blitz women have, nor has the media paraded male celebrities with eating disorders. If a man has anorexia, denial is part of the program. If he's bingeing, an eating disorder isn't the first place his mind goes to explain his excesses. Bingeing can be dismissed as a guy thing. Men with bulimia are less likely to purge in obvious ways, like by vomiting or using laxatives. They're more likely to restrict or exercise compulsively. The bottom line: A man can easily remain clueless about his own eating disorder for a long time.

- ✔ **Family and friends:** These are often the people who challenge women they love with eating disorders to recognize the problem and get treatment. Men are less likely to share weight and eating problems with family or friends, as women frequently do.

- ✔ **Medical professionals:** Studies have shown that doctors are likely to explain visible symptoms, like weight loss, in ways other than an eating disorder. Depression, drug abuse, and AIDS are more common explanations.

The point here isn't that anyone is being negligent or uncaring. Male eating disorders simply haven't yet made it onto our collective radar screens. When you start trying to account for symptoms or behavior changes in yourself or a man you know, eating disorders aren't likely to appear in your mental repertory of possible causes.

Another reason men may go undiagnosed for their eating disorders is that they're hesitant to come forward and admit them when they do realize what's going on. The popular view is that eating disorders are women's disorders. Men often fear ridicule or being pegged as weak or homosexual if they have a "women's disorder." These fears just amplify the usual shame and secrecy associated with having an eating disorder.

Being male in a treatment world set up for women

If you're a man with an eating disorder and you overcome the obstacles of shame and ignorance regarding the need for treatment, you step into a world that's been set up for women. This is true for just about any group-based component to your program: residential treatment, partial hospital, intensive outpatient program (IOP) group therapy, or a support group.

Some of these programs literally exclude men. In the others, a man is certain to be a minority. This means by tradition and by numbers, the female perspective, which is so crucial to understanding female eating disorders, is going to get a lot of air time. In female-dominated groups, some men feel like outsiders at the very time they most need to feel shared understanding.

Some argue that the underlying issues are more similar than different for men and women with eating disorders. By this argument, sharing recovery work is okay and even beneficial — men and women need to understand each others' points of view.

Others argue that being a man with an eating disorder involves gender-specific issues — issues such as body image, uniquely male physical effects of eating disorders, sexuality, and the like — that men can more easily talk about in an all-male group or program. This argument is largely moot because such programs hardly exist. However, as male eating disorders come increasingly into focus, hopefully more services will become geared specifically to men in the future.

Chapter 16

Athletes and Eating Disorders

*T*o be a good athlete requires qualities such as a high level of discipline, perfectionism, a drive to excel, and a commitment to exercise. Sound familiar? These same qualities can also make a person vulnerable to developing an eating disorder. In fact, athletes appear to suffer eating disorders at a greater rate than non-athletes.

Not every nook and cranny of the sports world presents the same level of risk for the eating disorder–vulnerable athlete. Some sports environments magnify the risk, while others buffer and minimize it. In this chapter you find out what the most important influences are. I also go over some unique qualities of the risks for women and for men, and I offer a list of warning signs to help parents recognize when their child athlete may be at risk for an eating disorder. I review guidelines for treatment, focusing on the question you most want answered: When can I compete again?

Running a Greater Risk for Eating Disorders

Over the last 25 years, weight and eating problems have been on the rise among athletes. This goes for everyone from the elite professional to the college or high school competitor, all the way down to the guy at the corner gym. How widespread is the problem and why is it worse for athletes? I explore the answers in this section.

Studies show that from 15 to 25 percent of athletes have eating disorders. Risk for bulimia appears to be greater than risk for anorexia. Estimates for disordered eating practices (fad dieting, fasting, purging, and so on) go as high as 70 to 80 percent in some groups of athletes. Certain qualities of the sports world and of athletes themselves increase the risk for individuals to develop disordered eating practices and full-blown eating disorders.

Magnifying cultural pressures for thinness

If you're an athlete, you're exposed to the same cultural pressures for achieving an ideal body size as the rest of us. Additionally, the hothouse of athletic competition has two particular ways of magnifying these pressures:

- **Sports that emphasize appearance:** These include figure skating, cheerleading, and gymnastics.

- **Sports in which the athlete or coach believes low body fat improves performance:** These include track, distance running, and swimming.

Imagine an athlete who's starting out with the kind of self-doubts that make anyone prone to an eating disorder. Now add an athlete's constant search for the competitive edge. Offer her either of the preceding two reasons for focusing on her weight and becoming dissatisfied with her body. You now have a very potent brew for disordered eating practices to control weight. These practices place a person at higher risk for developing a full-blown eating disorder.

Thinness does not equal fitness. Evidence does not support the notion that lower body fat always promotes better sports performance. Thinness can even impair performance in some instances.

Tipping positive traits into bad results

Many of the same qualities that help you become a competitive athlete are surprisingly similar to traits associated with eating disorders, particularly anorexia. These include

- Discipline, persistence
- Perfectionism
- Self-sacrifice (taking one for the team, putting your own needs aside)
- Compliance (for example, with coaching)
- Exercise commitment

As researchers point out, coaches and others see these traits as assets in an athlete. This view makes it that much harder to identify when these traits actually signal an underlying eating disorder.

Identifying higher-risk sports

Some sports present a higher risk for developing disordered eating and eating disorders than others. The following sports present the highest risk:

- **Endurance sports:** Examples include running, swimming, and cycling.
- **Judged sports:** In these sports, appearance may enter into the judges' scoring. Examples are figure skating, gymnastics, and diving.
- **Sports with weight categories:** Examples include wrestling, horse racing and rowing.
- **Sports in which clothes reveal the female body:** Examples are figure skating, tennis, and gymnastics.
- **Sports that emphasize an ideal appearance:** Examples include gymnastics and bodybuilding.

A study suggests that refereed sports, such as volleyball, basketball, and soccer, may actually have some protective effect on the body-image concerns of participating athletes. In these sports, appearance has no effect on outcome.

Boning up on bodybuilding

Bodybuilding appears to be a sport that acts like a magnet for men and women who already have eating disorders or who run the risk of developing them. The lure is to use the sport to sculpt the body to an ideal shape. It's irresistible to many people at both competitive and noncompetitive levels who are preoccupied with body perfection as a measure of worth.

Dieting is extremely common among bodybuilders. It may get even more emphasis because you do a lot of standing still instead of aerobic running around that burns off calories. Dieting, combined with body-image preoccupation, perfectionism, and a drive to be thin, makes a lethal brew for eating disorder development. All these ingredients are present with dedicated bodybuilders in a sport that aims at perfecting body shape and size. Male bodybuilders can also develop preoccupations with bulking up to build a perfect muscular physique. Bodybuilders of both sexes show high rates of disordered eating behavior.

Focusing on Female Athletes

If sports magnify cultural pressures for thinness, they also magnify the fact that these pressures still fall most heavily on women. Studies suggest a female athlete is about nine times as likely to develop an eating disorder as a male athlete. Sports that emphasize having a lean body, such as swimming, distance running, and gymnastics, contribute more than their fair share. At least twice as many women participating in these sports end up with eating disorders as those participating in non-lean sports, such as basketball.

If you're a female athlete, you face some uniquely female health risks from combining athletics and disordered eating. These risks are collectively called the *female athlete triad*.

Falling victim to the female athlete triad

The *female athlete triad* describes what many consider to be a *subclinical* eating disorder — one that doesn't meet the definition of a full-blown disorder — with the female athlete's name on it. The triad includes

- **Disordered eating:** Risky eating practices, like fasting, grapefruit dieting, or purging, are considered disordered eating. The female athlete may turn to these practices as a remedy when she's faced with outside pressures to lose weight and/or internal fears about the effect of weight on her looks or performance.

- **Loss of menstrual periods (amenorrhea):** This signals too little of the sex hormones, like estrogen, necessary to produce a menstrual cycle. (Your reproductive system just shuts down when your body's energy supplies fall too low.) *Note:* Estrogen is also necessary to build new bone.

- **Osteoporosis (loss of bone density):** When bones lack the material to rebuild themselves, they become porous, weak, and prone to fracture.

Recognizing the results of the triad

If you're failing to resupply your body's energy needs and/or you're purging, you're going to see your sports performance fall off eventually. This is due to

- Loss of muscle mass, muscle strength
- Weakness, fatigue, lowered pulse
- Stress fractures and other injuries
- Heart irregularities, heart failure
- Dehydration

Some athletes, through sheer grit, can overcome these effects for a time. But this only feeds the fantasy that you can rob your body of nutrition indefinitely without damage. (I discuss the physical effects of starvation and purging in more detail in Chapter 6.)

Losing the body's natural rhythms

Loss of menstrual periods has been mistakenly taken by many female athletes and their coaches as a sign of well-disciplined training. It's not. It's a warning sign of something wrong with your body. Loss of menstrual periods may be sports-related — due to overtraining, an energy drain caused by disordered eating, or stress — or it may have other causes, such as pituitary or adrenal problems, even tumors. Just because menstrual loss is common doesn't make it safe. If you've lost your periods, see your doctor.

Losing bone mass

Osteoporosis is usually a postmenopausal woman's problem. When a young woman doesn't eat enough, her body robs minerals from her bones and osteoporosis can develop early. The big problem with this arrangement is that it occurs in female athletes during what should be peak years for building up bone density. The years from age 12 to 30 (on average) are bone-banking years for women. You create a large account you can draw on later when your body starts producing less estrogen. If you're suffering from the female athlete triad, you're drawing down your account just at the time you should be building it up. There's no replacing it later.

Measuring Risk for Male Athletes

Do the same sports create eating disorder risk for male athletes as for female athletes? Generally speaking, the answer is yes. (However, one sport, wrestling, is snaring surprising numbers of male athletes into disordered eating practices and eating disorder risk. See the sidebar "Wrestling: Where disordered eating is part of the drill" for details.)

Male athletes are at risk for sports-related weight and eating problems just like females, even if in smaller numbers. An Australian study found that 5 percent of men participating in "thin" sports, such as cross country or swimming, showed full-blown eating disorders. Experts believe the numbers of male athletes with eating disorders is actually far underreported.

Men, like women, are likely to diet restrictively, fast, or purge in order to look better or perform better in sports that emphasize thinness. Male athletes also binge, sometimes after a period of restricting or as a way to manage the stresses and disappointments of competition.

Wrestling: Where disordered eating is part of the drill

Wrestling is a high-risk sport for male athletes when it comes to eating disorders. It has actually claimed lives at competitive levels due to athletes' extreme weight loss efforts. Most of the risk comes from a common practice called *cutting weight.* Cutting weight means shaving off several pounds or more before a match weigh-in. The idea is to qualify for a lower weight category so you can compete against a smaller guy and have the advantage.

Wrestlers use every kind of disordered eating practice to cut weight before a match (not to mention "thermal" methods like exercising in rubber suits to sweat off more pounds). As a result, they can face potentially fatal heart and kidney problems from dehydration and the muscle-wasting effects of rapid weight loss.

Many wrestlers follow the deprivation of "cutting" with bouts of bingeing. A wrestler might cut and binge repeatedly during a wrestling season. Most wrestlers can return to normal eating during the off-season. But many can't. Those who can't are at high risk for developing eating disorders.

Women who wrestle engage in disordered eating practices to cut weight before matches, too; thus, they're as likely as men to be at risk for developing eating disorders. So far, women aren't wrestling in numbers that put the sport high on the list of female athlete eating disorder risks. In contrast, wrestling may produce nearly three quarters of the eating disorders that occur among male athletes.

Recognizing an Eating Disorder in a Child Athlete

Food and exercise routines are common elements of sports training. You expect them to be different than the routines of non-athletes, especially at higher levels of competition. Knowing when a special routine becomes a dangerous and disordered one isn't always easy for parents, trainers, and coaches. Here are some signs to look out for:

- **Chronic dieting:** Dieting behavior always poses a risk. When it becomes a way of life, it's a sign of high risk.

- **Excessive weight loss:** Small weight losses can be a normal side effect of starting a sport. Let your pediatrician guide you if you're concerned.

- **Constantly moving the weight loss goal posts:** If no amount of weight loss is ever enough, consider this an eating disorder red flag.

- **Excessive exercise:** Exercise that interferes with other activities, results in fatigue or injury, takes up more and more of each day, or can't be put off for illness is excessive.

✔ **Compensatory exercise:** This is exercising to make up for eating — even normal eating.

✔ **Delay or loss of menstrual periods in girls:** Missing periods always warrant medical evaluation. Malnutrition, stress, and excessive exercise are common causes in female athletes.

✔ **Frequent sports-related injuries:** These are a sign that something's wrong; they're often a sign of malnutrition and/or excessive exercise.

✔ **Frequent leg cramping in practice or competition:** Muscle cramps are often a sign of dehydration due to insufficient nutrients or purging.

✔ **Evidence of purging:** Evidence may include signs of diuretic or laxative use for weight loss. Making a beeline for the bathroom (to vomit) after eating is another sign.

Scoring with the Right Coach

Sports experts agree that the person with his finger on the pulse when it comes to athletes and eating disorders is the coach. A coach advises the athlete what she needs to do to achieve. He tells her how to think about herself in relation to her athletic accomplishments. His voice carries special weight in the lives of young athletes.

The qualities of different coaching styles appear to have the biggest effect on athletes when it comes to risk for developing or avoiding eating disorders. Consider the styles of the following types of coaches:

✔ **The weight-critic coach:** This is the coach who makes open comments, usually in front of teammates, about individual weight. He uses humiliation as a motivator. These tactics match the way a person with an eating disorder, or someone at risk for one, already views herself.

✔ **The win-focused coach:** This is the coach who conveys to the athlete that winning is everything. The athlete who's a perfectionist, struggling with self-worth, is already at risk for harming herself, and she's even more likely to do so if she thinks it's required in order to win.

✔ **The accentuate-the-negative coach:** This is the coach who only notices what's wrong in an athlete's performance. This just reinforces eating disordered thinking, whereby you're only okay when you get it right.

✔ **The athlete-focused coach:** This is the coach who's most interested in helping individual athletes develop their fullest potential. Safety and well-being come before winning. This is the opposite of eating disordered thinking.

✔ **The eating disorder–informed coach:** This is a coach who

• Recognizes that low weight and low body fat are unproven as performance enhancers.

• Recognizes the signs of disordered eating and eating disorders.

• Understands the risks of disordered eating behaviors and the severe consequences of eating disorders.

• Knows how and when to refer an athlete for help.

Tackling Special Issues for Treatment

The biggest issue added to your plate if you're an athlete facing eating disorder treatment is whether your sport and your treatment can go on at the same time. The most basic answer is: not if sports participation compromises your eating disorder recovery.

In their book, *Helping Athletes with Eating Disorders*, Ron A. Thompson and Roberta Trattner Sherman offer guidelines to help decide when participation for the eating disordered athlete is okay. For example:

✔ An athlete who refuses evaluation or recommended treatment should be suspended.

✔ An athlete whose weight is less than 90 percent of the recommended weight should not compete.

✔ When training practices compete with treatment, treatment comes first.

✔ Sports activities that put the athlete's physical or psychological health at risk are out of bounds.

✔ If some lower level of participation is possible for the athlete who has been sidelined, this can help her hold onto her sports identity, pride, and sense of belonging.

Thompson and Sherman make this important additional point about being an athlete in eating disorder treatment: Many of the same qualities that make for eating disorder vulnerability and sports success — determination, discipline, focus, follow-through — can also make for recovery success.

Chapter 17

Eating Disorders on the Stage, Screen, and Runway

. . . .

In This Chapter

▶ Reviewing the risk for eating disorders among dancers, models, and actors

▶ Understanding how professional requirements for thinness promote eating disorders

▶ Recognizing the importance of reducing environmental pressures for thinness

. . . .

*F*emale dancers, models, and actors run elevated risks for developing eating disorders. Is there something about the training and the professions themselves that create this elevated risk? In this chapter I explore how the qualities necessary for success in these fields often overlap with qualities that contribute to greater risk for eating disorders. An even bigger problem is that being abnormally thin is often necessary to advance and get jobs. This magnifies ordinary environmental pressures to be thin many times over.

Tragic eating disorder–related deaths have led to a close look at contributing pressures and practices within each field. I go over some of the steps aimed at reform along with some expert recommendations for further reducing eating disorder risk. Finally, I suggest some ways parents of child dancers, models, and actors can magnify or buffer the excessive pressures for thinness to which their children are exposed.

Discovering the Risks Behind the Scenes

Performing artists face more intense pressures to maintain exceptionally thin or fat-free bodies by the very nature of their craft. For too long, the industries surrounding dancers, models, and actors have turned a blind eye to this serious problem. This effect is amplified by teachers, audiences and sometimes families taking the same position. As a result, the numbers of performing artists affected by eating disorders are staggeringly high.

Facing daily pressures to be thin

Dancing, modeling, and acting each have their own special twist on the way the pressures for being thin come up. All have an effect on the lives of both aspiring and working participants in these fields.

Dancing on thin ice

Dancers usually begin rigorous training in childhood, preparing their bodies to become precision instruments. Dancer/therapist Linda H. Hamilton, PhD, says that puberty throws a monkey wrench into the precision by adding a surge of extra fat for girls.

Why does normal fat have such an adverse effect? First of all, the dance world, particularly ballet, prefers a curve-free preadolescent body. Second, with her new distribution of fat, a dancer has to relocate her center of gravity and relearn how to be in carefully balanced positions. Third, she has to worry about how added weight affects being lifted by another dancer. Adolescence is already a time of higher risk for anorexia. Effects of weight on performance and appearance, and thus success, make the risk among adolescent dancers that much greater.

Modeling size zero

The last word on a particular modeling job comes from the designer and the size of the sample she's made to be worn down the runway. If it won't zip on your body, your body isn't going down the runway in it. Just how small can sample sizes go and what will the effect of microscopic sizes be?

These questions have been called the "size zero problem." It refers to models so small they fit into size zero clothing and to the way their images affect an ordinary woman's desire to become that small as well. (The main effect is to make her very unhappy and possibly more prone to an eating disorder.) But it seems to be an effect that boomerangs right back into the industry. As soon as enough ordinary women decide that size zero is the perfect size to be, it guides many a designer's hand, and more and more models are presented with impossibly small samples to fit into. (The industry is taking a close look at banning actual size zero models from runways.)

Even if size zero is banned, other weight pitfalls exist. Many models work internationally. Those who do can find themselves in weight zones that change along with the time zones. Weight that's fine in one city and country can be considered too heavy in another. No one says, "I'm too heavy to work in that country." Instead, models try to shed the weight to get the job. Eating disorder risk can bloom under these conditions.

Acting out the role of thinness

For actors just getting into the business, the *ingénue* role is often the plum female part. The ingénue is the young innocent. Directors, producers, and audiences seem able to imagine her only as thin and attractive. Thus, the role thinness plays with regard to aspiring actors is similar to the role it plays with dancers. Thinness takes on career meaning at a time when young women are already most likely to develop an eating disorder. A slightly older actor who has paid the rent from ingénue roles but is starting to age out of them often depends on maintaining an adolescent-thin body to help keep those parts coming well into her twenties.

Even among established actors, gaining or losing significant amounts of weight is sometimes required for a part. When an actor pulls this off, the public tends to view it as a bit of acting heroics. But more than one actor has later reported how making such a drastic change resulted in serious eating problems and disordered eating behavior. If you put an actor who's already at risk for an eating disorder through such an experience, you can have a perfect storm.

Seeing more and more artists impacted

You'd think in this age of too much celebrity information, there'd be no end of data about the prevalence of eating disorders among people in the performing arts. In reality, only the dance world has been exposed to much in the way of formal study. What the public knows about the rest relies more on the reports of individual performers and, of course, on what it sees with its own eyes (for example, gaunt models peering out of magazines or rail-thin starlets on TV and movie screens).

Dancing into danger

According to dance expert Linda Hamilton, *one in five* female dancers is likely to develop an eating disorder! Nearly half of female dancers have some type of weight or eating problem. Eating disorder rates are highest in traditional ballet compared to modern or jazz dancing, which are somewhat more forgiving for body size. A well-known study of ballet students by David Garner and Paul Garfinkel found a mouth-dropping 25 percent to have anorexia. That's compared to a rate of 1 percent for anorexia in the general population. Patterns of disordered eating that didn't quite meet the strict criteria for anorexia or bulimia showed up in another 11 percent of these young dancers.

Modeling risky behavior

While no large-scale studies have been done with regard to eating disorders among models, the profession presents all the elements of a high-risk group (see the following section, "Considering Eating Disorders as Part of the Job"). In a very small-scale study, researchers found that the models they surveyed were engaging in disordered eating practices at rates higher than women in the general population who were diagnosed with formal eating disorders.

Acting on confessions

Celebrity confessionals still substitute for actual research when it comes to data about the stage and screen. Some actors, such as Jane Fonda, Tracey Gold, and Jamie-Lynn Sigler, have been candid about their eating disorder histories, often hoping to help others by sharing their experience. Most often, as rumors abound about an actor or actress struggling with eating disorders, denials are the byword of the day, in spite of photos that seem to imply a possible problem.

Considering Eating Disorders as Part of the Job

If you're already vulnerable to an eating disorder (for example, because of heredity or personality characteristics), environmental pressure makes for important added risk. If you're a dancer, model, or actor, you know that pressures to be thin come from everywhere in your environment. The biggest pressure, when all is said and done, is that you must be thin to get the job. These pressures for thinness are woven into the professional lives of dancers, models, and actors, creating high risk for eating disorders.

Focusing too much on the body

Excessive body preoccupation is part of having an eating disorder. But how do you get away from it when your body is your professional equipment? This is the dilemma in several ways for dancers, models, and actors. For starters, people are intended to look at you. You might say being looked at is what you do for a living. Second, before you ever do that first pirouette, strike that first pose, or deliver that first line, your body is what the audience sees first. Audiences usually have an opinion about what that body should look like (hint: not overweight or average). Third, if you're a performer or model, you have to stay tuned-in constantly to your body shape and size. These factors affect your performance if you're a dancer, your "look" for potential parts if you're an actor, or your ability to fit the clothing if you're a model.

Being surrounded by thin role models

Every profession is its own small universe of norms, standards, and expectations. People coming into a profession are guided and inspired by others who have already made it. These people become role models for what is acceptable and what gets rewarded in their field. If you're a dancer, model, or actor, most of what you see modeled in your chosen field is thin — especially at the more successful end.

Not only are role models thin, but so is most of the competition. When you have a lot of people competing for a limited number of slots, competition cranks up to high gear. Anything that may give one person the competitive edge over another becomes a source of comparison and anxiety. Insiders describe a kind of contagion effect created by thin bodies and weight loss practices. Once one person is known to be using an extreme diet or purging behavior to lose weight, for example, a chain reaction of anxiety can result: Should I be doing that, too?

Equating eating disorder qualities with success

In professions as demanding and competitive as dancing, modeling, and acting, the following personal qualities may make the difference between success and failure:

- **Perfectionism:** Only the best performance will do.

- **Being driven toward a goal:** This means seeing where you want to land and letting nothing stand in the way, no matter what the personal cost.

- **The ability to ignore personal discomfort in order to reach a goal:** Being able to switch off the connection to physical or mental discomfort is often a requirement.

- **A desire to please others:** Instructors, casting directors, film directors, and audiences all appreciate this ability to tune into and deliver what another person wants.

Unfortunately, these very qualities, when combined with an environment that strongly promotes exaggerated thinness, can be a recipe for developing an eating disorder. If you're a dancer, model, or actor who possesses these qualities, you also need to have offsetting qualities to buffer yourself from eating disorder risk. These include a strong sense of yourself, recognition of your worth apart from what you do, and the ability to set a priority on your health and well-being. Without these offsetting qualities, your risk for developing an eating disorder sharply increases, even though you may be helping your career in other ways.

Getting direct pressure to be thin

Instructors, coaches, trainers, and, for that matter, agents and managers, know the professional environments their artists or models are competing in better than anyone. Many consider it part of their responsibility to help the individual achieve the weight she needs to succeed. Some instructors are famous for making weight commentary a humiliating part of class ritual.

In this environment, the teacher, coach, or other authority who bucks the trend and provides a more moderate voice is truly valuable. As more information about eating disorders makes its way into the performing and modeling industries, more such enlightened authorities are springing up. Sometimes it only takes one person to say the emperor has no clothes.

Making thinness a requirement to get jobs

If you're a dancer, model, or actor, it's a fact of life that in many cases the part or job goes to the person with the slim body. Often it goes to someone with a too-slim body, one well below what's considered ideal weight. Putting career success or failure into the mix takes environmental pressures to be thin to another level. Studies have shown that athletes whose careers depend on being thin, like jockeys, have sharply elevated rates of eating disorders. It's no stretch to imagine performers and models being affected similarly.

The lucky person who dreams of being a dancer, model, or actor was born with the slim body type these industries favor (and hopefully some talent, to boot!). The unlucky person has the same dreams but was given a body that doesn't naturally fit the mold. Imagine such a person also has personality characteristics which make her vulnerable to an eating disorder. Add to that respected voices in her field telling her a few pounds are all that stand between her and her dreams. This performer or model is highly likely to do whatever she thinks it takes to get the "extra" pounds off. Some in this situation achieve their weight goals, but only at a terrible cost to their health and well-being. Others find their bodies simply won't be tortured into the desired size or shape, no matter what measures they take. In both cases, chances for an eating disorder are sharply increased.

Spotlighting Special Issues for Treating Performers

As a group, dancers, models, and actors face the same personal obstacles and have the same assets to help them overcome eating disorders as anyone else. The biggest problem for recovery related to being in one of these fields is that a person's success and very livelihood may depend on being too thin. As part of an optimal recovery package, the environmental demands for thinness need to be reduced. The entertainment and modeling industries are responding to pressures for related changes. Parents of child dancers, models, and actors need to be especially involved with their child performer.

Improving the work environment

People can and do recover from eating disorders in spite of overwhelming environmental pressures. But in order to do the most to reduce eating disorder risk for these groups and enhance chances for eating disorder recovery, the environmental level is the place to start. The focus needs to be on reducing the relentless pressure for thinness to which young dancers, models, and actors are exposed.

Tragedies in the dance and modeling worlds have led to just this kind of focus and the beginnings of change. Two high-profile runway models died as a result of their eating disorders. A promising young ballet star may or may not have died from the effects of her eating disorder. Unfortunately, it often takes tragedy to trigger overdue change.

After the death of the second model, several centers of fashion took action. It started with regulation of the Madrid and Milan Fashion Week runway shows. Models now have to show a minimum *body mass index* (*BMI*). (BMI is a measure of body fat compared to height and weight. You can find a BMI chart and an explanation for its use in Chapter 20.) Medical certificates showing BMI are now a requirement to work.

The British Fashion Council set up an expert panel in 2007 to look at the effect of industry working conditions and pressures on young models. They were especially interested in what may cause greater risk for eating disorders. Most of their recommendations had to do with raising awareness about eating disorders among all the people a model has to deal with. They include parents, managers, casting directors, agents, designers, and so on. The panel also recommended some form of licensing for models that would include certification of good health in order to work.

In 2007, New York State authorized creation of The Child Performers Advisory Board. The job of the board is to recommend

- ✔ Educational materials that raise awareness about eating disorders among child actors and models and their families
- ✔ Guidelines for identifying child actors and models at risk for eating disorders
- ✔ Ways for at-risk child actors and models to be ensured access to treatment.

Developments in the dance world haven't been so official. Change is happening more at the level of individual schools, companies, and instructors. As with models and actors, increased eating disorder awareness among all parties is a priority. Experts encourage instructors to be cautious with negative comments about body size and weight. Expert Linda Hamilton suggests that schools and companies can take the following actions:

✔ Set minimum weights for performers.

✔ Require physician's letters for dancers whose weight is in doubt.

✔ Refer dancers with eating disorders for treatment.

While it's hard to detect any signs of regulation in the acting industry, one company employing actors at least put a toe in the water. A major U.S. product manufacturer decided to set a minimum BMI for models in its advertisements. They also applied the minimum to any actors hired for company advertisements. This isn't a lot to report, but it's a start.

Helping child performers

In Chapters 18, 21, and 22 you find lots of general information about how you can help a child with an eating disorder. Here are a few things you may want to keep in mind if you have a child dancer, model, or actor:

✔ **Check the effect of your own aspirations for your child's success:** Are you consciously or unconsciously messaging your child to get or stay thin to succeed?

✔ **Stay on top of the kinds of pressures about weight your child is being exposed to from other sources:** You may have to step in with trainers, teachers, agents, and so on. Where you can't have a direct influence (for example, with casting directors), at least you can help your child put weight judgments into perspective.

✔ **Be realistic about your child's natural body size and shape:** Your child simply may not have the body type required for the niche you and she are dreaming of. If this is true, she needs you to be able to be realistic and accepting about it if she's going to become realistic and accepting herself.

Chapter 18

Eating Disorders in Children

*N*ormally, adolescence is when eating disordered behavior begins to sur-face. Heartbreakingly, worries about fat and pressure to diet are show-ing up at earlier and earlier ages. First-graders are unhappy with their bodies and think they better do something about it. These ways of thinking and behaving are known risk factors for the development of eating disorders.

Food and eating *disturbances* (which are not disorders) are pretty ordinary in childhood. It's not unusual for kids to be fussy about what they will and won't eat. Actual eating disorders in children are more unusual. There are few stud-ies of these disorders in children, so nobody knows exactly how widespread they are. But it's important to be able to recognize the symptoms. Left untreated, eating disorders can have big psychological and physical conse-quences on a child's overall development.

Children who get eating disorders are a lot like teens and adults who get them — and also a lot different. Kids also have disordered ways of interacting with food that aren't about weight worries. Nonetheless, they can spell med-ical and psychological trouble if allowed to go on too long. In this chapter I alert parents and others what to look for in children and preteens that may indicate a developing eating disorder. I also review special issues to keep in mind when seeking treatment.

Becoming Informed about Childhood Onset Eating Disorders

Kids have so many things they can do with food, besides just eat it and go out to play. They can reject it, gag on it, choke on it, become terrified of it, eat some things but not others, eat some things some days but not other days . . . you name it. Frankly, most of this may be all in a day's work if you're the parent of a school-age child. Cause for worry begins only when these behaviors gel into a fixed pattern and you can't help your child find a way out. A fixed pattern of disturbed eating that has no physical cause is a childhood onset eating disorder.

Children get two kinds of eating disorders: the kind familiar to teens and adults, and the kind that only kids get. Among the more familiar eating disorders, children appear to get only anorexia. Bulimia and binge eating mostly wait for adolescence. Among the kids-only disorders, the most common ones are *food avoidance emotional disorder* (*FAED*) and *selective eating*.

Food avoidance emotional disorder (FAED): When food is scary

Here are the major symptoms of *food avoidance emotional disorder* (*FAED*):

- ✔ Refusal to eat
- ✔ Weight loss or failure to gain weight
- ✔ Slowed growth
- ✔ Mood disturbance (depression or anxiety)

Unlike the kids with childhood onset anorexia I discuss in the section "Recognizing the 'Grown-Up' Disorder of Anorexia in Kids," kids with FAED aren't preoccupied with their body size, aren't afraid of fat, and aren't trying to get thin. They are children who are so emotionally upset, they literally can't eat.

Many kids with FAED focus their distress on the food itself. They fear it can choke or poison them or otherwise harm them. Experts say that often such a kid has had some upsetting experience with food in the past, through illness or accident, and is afraid it will happen again. Children with FAED usually have fears and phobias about other things besides food. They handle these other fears by avoiding, just like they do with food.

Selective eating disorder (SED): When food has to be just right

Selective eating disorder (*SED*), often called picky or fussy eating, is known as the childhood onset eating disorder that mostly drives parents crazy without doing a lot of physical harm to the child. The child with SED

- ✔ Sticks rigidly to a narrow range of foods (for at least two years), usually relying heavily on carbohydrates
- ✔ Refuses to try new foods
- ✔ Maintains normal weight and growth (even though you're certain she can't, based on what she's eating)

Often kids with SED gag when you offer an unwanted food. Most are responding to textures and tastes they can't tolerate. They are not trying to lose weight. Many become embarrassed by their limitations when they are old enough to socialize. Just "growing out of" SED doesn't seem to be a solution. (For alternatives, see "Getting Treatment for Kids," later in this chapter.) In fact, a tiny minority of SED kids take their disorder into adulthood.

Less common childhood food disorders

The following disturbed childhood eating patterns, taken together, account for the other 10 percent (or less) of the problems for which parents seek help:

- ✔ **Food refusal:** Unlike FAED, refusing to eat is a once-in-awhile thing, maybe occurring only in certain situations or around certain people. There may be mood problems behind the refusal to eat. Weight is not a preoccupation.
- ✔ **Restrictive eating:** These kids don't have much of an appetite and just aren't very interested in eating. They aren't worried about weight but may have other emotional concerns.
- ✔ **Functional dysphagia:** This is a phobia — that is, a morbid fear — of choking, vomiting, gagging, or being poisoned by swallowed food. Often the child has had some experience that set off the fear or planted the idea. It has nothing to do with trying to lose weight.

These disorders involve behaviors that are pretty common among preschoolers and don't necessarily suggest emotional problems. They become cause for concern when they continue into or start up in school-age years. If your school-age child is showing these symptoms and not responding to your efforts to help, don't hesitate to get an expert evaluation.

Studies suggest anorexia accounts for more than 40 percent of childhood onset eating disorders. FAED may account for 30 percent, and selective eating another 20 percent.

Boys take a much bigger part in childhood eating disorders than older males do in adult disorders. Studies show that a little more than a quarter of the children with anorexia and most of the children with FAED are boys. In comparison, only 5 to 10 percent of adults with anorexia are men. (You can read more about men and eating disorders in Chapter 15.)

Recognizing the "Grown Up" Disorder of Anorexia in Kids

As hard as it is to imagine school-age children becoming preoccupied with weight or going on starvation diets to be thin, kids as young as 4 to 7 have been reported to do so. Eating disorders in children can lead to long-term consequences in their development. What puts a child at greater risk for developing anorexia in the first place? What are the signs that your school-age child may have already developed anorexia? Understanding the psychology behind what can make a child susceptible to an eating disorder is helpful in assessing your child. Parents can also consider risk factors as they review the behavior of their child to help determine whether food-related issues are merely fussiness or something more.

Physical impacts in children

If you combine numbers for the most common childhood eating disorders, you find that refusal to eat is the main eating disorder symptom for kids. Starving or being undernourished for a long time is dangerous for anyone. It presents particular problems for kids. These include

- **Effects on heart and organs:** Chronic undernourishment damages heart and organ functions and interferes with the brain's ability to think and concentrate. (I discuss these effects of starvation in detail in Chapter 6.) Effects on children may be more severe because they have less fat to work with than teens or adults. Kids particularly seem to run a greater risk for life-threatening damage to their hearts.

- **Effects on growth:** Just when the body needs plenty of nourishment to fuel growth, food-refusal eating disorders are cutting off the source of supply. Kids who don't return to normal eating see their growth and height stunted and puberty delayed. Fortunately, resumption of normal eating overcomes these effects.

Psychological overview

The usual age of onset for these disorders ranges from 7 to 13. (After this, kids are grouped with adolescents.) It probably won't surprise you to learn that what's on the minds of kids with these disorders is less complicated than their teen counterparts. Teens are busy using their eating disorders to work out issues of self-esteem, identity, coping with life, and making the transition out of childhood.

Kids who develop eating disorders are usually anxious or depressed and lack any other language to express it. Many times they're responding to families who are in their own distress, or they're mirroring other family members who are upset and preoccupied with food and weight. Similar to teens and adults with eating disorders, these kids are urgent about issues of control. Also like teens and adults, they tend to be obsessive and to be perfectionists.

Reviewing the risk factors

From what's known so far, the following factors appear to create the greatest risk for developing childhood onset anorexia:

- **Body dissatisfaction:** Among the risk factors for anorexia, body dissatisfaction is the one that most strongly predicts developing the disorder. Once a preoccupation for grown-ups and teens, "feeling fat" has now become a way for kids to dislike themselves, too. For example, statistics show that one-third to one-half or more of primary and elementary school girls and boys are unhappy with their bodies and think they need to lose weight.

- **Dieting:** Like body dissatisfaction, dieting is showing up at younger and younger ages. According to statistics, fully one-third of kids report dieting by the time they've reached the fourth grade.

- **Family conflict:** Children who eventually develop anorexia are often trying to cope with their distress in an environment of chronic parent or family conflict.

- **Family over-involvement:** Compliant children often don't know how to have a separate "me." If a parent's voice is very strong or the family emphasizes togetherness at the expense of separateness, food and weight may become a child's last-ditch stand for control.

- **Family weight talk:** If you talk negatively about your own weight or your child's weight, the risk for an eating disorder in your child increases. This is most likely if you're the mom and your child is a girl.

✔ **Triggering events:** Kids are more likely than teens or adults to respond to an upsetting life event by developing anorexia. Such events can include loss of a family member or friend, parents' separation or divorce, parent's job loss, medical illness in the family, a move, and so on.

✔ **Anxiety:** Anxiety is very common in kids with childhood onset anorexia. The eating disorder can be an attempt to cope.

✔ **Personality characteristics:** Some studies suggest that overly compliant, rigid, perfection-oriented kids are more vulnerable to developing childhood onset anorexia.

✔ **Early feeding problems:** Research shows that kids who have problems with feeding in infancy or toddlerhood are more likely to develop anorexia in later childhood.

Knowing what signs and symptoms to look for

The symptom profile of a child with anorexia is pretty much the same as the symptom profile of a teen or adult with anorexia:

✔ Desire to lose weight, drive to be thin

✔ Phobic fear of fat

✔ Refusal to eat

✔ Weight loss

✔ Distorted view of body shape and size, seeing self or certain body parts as larger than others do

✔ Obsessive thoughts about weight and calories

✔ Excessive activity to lose weight or offset calories consumed

There are also ways in which the symptoms of a child with anorexia look different from those of an older person:

✔ **Loss of menstrual periods is not an issue:** Studies of childhood eating disorders cut off at the onset of puberty.

✔ **Failure to gain weight:** Though many kids with anorexia lose weight like their older counterparts, not gaining in childhood is also a symptom. Kids are supposed to keep getting bigger!

✔ **Fluid refusal goes with food refusal:** Refusing fluids puts a child at increased risk for dehydration, which can lead to heart and organ malfunction. (I discuss the effects of dehydration in detail in Chapter 6.)

Parents and kids often have different views when it comes to identifying the presence of eating disorder symptoms. One study found that parents were better at noticing when their kids had body preoccupation and mood disturbances (like depression). However, kids reported feelings inside like fear of fat that their parents had no idea of. The conclusion? To get the fullest picture, including both parents' and kids' views is best.

Getting Treatment for Kids

 When patients are very young, the emphasis in eating disorder treatment shifts in a couple of ways. The urgency for an early diagnosis is even greater, and the need for family therapy moves from optional or adjunct to mainline. Here are the key points for you to keep in mind:

- **Get your child evaluated without delay!** Childhood onset eating disorders can throw a child's physical and psychological development off track. The longer the child has the disorder, the more difficult catching up becomes. Prognosis for recovery is best when you intervene early.

- **Find an expert who knows kids and eating disorders.** You may need to override your pediatrician's initial impressions and seek an eating disorder specialist to evaluate your child. Childhood onset eating disorders are a relatively new focus and not yet on the radar screens of many otherwise competent physicians. (You can use the "Resource Guide" in the back of this book to start your search for an eating disorder expert.)

- **Put together a treatment team that includes psychological and medical experts.** Childhood onset eating disorders have psychological origins but medical consequences. Both need to be treated. If your child is starving herself, treating the physical effects of starvation comes first and may include hospitalization. (These treatment decisions are the same as for teens and adults. I go over them in detail in Chapter 9.)

- **Think of family therapy as a must-have.** The younger the child, the more important this is. Here are the main reasons:

  - **Your child is too young to be completely responsible for making the changes necessary to get better.** Young children can't just think their way out of psychological problems. They need their families to help them make changes or for their families themselves to make changes for things to get better.

  - **You need support and guidance for helping your child change disordered eating patterns.** It can be a big relief to work with someone who's seen these problems many times before and can offer you suggestions to help the situation improve.

Troubles for tots; problems for preschoolers

Feeding and eating disorders of infancy and early childhood is the official name for eating disorders that show up in your child before age 6 and last for at least a month. These disorders include

✔ **Pica:** Regularly eating nonfood substances beyond an age when you'd expect it and when it has nothing to do with cultural practices. (Pica came to everybody's attention when inner-city kids with the disorder were eating lead-based paint chips and suffering lead toxicity as a result.)

✔ **Rumination disorder:** This involves bringing back up partly digested food, rechewing it and reswallowing it, or spitting it out. It occurs mainly in the first 3 to 12 months of life, although people of all ages can have rumination disorder.

✔ **Feeding disorder of infancy or early childhood:** Diagnosed when a child fails to eat enough to grow or gain weight normally (or even loses weight).

Parents need to understand that these disorders aren't phases (that is, your child isn't likely to just grow out of them), and their causes aren't anything physical. They may create increased risk for eating disorders in childhood or adolescence. Parental counseling and behavioral treatment can be helpful.

- **There may be things happening in your family that are upsetting your child and fueling the eating problems.** Kids who develop eating disorders are often upset about family or marriage conflict and have no other way to express it. Sometimes part of the "medicine" for an eating disorder is finding ways to make things better in the family.

- **Your child may be responding to other family members who are upset about their own weight and eating.** Your child picks up everything you say about weight, appearance, and eating. These become the guidelines she applies to herself. Counseling for yourself can be a big help if you're having trouble with an over-focus on weight and appearance.

- **You may need to develop some new ways to relate to your child.** Childhood onset eating disorders often occur when parents are having trouble letting go of the reins a little to give a child more independence. An anxious kid can make this even harder. Having the support of a family therapist can make those first steps less hair-raising.

The input you get may be more in the form of parent counseling, or it may include everyone in the family. Or some of both. You can expect advice from a family therapist about what's likely to work best in your situation. She should also be able to advise you whether individual therapy for your child is a good idea. (You can read more about family therapy in Chapter 11.)

Chapter 19

Eating Disorders Later In Life

*W*hile it's generally true that the vast majority of people with eating disorders are younger women, middle-aged women are showing up at eating disorder programs in surprising numbers.

Some of these women are experiencing a second round of eating problems, having battled an eating disorder earlier in life. Others are experiencing their first bout. Senior women and men (those 65 and over) also develop eating disorders (mostly anorexia) more frequently than you or most of their professional caregivers may think.

In our weight-obsessed culture, neither middle-aged nor senior women (nor men) are exempt from pressures to be thin (or buff). In this chapter I go over what makes these pressures unique in midlife and later years and how an eating disorder often feels like a solution to coping with those pressures. I discuss special treatment considerations for each group, including the need to distinguish anorexia from more usual causes for loss of weight and appetite in elderly people.

Getting Older and Trying to be Thinner

Our culture is not deeply interested in what older people are doing. Beautiful young people wasting away or secretly bingeing and purging are more likely to grab our attention. Not much research has been done into eating disorders among those who are middle-aged and older, so nobody knows exactly how widespread their eating disorder problems are. However, by looking carefully at some "back door" sources of information connecting eating disorders with those over 30 — such as studies showing high rates of risk factors, increasing rates of requests for treatment, and death rates due to anorexia in the elderly — it becomes easier to see that you're never too old to acquire an eating disorder.

Seeking treatment later in life

If you go by the trends being seen in eating disorder treatment programs, eating disorders among women in their 30s, 40s, and 50s are definitely on the rise. Residential programs report that admissions of people in midlife have doubled and even tripled in the last decade. Admissions for women over 30 account for as much as 25 percent of program populations.

A big question on everyone's mind when it comes to people at midlife is whether eating disorders are actually on the rise or whether these people are just seeking treatment in greater numbers. The answer is probably some of both. Baby boomers have come a long way toward taking the stigma out of seeking psychological help. This has gone hand in hand with increasing public awareness about eating disorders. But this generation is also experiencing pressures for thinness in ways that grandma never thought of. Social pressures to be thin are big risk factors for developing an eating disorder. (I discuss this in the next section, "Fighting the Loss of Youth and More.")

In the *International Journal of Eating Disorders* (2006), researchers reported on a sampling of senior women who weren't seeking treatment. Just under 4 percent of these women had some kind of formal eating disorder. (Estimates for the general population are in the neighborhood of 10 percent.) Another 4 to 5 percent of these women had at least one eating disordered symptom. Though disturbing, the numbers don't spell a runaway epidemic. A California State University study found that while elderly women are just as dissatisfied with their bodies as middle-aged women, they are less driven as a group to do something about it.

Dying a little later, but still too soon

Unfortunately, one thing that's not hard to count is death certificates. When researchers at the University of British Columbia did just that, they found that while anorexia occurs most in younger people, it takes its biggest death toll in older people. Almost 80 percent of anorexia-caused deaths occur in people age 45 and older. Most think the higher death toll is because older bodies are less able to withstand the physical assault of prolonged starvation. Death rates due to anorexia continue to rise until sufferers are in their 80s.

Interestingly, more than 20 percent of these older people with anorexia are men — twice the number among younger men. (You can read more about men with eating disorders in Chapter 15.)

Fighting the Loss of Youth and More

Midlife is not necessarily a walk in the park for many folks, emotionally or practically speaking. But it seems in this day and age we've found a way to notch up the stress for women. Many think a direct connection exists between the added stresses of aging and an apparent upsurge in eating disorders among middle-aged women. Unique pressures can push older people into an eating disorder.

Experiencing midlife crisis is no joke

Undoubtedly, for many men and women, midlife can be a satisfying time filled with long-worked-for accomplishments, retiring to enjoy well-developed interests, and embracing the simple joy of spending more time with loved ones. But for far too many, midlife becomes a time mainly of being overwhelmed by multiple competing demands, experiences of loss, and the sense of being less and less worthwhile as judged by cultural standards.

Entering the "sandwich generation"

Those in midlife have been dubbed the "sandwich generation" because they are often caught in the middle between caretaking responsibilities for dependent children and newly dependent aging parents. Now, add to this being in peak years for financial responsibilities: paying the mortgage, health premiums for an entire family, saving for college, and so on. Maybe you're just hitting your stride in your career or trying to re-enter the job market after raising kids. Perhaps you're one of the growing number of women having their first kids at 40, and you're just entering those labor-intensive early years. The point is that you're unlikely to experience another time in your life when you're stretched in so many directions at once. And, of course, like pulling a rabbit out of a hat, you're expected to make it all work.

Finding that everything seems to be about loss

At the same time the demands are mounting, your supply of resources may be dwindling. Midlife can be a time of major loss, sometimes many losses. Coming to terms with them may place an extra strain on you and your sense of yourself. Here are some typical losses people experience in midlife:

- ✔ **Death:** Usually you think of losing parents during midlife. But for many, it's also a time of first losing friends to death.

- ✔ **Divorce:** Whether you're the one who wanted it or you got stuck with it, divorce tears your life apart at the seams. It doesn't mean you can't eventually land on your feet, but you're in for a period of confusion and turmoil. If you wanted your marriage to continue, you have a lot to grieve. The loss can be quite practical as well: On average, women drop to a lower standard of living following divorce.

- ✔ **The "empty nest":** For some, seeing the last kid out the door is freeing; for others, it's devastating. Either way, it requires some major redefining of who you are and what your role is in life.

- ✔ **Youth, youthful dreams:** One of the jolts of reality in midlife is that you are not immortal after all and you don't have endless time to do everything you had in mind. Some of your goals and dreams aren't going to be, and you have to put them to rest.

- ✔ **Physical strength:** At midlife you may have to come to terms with physical limitations to what you can do. Realizing that you can't exercise your way into a body with the capacities of a 20-year-old is another jolt of reality.

- ✔ **Fertility:** Even if you aren't interested in having (more) babies, to many women this is an important part of feeling womanly. It takes some time and internal effort to invest those feelings elsewhere.

- ✔ **Physical beauty — as defined by the culture:** Some people may age gracefully, but not all. Even if others view you as attractive as you age, you may not perceive yourself the same way, especially if you measure yourself against cultural standards of youthful beauty.

Getting wrinkles in a culture that has no place for them

No matter what you eat, how you exercise, or what kinds of lotions and potions you apply, some physical changes are going to happen in midlife (and beyond) that aren't going to be what you signed up for.

In women, hormonal shifts related to menopause result in

- ✔ Easier weight gain; more difficult weight loss

- ✔ A shift of fat deposits to your belly (while managing to find plenty to leave on your thighs!)

- ✔ Loss of skin elasticity (in other words, wrinkles)

When baby boomers face these normal changes of midlife, they do so in a culture insisting as never before that giving in to them is failing. Fifty is the new forty (or maybe even thirty — but no pressure!). Normally developing wrinkles, accumulating fat, and weakening muscles are viewed as flaws and reasons to see the plastic surgeon — as many times as it takes. Though men are beginning to feel some of this heat, the culture has mainly focused its disdain on the aging female body.

(Re)discovering the control cure

If you're seeking eating disorder treatment at midlife, you may have already overcome an eating disorder when you were younger. You may be experiencing a relapse as your personal blend of vulnerabilities runs into all the things that can make midlife women feel out of control. Or maybe you've lived with your vulnerabilities all these years, but you've managed to escape an eating disorder up until now. Midlife pressures may have become your tipping point.

Being overwhelmed by competing demands, enduring multiple losses, going through normal physical changes and being judged less valuable because of them — any of these experiences can leave a person feeling out of control. A woman who's achieved a certain amount of personal resilience doesn't blame herself, seeks support, knows certain things are temporary, grieves her losses, and focuses on what she can control.

However, for a certain number of vulnerable women, feeling out of control in one or more areas of life can instead start an emotional domino effect. *Everything* feels out of control. Life's changes are terrifying and shaming. They're a clear sign of personal failure. These emotions can become overwhelming.

If you have this kind of shaky self-esteem, urgency for control, and difficulty handling your feelings, you were a candidate for an eating disorder back in your teens and you're a candidate for one now in midlife. Food and body weight always seem like something convenient to control — and everybody applauds when you do. But pitfalls are unavoidable. (See Part I for a thorough discussion.)

Eating Disordered Over 65

Although theoretically, seniors can develop any of the eating disorders, the one they're actually most likely to develop is anorexia. While unique triggers can cause seniors to develop the disorder at this stage of life, other common reasons for food refusal and weight loss in older people have to be ruled out before anorexia can be considered as a diagnosis.

Triggering anorexia in seniors

Older people who develop anorexia often do so for the same reasons as younger people: Life feels uncertain and out of control. Focusing on eating or not eating makes things seem simple and controllable again.

Actually, "seniors" span quite an age range. Eating disorders at the younger end of the range, closer to age 65, are probably going to look different than those found in people in their 80s or older. Younger seniors may still have concerns pretty similar to people in midlife. Some may still be compulsively exercising and using strange diets. For the older senior, it may all come down to simple food refusal. She may not even be focused on weight loss anymore, although she shows the classic denial that she's losing weight or that it matters if she does. Seniors typically develop anorexia for the following reasons:

- **Loss of a partner or other family or friends:** Loss is one of the major causes of feeling out of control in later years.

- **Loss of control over key aspects of life (for example, where you live):** This gets worse as a decline in health and mental capacities may make you more and more dependent on others.

- **Fear of aging:** Uncertainty about what future losses, pain, or indignities may be in store may make you feel very out of control.

- **Social pressures to remain sexually attractive:** Comparing yourself to the prized people in the culture doesn't stop automatically when you start getting Medicare.

Seeing other reasons for diet problems

Seniors stop eating and lose weight for many reasons. You really need to be certain to rule out everything else before deciding the reason is an eating disorder. Most of the other reasons can and should be treated in some way. Here's a roundup of the usual suspects:

- **Depression:** Although people with eating disorders are often depressed, you can be depressed and not have an eating disorder. Depression is a major cause for loss of appetite among older people.

- **Social isolation:** Being isolated can lead to depression. It can also make eating and food preparation feel kind of empty and meaningless to some.

- **Biological changes:** Your body's energy needs slow down as you age. Appetite-stimulating hormones slow down with it. Your body doesn't fight so hard to hold onto its fat reserves anymore. By age 70, losing some weight and having less of an appetite are normal.

- **Medication effects:** Medication side effects may include suppressing your appetite or causing involuntary weight loss.

- **Illness, pain:** So-called *wasting illnesses,* such as cancer, cause weight loss by definition. Nausea and pain caused by other illnesses knock the stuffing out of appetite.

- **Food phobias:** An incident of choking or even a seemingly unrelated experience can make a vulnerable person afraid to eat again.

Distinguishing involuntary reasons for weight loss, like those in the preceding list, from anorexia may be difficult. When the cause of weight and appetite loss is something other than anorexia, the following typically apply:

- **The person doesn't deny she is losing weight:** If she acknowledges that she's losing weight, this means she recognizes there's a problem. She's not in a state of denial or trying to cover up what's happening to her body. This is because the weight loss or food refusal isn't serving a psychological purpose such as trying to feel in control.

- **The person doesn't deny that there are problems associated with weight loss:** Acknowledging that weight loss can lead to other health issues is not something a person with anorexia is likely to do. A person with anorexia sees only positives from weight loss, even if the loss is severe and life threatening.

Treating Eating Disorders in the 30+ Set

While the basics of eating disorder treatment remain the same regardless of age, some special issues come up in relation to people who come for treatment at midlife and as seniors.

Treatment issues at midlife

If you're a middle-aged woman seeking eating disorder treatment, chances are you're bringing both some important liabilities and some important assets to the process. Some practitioners emphasize the liabilities, others the assets. An ability to see both clearly is important. That way you feel understood and you and your therapist can make the best plan for treatment.

For example, if you've struggled with an eating disorder for many years already, your disorder is very ingrained by now. Eating disorders are easier to treat when people haven't had them for very long. The same can be said for the personality characteristics that fuel them, like perfectionism, black-and-white thinking, or the need to please others at your own expense. On the other hand, you are now coming on your own, not because your parents, coach, or school made you. You know that you need to get better. You have motivation working for you in a way that many younger patients don't.

A long-term battle with an eating disorder or underlying personality dynamics may have left you a little battle-weary. Your mind, body, and spirit may all feel a little worn out. On the other hand, entering treatment at midlife, you bring some life resources to the table you didn't have at 15 or 20. You have life experience and — this is a big one — you have *perspective*. You know more about how things work and what really matters. These are important assets for your recovery.

Treatment issues for seniors

The evaluation stage is really crucial with older people for two reasons. The first is to rule out the many other things that can cause seniors to stop eating and lose weight. (See the previous section "Seeing other reasons for diet problems.") Medical causes need to be diagnosed and treated. Medications should be evaluated and any relevant adjustments made. It's especially important to look for signs of depression. Depression can look like anorexia and often goes untreated in elderly people.

The second reason a careful evaluation is crucial is that physicians and caregivers don't expect eating disorders in the elderly, so they aren't on the lookout for them. This is similar to the situation faced by men and kids. If you think a senior you love may have anorexia, you may need to ask specifically for her treatment team to consider it.

If a *senior* senior receives a diagnosis of anorexia, control issues are almost certainly part of the picture. But they aren't the same as for a younger person. It's one thing to *feel* your life is out of control. It's quite another to hand over the keys to the car, leave your home of 45 years for assisted living, and have someone who could be your grandchild telling you when you're going to go to bed. Anorexia, under these conditions, is often a way of saying, *Enough! I still decide some things!* A therapist and others who want to help need to take the painful losses of control that go with this life stage into account.

Chapter 20

Eating Disorders and People Who Are Obese

*O*besity isn't an eating disorder! And it doesn't automatically signal other emotional problems, for that matter. On the other hand, social misconceptions and prejudices can contribute to the development of eating disorders in people who are obese.

In this chapter I go over these issues and take a look at the particular landscape of eating disorders among people who are obese. You find, for example, that if a person who's obese has an eating disorder, it's most likely to be binge eating disorder (BED) and that increasing obesity increases the likelihood of developing BED. I also take up special treatment considerations for people who are obese and have eating disorders. Quite a controversy is brewing about what the proper treatment should be. I take you through both sides of the issue and make some recommendations about other aspects of treatment.

Being Obese and Eating Disordered

If you're obese and have an eating disorder, you most likely have BED. How widespread is BED among people who are obese? Does it differ from BED in people who are of average weight? Do people who are obese and have eating disorders differ from obese people without eating disorders? I answer these questions in this section, but first I define what obesity means.

Defining obesity

For research purposes, *obesity* has a specific definition. It's defined by the body mass index (BMI), a ratio that combines weight and height. Obesity is officially defined as having a BMI of 30 or greater (several versions of the BMI can be found online simply by searching on "BMI"). You should know that the BMI chart, like the height-and-weight charts that came before it, did not come down from Mount Sinai. Somebody made them up. They involve as much social opinion as science. I leave it to you to decide for yourself whether this chapter is relevant for you.

Seeing how BED differs in people who are obese

The biggest difference between BED sufferers who are obese and those who aren't is the role dieting plays in their lives. Nearly all people who aren't obese report the familiar yo-yo pattern (going on and off diets) that cycles with their bingeing, with dieting playing an important role in how they started bingeing in the first place. In clinical studies of those who are obese and have BED, only half reported the same cycling pattern with dieting, while the other half didn't. The differentiating factor? Those who are obese with BED but don't yo-yo diet started bingeing before they ever started dieting. (You can read more about the cycle of dieting and bingeing in Chapter 4.)

Emotional upset is likely to trigger overeating episodes in both obese and nonobese people who binge. So-called *disinhibiting* triggers — things that lead you to let down the controls — also result in bingeing. Alcohol is an example of a disinhibiting trigger, as is being in the presence of lots of food or really great-looking food.

Being a person who's obese with BED

If you're a person who's obese and you have BED, you're likely to have more psychological problems than people who are obese but don't have BED. In particular, you're more likely to be depressed and have a history of depression and other mood problems, like anxiety.

An interesting study by researchers in Toulouse, France, compared overeating in women who were obese with and without BED. Both groups overate when stressed or emotionally upset. But a lot more emotional overeating went on in the BED group. The researchers found it was because of missing skills: the ability to identify and express emotions. (When you're missing these skills, you have a condition called *alexithymia.*) The researchers rightly concluded that developing missing emotion-related skills is crucial to eating disorder recovery for these women.

About 2 to 5 percent of people who are obese in the United States are estimated to have BED. These rates are similar to the overall population. Taken from another angle, about 8 percent of the people who have BED are obese. The more obese you are, the more likely you are to have BED.

Among people who seek treatment for obesity, binge eating is an extremely common symptom. Up to one-third of treatment-seekers report some degree of binge eating, although they don't necessarily have full-blown BED.

Highlighting Special Issues for Treatment

If you're a person who's obese, much of your eating disorder treatment is the same as for people of other sizes. However, in one way or another, your weight is going to be part of the issue, even if you decide *not* to make it an issue. Most likely, you need to address the effects of social stigma and work through dealing with both weight and BED issues.

Night eating syndrome and nocturnal sleep-related eating disorder

Night eating syndrome is the name for a combined eating and sleep disturbance found mostly among obese people and its features include:

✔ Eating little during the day

✔ Eating most of your day's calories in the evening and/or at night, often after having gone to sleep and then reawakening

✔ Being fully conscious while eating

✔ Being triggered by stress and depression and getting better when these are alleviated

People who have been identified as having night eating syndrome appear to have several hormonal abnormalities which researchers think may help explain their symptoms:

✔ *Melatonin,* a hormone involved in sleep, is lower than average.

✔ *Leptin,* a hormone involved in appetite control and weight regulation, does not peak at night as it should.

✔ *Cortisol,* a so-called stress hormone, is elevated.

Treatment for night eating syndrome is essentially the same as treatment for any kind of emotional overeating — finding out how to cope with stressful feelings in more productive ways. This has to be a good thing! Zoloft, an SSRI (a class of medication with antidepressant and anti-anxiety effects), has been found helpful in the treatment of night eating syndrome.

Treating the effects of social stigma first

Women generally feel pressured by a culture that worships thinness, but this pressure can be a lifetime nightmare for women who are obese. Few obese people of either sex reach adulthood without their unfair share of cruel or discriminatory experiences. A steady diet of such experiences can take a toll. It's likely to affect self-image, mood and outlook, and a person's sense of possibilities (or lack thereof) in life.

As with any stigmatized minority, a few hardy souls seem to have such natural or cultivated resilience that they manage to hold on to their good image of themselves despite all the battering. Most people, however, can't. If you're part of the majority who feel the painful effects of cultural battery, you need to make sure that whoever you work with understands the issue of discrimination and can talk with you about it.

Talking about size discrimination early in treatment is usually a good idea. First, if you don't, it tends to be that famous rhinoceros on the table — the big, obvious thing everybody's ignoring. Second, for some people, just identifying the cultural causes of their bad feelings about themselves can go far to alleviate depression and lift self-esteem. Validating this part of your experience is an essential first stop — and worth trying before you work on your feelings from other angles.

Treating obesity versus treating BED

The treatment world is divided with regard to how you should be treated if you're obese and have an eating disorder. One group says your obesity should be treated first, and your eating disorder should come second. Another group says your eating disorder should be treated first, and other decisions should be made thereafter. I review the arguments of each so you can decide for yourself.

Treating the obesity first

When experts talk about treating obesity first, they mean you should diet and lose weight (or use as-yet-unproven weight loss medications or bariatric surgery). This group believes that sound and solid weight loss programs, overseen by professionals, don't trigger your eating disorder symptoms — at least not like the bad and crazy diets you try on your own.

The biggest argument this group makes is that the health risks of obesity are simply too great to safely postpone weight loss. Maybe your doctor and your mom tell you the same thing. They point out statistics about the increased risks for diabetes, high blood pressure, heart attack, and stroke among people who are obese. They remind you that your health improves with just a 10 percent loss of body weight, and that you don't have to overwhelm yourself with impossible goals.

Treating the eating disorder first

Proponents of treating the eating disorder first point to the fact that eating disorders always require treatment. Obesity doesn't. *The first thing that needs to happen when you consult a professional is a conversation about whether you even want treatment for obesity.* I know; it's probably what brought you into treatment in the first place. But — just like being overweight — trying to lose weight is full of physical and psychological pitfalls. At the very least, it should be treated by you and your professional team as a choice and not a duty!

Your decision about treating your obesity may be influenced by some of the following arguments, which present reasons for treating your BED first even if you decide to take on weight loss as a goal:

- ✔ **Dieting doesn't work:** Never has there been an activity that's failed so frequently yet gotten so many second chances. Ninety-five percent of people who lose weight through dieting regain it — often with a little extra to boot. Yet people keep trying, if not this diet, then the next. And professionals keep recommending them.

    How do those state-of-the-art weight loss programs suggested by the "diet first" group fare? People who participate lose an average of 10 to 15 percent of body weight. But they regain an average of 75 to 80 percent of their losses within 5 years of ending treatment. If you do the math, this doesn't put you in the health benefits range of a net 10 percent loss. And it doesn't put you much ahead of your own dieting devices (except I bet the program is much healthier).

- ✔ **Dieting triggers eating disorder symptoms:** The argument that a sound, sensible program doesn't trigger eating disorder symptoms is based on how well BED participants do during the dieting phase. Anyone with BED can tell you that the dieting phase is when they're likely to do well, especially with structure, but there's no telling how long that phase will (or won't) last for a particular person. You may last until the end of the day, the end of the week, or the end of the diet. But at some point, being on a diet is likely to trigger bingeing.

- ✔ **The health risks of obesity are exaggerated:** This may surprise you: It's already been established that your health risk is *less* if you are in the preobese *overweight* range than if you're underweight or average. An increasing number of medical experts are questioning whether obesity is actually the culprit when it comes to so-called obesity-related diseases.

    First of all, it's hard to separate the effects of obesity from the effects of a no-exercise lifestyle. One way to tell them apart is to test obese people who are also fit. When researchers do this, they find that the fit obese people not only show reduced risk for diabetes and heart disease, they have lower overall mortality rates than unfit slim people.

Second, if excess fat is a problem at all, it seems not to be overall body fat that causes you trouble. Rather, it's *belly fat* that appears to make all the mischief with your blood sugar and arteries. You do have to exercise to get rogue belly fat cells in line. But a good exercise program (like daily walking) is usually enough and doesn't make your eating disorder go bonkers.

✔ It's hard to lose weight *and keep it off* without treating the underlying eating disorder: Even if you're still holding onto a plan to take off weight, tackling your binge eating disorder first is probably the best way to go. Otherwise, relapse can undo a lot of hard work. Interestingly, studies have shown that when binge eating disorder was treated successfully, a little bit of weight loss was a side effect for a quarter of their participants. The weight loss held up at the one-year mark.

Treating the whole person

If you focus only on weight loss or only on controlling bingeing, you miss the most important point — you! Eating disorder recovery is always a time for focusing on the whole person. But there are some particular things to keep in mind if you are obese and have BED:

✔ **Depression:** You and your therapist need to sort out where your depression comes from. If it's mostly a response to living in a discriminatory culture, your "medicine" may involve raising your consciousness about it and participating in some antisize discrimination activity, if it feels appropriate.

Many people of all sizes with BED suffer from depression. Often people with BED eat to cope with their depression. Treating any depression you're experiencing is important to your recovery. You may find that talking therapy and/or medication are helpful with the noncultural sources of your depression.

✔ **Alexithymia:** *Alexithymia* refers to a condition in which you lack the skills for identifying or communicating your emotions. This leaves you more vulnerable to turning to food. Because you're more likely to suffer from alexithymia if you're obese and have BED, your recovery requires a healthy dose of emotion skills training. This is true for everyone with an eating disorder, but you may need to start with the basics: How can you know what you're feeling? Can your feelings be put into words?

✔ **Body acceptance:** Body acceptance is an especially big hurdle when an entire culture is telling you that your body is unacceptable and the only solution is to change it. If you're done trying to change your body, you may need extra support for your decision. Make sure you know who you can count on among family, friends, and co-workers. Tell them what kind of support you need. People don't always figure these things out on their own. Besides, what you need may differ from one person to the next.

Part IV

Advice and Help for Families and Others Who Care

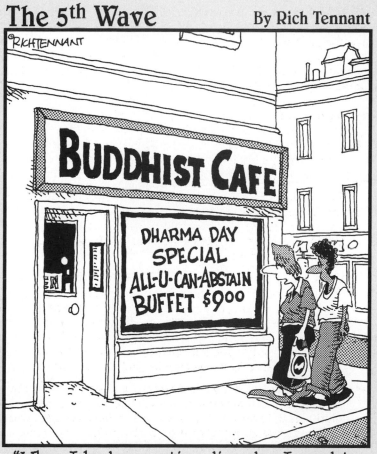

The 5th Wave   By Rich Tennant

BUDDHIST CAFE

DHARMA DAY
SPECIAL
ALL-U-CAN-ABSTAIN
BUFFET $9⁰⁰

"When I had my eating disorder, I used to come here all the time."

In this part . . .

1 address families and other people supporting someone in recovery. I especially take into account parents who are responsible for minor children with eating disorders. (Where your situation requires a different approach — say you're dealing with an adult, you're a spouse, a friend, or an employer — I give separate advice and guidelines.)

I give special attention to situations in which you need to confront the person with the eating disorder. I talk about how to prepare yourself, including gathering information and planning for pitfalls. I go over a list of do's and don'ts for the actual encounter and discuss how to handle anger and denial. I then skip forward to managing day-to-day living with that same person once she's in recovery. It may be no bed of roses, but there are ways you can all survive. I review some approaches to nourish and others to avoid. Finally, I discuss the wear-and-tear on you, the caregiver — how to know when it's getting to be too much and how to find the kind of help you need to get you through.

Chapter 21

Forming a Plan to Help the Person with an Eating Disorder

Maybe you fantasize about having a really simple first conversation with your child or another person you care about who has an eating disorder. In your fantasy, she approaches you, tells you she has a problem, and asks you to help her get treatment. Then, together, you walk off arm in arm to the therapist's office.

This chapter assumes that your situation is more complicated and more real than a fantasy scenario. Your child (or the person you're concerned about) isn't bad; rather, she faces a lot of factors that make her want to deny having an eating disorder or avoid talking about it.

In this chapter I focus on getting you ready for that first real conversation. (In Chapter 22 I walk you through implementing your plan.) Think of yourself as being in training. You want the scenario to go as well as possible. Complicated matters tend to go better when you're prepared. You also want to feel grounded in your own knowledge and support if your child's first reaction isn't so great. Preparation doesn't make conflict easy. But at least it gives you a leg to stand on.

By reading this chapter, you actually end up with two legs to stand on: a practical one and an emotional one. I give you lots of information about how to shore up each leg in "training." I divide this practical and emotional advice into three areas:

✔ Information

✔ Treatment resources

✔ Support

You want to prepare yourself by getting enough of each of them. This chapter tells you what you need to know, why you need to know it, and how to go about training for the best possible result.

Becoming Informed About Eating Disorders

Many good reasons exist to stop and get as much information as you can right now. This is especially true if you're going to be an ongoing part of the support system for the person with the eating disorder. The more you know, the more helpful you can be.

Becoming informed can also help you with what you're going through right now. Your head may be swirling with images and myths that have little to do with eating disorder reality. Getting the facts, ruling out the folklore, and seeing what you need to do can be very calming.

In this section, I go over three basic questions about eating disorders you want to answer before you start talking with the person you know who has an eating disorder:

- ✔ How do you recognize the signs that someone you care about has an eating disorder?
- ✔ What's an eating disorder about, and why do people have them?
- ✔ How do people with eating disorders get better?

Knowing the answers to these questions helps you keep in mind a bigger picture about the disorder and what the person you want to help needs. The person with the eating disorder can't be expected to comprehend this right now, so you may temporarily have to think for both of you.

Recognizing visible signs of an eating disorder

In Chapters 2, 3, and 4, I describe the major eating disorders the way a person may be experiencing them from the inside. In this chapter, I review the same eating disorders from your perspective, that is, by looking at them from the outside. From that outside perspective, eating disorders can be mighty confusing! So many people put an exaggerated emphasis on weight and dieting these days. What clues do you look for to tell you they've become more than that for the person you're worried about? The following sections flag the main warning signs.

General warning signs of an eating disorder

Some warning signs are common among all the eating disorders. These universal caution flags include the following behaviors with regard to the person who has an eating disorder:

✔ Preoccupation with weight and dieting

✔ Belief that she can only be worthwhile or okay if she's thin

✔ Depressed mood when she's not happy about her weight or how she's eating

✔ Severe self-criticism when she doesn't get things right

Signs specific to anorexia

The following symptoms may be an indication of anorexia. (**Note:** The person you suspect may have an eating disorder may show symptoms of both anorexia and bulimia, because sometimes these disorders have symptoms in common.) Be on the lookout for the following:

✔ Losing a significant amount of weight not explained by illness

✔ Losing normal menstrual periods

✔ Believing that she is fat, regardless of her weight and regardless of what you say

✔ Developing narrow, sometimes weird, food preferences

✔ Refusing to eat in front of others

✔ Cooking eagerly for others, but eating none of the food she prepares herself

✔ Wearing baggy clothes or layers of clothing to hide her size and shape

✔ Overdoing it with exercise (exercising too much, being upset if she has to miss a workout)

✔ Feeling too cold, even in warm temperatures or when warmly dressed

✔ Feeling dizzy or faint

Signs specific to bulimia

The following symptoms are common among people who have bulimia. If you suspect bulimia, be on the alert for these indicators:

✔ Binge eating (usually done in secret; your evidence may be missing food or a bread-crumb trail)

✔ Finding excuses to leave the table after a meal

✔ Signs of vomiting in the bathroom

✔ Evidence of excess laxative or diuretic use

✔ Swollen glands, so-called *chipmunk cheeks*

✔ Excessive exercise

✔ A pattern of weight fluctuations, usually in a 10- to 20-pound range

✔ Withdrawal from social activities

Signs specific to binge eating disorder

Some symptoms of binge eating disorder are similar to those of bulimia, which also involves bingeing behavior. You may notice the following:

✔ Binge eating (usually done in secret; your evidence may be missing food or a bread-crumb trail)

✔ A succession of various dieting attempts

✔ A pattern of small or large weight fluctuations

✔ Refusal to participate in social activities when she thinks she's too fat

Understanding what an eating disorder means to the person who has it

When you observe the person you know with an eating disorder, you may see someone who seems incredibly stubborn, out-of-control, sneaky, or dishonest. All these characteristics may actually be true on one level. But that's all the more reason for you to understand that life has come to feel completely unmanageable to her in many ways. Strange as it may seem, she is trying desperately to cope. Her eating disorder is her chief coping strategy. (But she doesn't know that.)

The person with an eating disorder feels woefully inadequate, although you may find this hard to believe. She may be a very high achiever, but inside she's always on the brink of failure in one way or another. She probably feels pressured by each new stage in life, whether that's adolescence, college, career, marriage, or parenthood. Her eating disorder may have started in response to the demands of one of these stages and worsened with each new one.

Dieting and weight loss are demands she understands. When the expectations of the outside world seem too big to handle, she can turn to a world where she feels a sense of control. She can feel in charge, or imagine being in charge, with the next diet. The same goes for pressures from the inside. The person with an eating disorder doesn't feel equipped to handle her emotions. So she turns to food and dieting for soothing and control. Maintaining this focus keeps her from feeling overwhelmed.

When you come in the name of health and healing, you recognize that the eating disorder is actually doing damage, but the sufferer feels threatened. What you offer are not strong motivators to her, because they appear to remove the very tools she relies on for coping and psychological survival! You need to stay strong and firm, especially in the early stages of recovery.

I discuss in detail how eating disorders serve as survival or coping strategies in Chapters 2–5. You also find this point of view in my discussion of treatment and recovery strategies, especially in Chapters 10 and 14.

Getting the basics of eating disorder treatment and recovery

Two factors are involved in the equation that comprises an eating disorder. In order to get those factors to add up to a successful recovery, both must be addressed. These two components are

- ✔ Reducing the eating disorder symptoms (dieting, weight loss, bingeing and purging)
- ✔ Developing the internal strengths and coping skills that reduce the chances of relapse.

If the eating disorder symptoms of the person you want to help are very severe and her health is at risk, the two parts of recovery need to come in this order: symptoms first, everything else second. Not only is survival at stake, but anorexia, in particular, also physically affects the brain in such a way that the sufferer's thinking becomes distorted. She may not be capable of addressing issues that require mental concentration until her symptoms are brought under control. (I discuss this in greater detail in Chapter 7.)

When symptoms aren't so high-risk, treatment doesn't always proceed in such an orderly fashion. The focus may be on recovery skills alongside symptom reduction, for example, with each improving a little at a time. Or a lot of recovery work may need to be done before you see a significant reduction in symptoms.

A key factor to keep in mind is that treatment is not a speedy process. The exception may be if you catch the eating disorder very early and the symptoms are very mild. Otherwise, be prepared to be patient. Even if symptom reduction goes fairly quickly (*quickly* being something like six months), recovery usually takes at least several years, and usually longer. What you get for your trouble, however, is more than just an eating disorder-free person. You witness the development of someone who's more resilient and better prepared to take on life's challenges.

In Chapter 9 I go over the various treatment options you may need to think about in the beginning. I explain how symptom severity guides choices about the right kind of intervention for the person with an eating disorder and the personnel you need to get the job underway.

Being Ready with Resources

You're better prepared to tackle and survive the initial conversation with the person with an eating disorder when you've already thought a few steps beyond the conversation to what needs to happen next. Knowing how to get started with a treatment process makes you more helpful to the person with an eating disorder when you finally speak. In this section I go over how resource preparation varies, depending on who you're dealing with, and I explain how to use this book to begin your search for treatment resources.

What's the hurry?

Maybe you're typically not a planner and you're thinking, "Why can't I talk to the person first, see how that goes, and then start thinking about treatment?" To answer the question, you may find it helpful to look to people with experience in helping families approach addicted members.

Is preparation the same for everyone?

Just what kind of resource preparation you need depends a lot on the age of the person with the eating disorder and your relationship to her. Here are a few guidelines:

- ✔ **If this is your preadolescent child:** Have a medical exam already scheduled or at least locate a doctor who can help you. Preselecting a family therapist and talking with her ahead of time is also a good idea. (Look ahead to the next section, "Gathering Support," for ways to get the most from this conversation.)

- ✔ **If this is your adolescent child:** Have some therapists' names on hand but also be prepared for some level of negotiation. (This, of course, depends on the severity of your child's symptoms. Your daughter's voting rights about treatment diminish if her situation is life-threatening!)

- ✔ **If you're dealing with an adult:** Come with a few referrals (therapists or treatment programs). Of course, the person with the eating disorder may or may not accept them.

Interventions

Interviews called *interventions* are a well-known motivational tool. Interventions bring together everyone significant in the addicted person's life to express their support and concern or fear. In the best-case scenario, an intervention ends by whisking the now-motivated addicted person into treatment. Space in a rehab program is ready and waiting, prepared ahead of time for this moment of increased motivation.

Even if your conversation isn't as dramatic as an intervention, the idea to hold on to is that when the person with an eating disorder expresses some willingness to seek treatment, you want to be prepared to act. Readiness can come and go when something feels this scary. Expect it to feel scary.

Where do I start looking?

Chapter 9 and the "Resource Guide" at the end of this book are two excellent places to start looking! In Chapter 9 I review how to search for community sources of treatment, such as clinics and hospital- or university-based programs, professional networks, or word-of-mouth resources.

In the "Resource Guide" you find names of a number of organizations that maintain lists of eating disorder specialists and treatment facilities on the Internet. The Internet has become *the* information resource for so many people these days that most programs and facilities have a page for you to investigate. This is less true for individual practitioners like doctors and therapists.

Gathering Support

Just what you need in the way of support depends a lot on your relationship with the person who has the eating disorder. If you're a parent or other family member who will be deeply involved in the treatment process over a long period, your needs are different from those of the concerned co-worker who may or may not have an ongoing relationship with the person who has the eating disorder. To reach your goal, you may need three kinds of support right now:

✔ **Help in getting the job done:** Other people may have as big a stake in the conversation you're facing as you do. Maybe these people can also be present. Or maybe they can help you think through how you want to handle the situation and supply moral support.

✔ **Advice about what to do:** Handling a situation like this may be above your pay grade. Sometimes talking to people who have more experience than you do is crucial — or at least helpful.

✔ **Emotional support:** Chances are you've already been through a lot of upset about this situation. You're worried about the eating disorder sufferer. You don't know exactly what you're supposed to do. You don't know how your intervention is going to turn out. This is a recipe for stress. (I devote Chapter 24 to the support you may need throughout the recovery process.)

In this section I focus first on families and the value of planning together how to talk to the person with the eating disorder. I then discuss the kinds of support you may need from outside the family. Last, I discuss the situations of people who are getting ready to bring up an eating disorder with a non-family member.

Making a plan with other family members

If the person with an eating disorder is a family member, there's no time like the present to rally the troops! An eating disorder affects everyone in the family, and everyone can contribute to making the situation better.

You may decide that a two-parent talk with your child is the best way to go. (Make that one-parent if you're raising your kids on your own.) This makes particular sense if your other children are quite small. Or maybe you're convinced the child with the eating disorder will feel ganged-up on rather than supported if everyone's along for the ride at this stage. On the other hand, you may decide your child with the eating disorder is most likely to respond to an appeal from everyone. (I go over specific strategies for this conversation in Chapter 22.)

My main point right now is less about who you finally include when you speak to your child with the eating disorder and more about beginning the process of bringing the family together for support and problem-solving. Your child with an eating disorder will need lots of help in the days to come. But so will you.

Finding support for yourself

A lot of potential exists for feeling alone and overwhelmed when you first take on a strange and upsetting disorder, especially when that disorder is afflicting your child! Make sure you don't become isolated as you work on becoming informed and finding resources for her. Be certain that the people you trust and rely on — family, friends, co-workers — know what you're going through, what steps you're taking, and how it's going. Let them care about you!

Sometimes the best support in the world from family and friends still doesn't meet all your needs. Two good reasons for seeking professional help now, before you've even spoken to your child are

1. You're so upset that your own emotions, such as anxiety or depression, are taking center stage.

   You're entitled to be upset. A child with an eating disorder is upsetting! But you probably want to be as calm and centered as possible when you speak to your child. If speaking to family and friends doesn't help you enough with your feelings, you have a perfectly legitimate reason to use professional services.

2. You're confused about the best way to proceed.

   You aren't expected to know how to handle an eating disorder. Some kids present bigger challenges than others. Maybe you already have hints that your daughter denies anything is wrong. Maybe she's angry and seems impossible to talk to, even about noncontroversial topics. You can go in armed with a few ideas from someone who's already been there.

Two experts you can call on now may be in your future anyway. The first is a family therapist. Family therapy is a very good idea for your daughter's treatment. You don't have to wait! A family therapist can give you guidance about your child at this planning stage as well as during treatment.

The second possibility is an individual counselor or therapist for yourself. I discuss this possibility in more detail in Chapter 24. The point is, you don't have to take care of everything for your child first. Making sure you're alright as this process begins is not only okay — it's a superior idea!

Seeking support in nonfamily situations

The person you're seeking help for may not be your child, but that doesn't mean you don't feel the need for support. The less out-and-out responsibility you have for the person with the eating disorder, the less solid ground you may feel you have to stand on to speak up. If the person you want to help is

✔ **Your friend:** Are you underage? You may want to get your parents' support. Not so comfortable with that? How about a school guidance counselor? Avoid speaking with the person's other friends. She may feel betrayed when she finds out. If you're an adult, you probably have friends who don't know the person. Speaking with them is okay.

✔ **Your roommate:** If you're in a college dorm situation, by all means, speak to the dorm's resident head. You don't have to be in this alone. You can also get advice and support from your college's student counseling services.

If this is a roommate in the adult world, enlisting the support of friends and family is a good place to start. How much more support you need depends on how dire your roommate's situation is and/or how much her behavior (such as stealing food) intrudes on you. You may appreciate some temporary professional counseling about high-risk situations. For instance, when is it okay to call in her family? How about emergency medical workers? When do you call it a day with the roommate arrangement, no matter how convenient it is or how fond you are of the person?

✔ **Your employee or co-worker**: Put this book down (just for the moment) and go speak to someone in your human resources department! You need to know company policy and procedure. You need a chance to vet your mission. Are you implementing policy? Are you there purely as an expression of personal concern? How does your professional relationship with the person with the eating disorder influence the answer to these questions? You need backup — perhaps legal, probably emotional — if you're going to be the point person for this conversation.

Chapter 22

Implementing Your Plan to Help

. . . .

In This Chapter

▶ Understanding what you're trying to accomplish

▶ Recognizing some useful do's and don'ts

▶ Knowing how to deal with anger and denial

. . . .

You're about to change things in your house. You're convinced of your child's eating disorder. You've been gathering your courage and preparing your plan (see Chapter 21). Now you're ready to break the silence. Maybe you'll end up feeling like you've temporarily turned your household upside down. Or, instead, you may feel like you've broken a spell hanging over it. But one thing is certain. You will have started the clock ticking toward your child's recovery.

In this chapter I outline what you can expect to accomplish, some guidelines on how to approach the person with the eating disorder, and some ideas on handling the very common responses of anger and denial. I write this chapter specifically for parents, but include a section at the end for other relationships, such as spouses and roommates.

Knowing What You're Out To Accomplish

You know those times when you've stored up what you wanted to say for so long that when you finally speak, every thought you ever had on the subject comes spilling out? That's not what you want to do when you have the first conversation with your eating disordered child.

A better approach is to focus on a few realistic goals for your conversation (see Chapter 21). You may find it reassuring to know that you don't have to get to the bottom of what may be causing your child's eating disorder today. Or figure out how to solve it today. Or even get a firm commitment to treatment today. Today, or whenever you plan to do it, you just need to have the conversation, for better or for worse.

Actually, for this conversation, small is big. I know that may sound weird, but I want you to really embrace this little truth. "Small is big" means that seemingly small steps can have big effects. What may not appear to be a very big outcome to shoot for can turn out to have significant results down the rocky road of recovery. Look at it this way: One teensy tiny positive thing (like having the first conversation) could be just the nudge that starts your child on the right trajectory toward recovery. And you will have started the process instead of feeling stuck where you are.

In this section I go over some reasonable outcomes to look for in a first conversation with your child about her eating disorder and the bigger effects they can have in the future.

Keeping your eyes on the small, reasonable goals can serve as your internal navigating system. When you're tempted to veer off course or the conversation actually does go off the road (it will!), you'll have a reliable guidance system to nudge you back on track.

Getting the problem out in the open

If everyone's been tiptoeing around the eating disorder, that famous rhinoceros on the table that no one speaks about, finally getting it out in the open can be a big relief. This is true even if the conversation doesn't go so well, merely because you've at least acknowledged that the rhino is there.

After you name the problem — anorexia, bulimia or binge eating disorder — you enter a new chapter. You may fight about it, cry about it, misunderstand each other about it, or problem-solve about it. But you won't be pretending about it anymore. Your child will ultimately respect you for having the courage to reach out, and she'll appreciate it one day. Because she isn't able to tell you this now, I am.

Starting the process of talking

By having this conversation with your child, you are setting an example. This small-but-big goal is especially meaningful if your family doesn't have a tradition of being out in the open about unpleasant things. Kids observe these patterns and take them as their parents' expectations. Your child may have even assumed you needed (or wanted) protection from a conversation like this.

You may not get very far today. But you've established that the eating disorder is something you're prepared to talk about. This is HUGE. There may be other obstacles to talking in the future, but your child now sees that you aren't reluctant to talk about them and tackle them.

Making your concern clear

Later in this chapter I offer some guidelines for the tone to set when you talk with your child about her eating disorder. You'll follow them imperfectly and say things you'll later wish you hadn't. But what your child will get, for all the fumbling, is that *it matters to you* that she's in trouble.

If you can keep just one guideline in your mind when you go to speak to her, remember that your caring and concern are what matter most to her. Set your internal navigator on this goal and you'll find a way to say what you need to that carries the message of your concern. And no matter what she says, she really does hear you.

For example, Carolyn and Pete Jones were sure they'd done everything wrong when they spoke to their 14-year-old, Samantha, to tell her they suspected she had anorexia. The conversation ended with Samantha screaming: "You just want to control me and ruin my life!" One night, six weeks later, the couple turned in to bed, worried sick like every other night. On one of their pillows they found an essay Samantha had written for her high school English class. The topic was "Modern Day Knights." Carolyn and Pete laughed and cried as they read about themselves as knights who'd ridden into the dragon's lair, knowing the dragon was Samantha's anorexia and not Samantha. Scribbled by hand on the back was the note: "Can we talk? No fire-breathing, I promise!"

Suggesting treatment

Most of the time, it's appropriate to at least put the suggestion for treatment on the table in your first conversation with your child. How this part of the conversation goes depends on

✔ **Your child's age:**

- **Preadolescent children:** This is usually a matter of explaining to your child the treatment that you've already arranged.

- **Adolescents:** You always want to look for some degree of choice you can offer. Whether getting treatment at all is a choice depends on how serious your child's symptoms are.

- **Adult children:** As with any other adult, you express your concern, and ask if your suggestions would be appreciated. (See the section "Dealing with Anger and Denial" for how to handle life-threatening situations where you have neither control nor your adult child's cooperation.)

✔ **The severity of your child's symptoms:** If the situation doesn't seem severe and your child accepts the conversation and suggests a reasonable plan of action that doesn't involve therapy, you may consider it. But don't leave it open-ended. Put your child's plan within a time frame that includes measureable milestones with positive results. If she misses deadlines or results are poor, then put your plan in place.

If you need to insist on treatment, look for other options you can offer. This week or next? Does she want to meet with the family therapist alone first? Any guidelines for picking her own therapist? However, the options should not be endless and must result in action.

✔ **How the rest of the conversation has gone:** If treatment is necessary but the conversation has really gone south (she's angry, overwhelmed, or in denial), table the treatment discussion for the time being. But make clear why you're postponing it and that you'll get back to it eventually. In fact, you may want to set a date to talk again.

Laying the groundwork for future conversations

Getting the eating disorder out in the open and establishing that it's something you're ready, willing, and able to discuss is, in itself, a huge accomplishment. Whatever progress you're able to make in the first conversation is good enough for that conversation. Sometimes it's useful to stop and let things percolate, let everyone calm and cool down if the talk becomes heated, and let everybody regroup if you reach an impasse.

Stepping back and letting what has been said sink in is a positive step. We all need time to consider new ideas. Initial resistance to even the tamest of new ideas is not unusual, and what you are suggesting is a big, life-changing deal to your daughter. But, most of us, given time, come around to new ideas once our emotions have settled and reason takes over. In fact, stepping back and letting your daughter take time to think about what you've said, even if she has yelled and screamed and nothing has been resolved, may help her be more receptive later on.

Once the conversation has started, you won't be starting from scratch the next time around. You'll be picking up conversational threads from your first discussion. If things didn't go so well the first time, picking a thread can actually be quite helpful. Starting with one of your child's threads the second time around can be a great way to show you were listening and to set in motion a possible repair process. For example, you can say something like the following:

✔ "You know, I've been thinking about what you said about some of our family's eating patterns and I think you make a good point."

✔ "I don't think I actually got what you were trying to say about feeling criticized. Could you try me again?"

✔ "If we did things the way you suggest, how do you think that would work out? What's your worst worry about doing it the way we suggest?"

By inviting her to continue the conversation in a nonthreatening way, you express your respect and genuine concern. Be sure to listen carefully and to seriously consider what she says.

Knowing Some Important Do's

It's always useful to have some positive behaviors to point yourself *toward*. In this section I review some "do's" to help you navigate that opening talk about your child's eating disorder. In fact, these are pretty much all-purpose "do's" that can take you through any follow-up conversations as well.

Do be calm and centered

Although you can't really instruct yourself to be calm and centered, you can aim to be. (By *centered* I mean having a certain confidence in what you're saying and doing, trusting where you're coming from.) What can you do to help yourself be more calm and centered? Here are a few things that have helped others:

✔ **Plan ahead what you want to say:** You probably won't be able to think of all your best points and how you want to say them in the heat of the moment.

✔ **Go over your plan with someone you trust:** You don't have to think of everything or anticipate every response on your own.

✔ **Write things down:** Some people organize their thoughts best on paper.

✔ **Alert your support system:** Make sure the important people in your support system know what you're doing and when you're doing it as far as this talk goes. You don't have to feel alone.

✔ **Reassure yourself:** Think of the parts of the conversation that worry you most. When have you successfully handled something similar?

✔ **Picture a successful outcome:** Even if what you picture is pie-in-the-sky, it allows you to feel calmer. (Try it out right now and see what happens.) Here's the bonus: The calm feelings will positively affect the way you speak to your child. Who's to say you won't get the outcome you want?

Do say clearly what you mean

"Say what you mean and mean what you say," is an old adage that works here. It may cause a lot more squirming now, but your child is going to trust you more if you put your cards right out on the table. You can say something like

- ✔ "We're more and more worried about your dieting. We don't think it's healthy. I'd like us to talk about it."

- ✔ "I've been finding empty laxative packages in the garbage. I read about purging. Is that what you're doing?"

- ✔ "When kids quit seeing their friends, it usually means something is wrong. You haven't been spending much time with us either. I think we need to discuss it. I want to help."

You're constantly setting an example of what's okay to say. Your child also takes what you say as a gauge for what you're able to tolerate hearing her say. If your child wants to avoid any confrontation with her eating disorder, your vagueness just helps her do so. She needs the example of your bravery to eventually find her own.

Do report your own reactions and concerns

The point of sharing your feelings, besides getting your concern across, is to give your child some feedback on how her eating disorder behavior is affecting you and other people in the family. For example:

- ✔ It frightens you that she's so thin and seems so unaware of it.

- ✔ It upsets you on her behalf to see her pull away from her friends and spend more and more time alone. She doesn't look so happy.

- ✔ It makes you angry to grocery shop one day, only to find the shelf half empty the next.

- ✔ Her brother and sister are complaining about the way they find the bathroom after she's been in there purging.

All these reactions and any more like them are important for her to hear. She's seeing through a much distorted lens right now. You're providing her with some reality. This includes the reality of what her family members can and can't tolerate in her behavior. It also includes the normal reactions of loved ones watching a family member being reckless with herself, possibly with her life.

Do make it clear that you don't expect your child to do anything about your feelings. You can take care of those yourself. You're providing information about how you see her eating disorder affecting her and what it's like to live with it.

Please notice that blame and accusation statements usually start with "you," as in, "You're a sneak and a liar." On the other hand, statements about your own reactions and feelings start with "I," like "I get angry when I think you clean out the cupboards after I shop and you don't tell me." Couples in treatment are frequently encouraged to use these so-called *"I" statements* to help manage conflict. "I" statements allow you to make your point without assassinating the other person's character. (Note: Saying "I'm angry that you're a sneak and a liar" is cheating!) Telling your daughter you feel terrified and powerless when she doesn't eat has the effect of reducing blame and putting the two of you on the same team to fight her eating disorder.

Do be prepared to listen

You may either have so much to say in this conversation or be so nervous about it or so fed up that it's hard to be open to your child's side of things. Slow down. Breathe. Write the following instructions on your wrist, if you need to: *Stop and listen.*

Listening is a profound sign of respect. Your child instinctively feels that respect. It goes far toward keeping her engaged in this difficult conversation. But — this is an important thing for you to know — the respect you're showing is for your child, not necessarily for what she is saying. Listening isn't an endorsement of what you hear. It's just listening.

What else do you get for your trouble when you take the time to listen to your child?

- **You model a good skill for difficult conversations:** You show your child that she can rely on you.

- **You may find out something:** Maybe you didn't know how badly she got teased last year for extra weight. All the dieting started because she vowed not to get the same treatment in high school.

- **You may understand your child better:** You may not have known that your straight-A child always feels like a failure and a fake about to be found out.

- **You may hear something important to take into consideration moving forward:** You had no idea she's depressed so much of the time. At minimum, her depression needs to be evaluated. It may be part of what needs to be treated along with her eating disorder.

Of course, hearing many of these things can break your heart. All the more reason to make sure your own support system is in place. (For more details, see Chapter 24.) A reminder: Your child can't be part of your support system!

Do be supportive

You want to be sure the things you say convey your support for your child. This may be easier if you remember that you're supporting your child, not her eating disorder. And you're certainly not supporting rude or disrespectful behavior. Support is not a message that *anything goes*. It's a message that you love your child and that you'll do everything you can to see her reach her highest star in life, *whatever that is for her.*

More specific to the eating disorder, your child needs to know you're in it with her to find solutions. And even if she can't see her way out right now, let her know that you have faith in her strengths. Remind her that she's done other hard things. She can do this. And she has you behind her.

Do encourage your child to take responsibility for her eating disorder

You may feel sorry for your child. You may be furious with her. You may see her as a helpless victim of something bigger than her. Nevertheless, you must start conveying your expectations that she be responsible for as much of her eating disorder as she can. She can't fix the fact of having an eating disorder. But right now she can

- Acknowledge having the disorder and the extent of it.

- Agree to necessary treatment.

- Be responsible for her eating disordered behaviors and how they affect others in the family. (For example: cleaning up after herself, replacing filched food, helping pay for binges, and so forth. I discuss this in more detail in Chapter 23.)

As you can see, some of these items can't be achieved in one sitting. For example, denial is part of having anorexia. And hiding symptoms in shame is part of bulimia and binge eating disorder. Expecting your child to become responsible is a stance. You and your child will work toward her meeting the expectation. Even if it takes a while, you're sending an important message of your faith that she can do the right thing.

All of these guidelines can seem pretty daunting, like a recipe for sainthood rather than a conversation with your kid. Remember, you won't get it all right and you don't have to. There will be other conversations on other days. And each will offer a chance for do-over and repair. Not a bad lesson for a child who thinks things have to be perfect, right?

Avoiding Some Important Don'ts

You know that old expression: "It isn't what you say; it's how you say it"? In this section I focus on some typical pitfalls that can easily derail your conversation right at the start. They relate to when not to speak, how not to speak, and what not to speak.

Don't choose a time when one of you is already upset

Don't sit down for that eating disorder talk when you or your child is already really upset about something else. Okay, this one is relative. You're probably kind of upset just because you're planning this conversation. But you can avoid times when some other argument or crisis is center stage. For example, maybe you and your child just fought about her grades, you just learned your mother has to be hospitalized, or you and your partner just had a major meltdown about the electric bill. These are not the best times to have your first eating disorder discussion.

If your family is like most, you could wait forever for a moment of perfect peace and calm. But on the other hand, it's okay to wait until the floodwaters from one storm have receded before you blow into town with another. Especially one that's bound to challenge the levees like your child's eating disorder.

Don't accuse or blame

Think of a time when someone — employer, family, friend — wanted you to change something and the conversation went well. Now think of a time when somebody wanted a change and the conversation didn't go so well. What was the difference? It probably had something to do with the way each person made you feel about yourself.

When you include blame or accusations in your conversation, your child starts out a leg down. She has to defend herself. Here are some examples of remarks that can easily slip into the conversation when you're under distress but are guaranteed to put your child on the defensive:

- "Don't you know how you're upsetting your mother?"
- "We can't enjoy ourselves anymore because of you."
- "You're all skin and bones!"
- "You're a sneak and a liar."
- "We didn't raise you to behave like this."

Here are the biggest problems with putting your child on the defensive:

- ✔ You unintentionally place yourself on the team opposing your child, when what you want is to start building teamwork between you. You want it to be you and her against the eating disorder.

- ✔ When your child is busy defending herself from accusations, she isn't hearing the more important parts of your message.

- ✔ If your child has an eating disorder, she already feels worthless. She'll just use remarks from you that sound blameful as more fodder for her own self-blame mill. (Even if she defends herself to you!)

Don't plead

Children with eating disorders already have very distorted views about their control in life. If your child has anorexia, she imagines she has ultimate control. If she has bulimia or binge eating disorder she feels completely out of control. Either way, she needs her parents to have better ideas than she does about how to be in control of the situation.

What does this have to do with pleading? When you plead with your child to cooperate or "stop having" her symptoms, you suggest that you have little to offer to help her. The responsibility for finding a way out is all on her. She's already demonstrated she doesn't know how to get out of this jam on her own. She needs to know you have more confidence and direction than she does (which is not the same as having all the answers!).

Don't threaten

Surprisingly, when you threaten your child, you sound just as out of control as when you plead. Threatening is the kind of thing you do when you feel helpless and don't have any other ideas. Whether your child can put it in those words or not, that's how your threatening comes across to her, too. And that makes her feel angry and frightened. No matter how she fights you, she needs to feel you're equipped to help her find a way out of her eating disorder predicament.

Don't ask whether it's your fault

The moment you ask your child if she blames you for her eating disorder, two things happen, and you don't want either of them.

✔ First, the conversation becomes about you. There's a place for your feelings. (See the earlier section, "Do report your own reactions and concerns.") But asking your child to manage your guilt feelings isn't part of that picture. It isn't her job, and she can't really do it for you anyway. Goodness knows, your feelings of guilt are a big part of this story. And you should take them seriously. But you want to look for adult support. (Chapter 24 focuses on how you can get the support you need.)

✔ Second, she reads it as you needing protection. That makes her less likely to share difficult feelings. And, just like with the pleading, she doesn't know whether she can lean on you. This doesn't mean you're not allowed to show you're upset. That would feel phony. It means you can't ask your child to fix your feelings. You need to let her know you've got that base covered. She can focus on getting better herself.

Dealing with Anger and Denial

You could avoid every "don't" and do every "do" and still meet with a tantrum or even, "I don't know what you're talking about." Back to the drawing board and square one? Not at all. Actually, your plan needs to include expectations of these angry or denying reactions. They're pretty common when you confront people with eating disorders. In this section I focus on your responses to them. First, I give you a little food for thought that may help you digest them better. Second, I offer some ideas for responding to your angry or denying child.

People don't easily give up their survival strategies

If you are shocked and furious at your child's denial or lack of cooperation, I don't have any magic that can make you feel okay. But I invite you to do the following tiny exercise:

✔ Think of the moment in that first encounter, or any other, that she most drove you up the wall. . . Picture her really vividly. . . Got it?

✔ Now imagine that you are witnessing someone who is fighting for her life. . . What effect does that have on what you see?

How do people behave when they are fighting for their lives? One thing I know for sure is that they don't easily surrender their survival strategies.

I advise you to do two things at times like these:

1. Spend some quality time with anyone and anything that reminds you you're a good person and a good parent. Your eating disordered child can't do that for you right now.

2. Go back to basics about eating disorders. Your child believes she'll be worthless if she can't control her weight with her eating disorder. You become the force of darkness if you threaten to take it away.

Keep the faith. Everyone is basically programmed for health and life, including your child. Kids haven't lived long enough to see the big picture, one that holds more options than an eating disorder as a way to feel worthwhile. You have to be the one who knows about that bigger picture until your child can see it too.

She hears you, no matter how she responds

The eating disorder is the face your child is showing to the world right now. It isn't all there is to her (thank goodness!) She's still capable of hearing the healthy and caring things you say. Your child is stashing your messages away, even while she rejects them to your face, like a squirrel stashing nuts for the winter. (If your child is an adolescent, try substituting "angry teen" for "eating disorder" in this paragraph. You've got both of them!)

The main thing to remember is that your child hears what you say, no matter how she responds. This isn't a recommendation that you simply keep talking at her while she continues with her eating disorder. You may have to take other steps, as I discuss later in the section "Deciding when you need to take action." But in the meantime, keep those healthy and caring messages coming! You'll want to make sure the messages are affirmations about her or your relationship unrelated to food or weight. (Read more about this in Chapter 23.)

Arguing puts the focus back on you

It's a good idea to know when a conversation is no longer useful — or not useful in its present form. Getting drawn into an argument is one of those not-useful times. Teenagers can be particularly skilled at using arguments to avoid a subject. It gets the focus off them and on you. For example, your teenager may say

✔ "Why are you always accusing me of things I don't do?"

✔ "How I eat is none of your business."

✔ "You should see the way Dad eats."

✔ "I defy you to find one girl in my class who isn't dieting. Nobody else's mom is making a big deal of it."

✔ "You're the one who told me I have to be disciplined about exercise if I want results."

If you're mad or feeling defensive, you can walk right into it. In fact, be certain that at least sometimes you will. The trick is to notice you're in it and get back on track. If you can do that within the same conversation, go to the head of the class! Sometimes it works to point out the maneuver:

✔ "You've done a good job of getting us to talk about me. Okay, now let's get back to the part about you."

This is where that idea of being centered — trusting your mission — can be so useful. Your knowledge or suspicion that your child is seriously harming her health and well-being may help you cut through a lot of flack. You can respond by saying:

✔ "I know this is hard to talk about. But we can't avoid it anymore. Your health is too important."

✔ "We can take up your complaints about me once I'm not so frightened about your health. Right now that has to come first."

Finally, you're not required to keep pitching once the conversation has become unproductive and there's no getting it back on track. You can tell your child you don't think the way the conversation is going is helping. Taking a breather can be framed as a useful strategy. You can also forecast getting back to it with a clear head and maybe some fresh ideas.

Deciding when you need to take action

Your first approach and follow-ups may convince you that you need to do more than have a heart-to-heart to move the ball up court. You may need to step in with parental controls to protect your child by

✔ **Insisting on treatment:** Some parents become so intimidated by their kid, their kid's anger, or by the eating disorder itself, they don't know that it's okay and often necessary to simply insist. Surprisingly, your child is often just waiting for you to do this.

✔ **Using leverage:** Don't be afraid to use the controls you have. You're not required to give your child access to all the goodies and experiences she wants if she's not cooperating with treatment. This includes going away to school. Some parents find this unthinkable. But consider: Would you send your child off to school with uncontrolled diabetes? Or a drug addiction?

✔ **Taking emergency measures:** If your child is refusing treatment and her health is in serious jeopardy, you can't wait. (I review the warning signs for emergency hospitalization in Chapter 9.) You'll want to involve your child's doctor. The nightmare for families is when police have to be called in for older teens or adult children. One encouraging note is that even people who are hospitalized involuntarily for anorexia appear to benefit from it.

Don't hesitate to seek out an eating disorder expert if you need support or advice for dealing with your child at this point. The best place to start is with a family therapist who specializes in eating disorders. Family therapy is probably going to be part of your child's treatment plan. The therapist is a good person to coach you through this early stage.

Chapter 23

Making Life Livable While Supporting Another's Recovery

*T*his chapter is about the day-to-day struggles of living with someone who has an eating disorder for the long haul of recovery. (I take the perspective of a parent working with a child, but the principles apply to other relationships as well.) The appearance of an eating disorder on your doorstep presents you with many dilemmas and demands for skills you don't find in the basic parenting manual. For instance, you need to master the delicate dance of disengaging from responsibility for your child's eating disorder symptoms while holding her accountable for the effects these symptoms have on you and other family members. You have to find out how to separate support for her recovery from control of her disorder. And, just as important, you need to start moving the eating disorder off the center stage of family life.

In this chapter I identify the skills you need to survive and thrive during your child's recovery. I discuss how to handle the common obstacles parents run into when trying to put these skills into practice. Finally, I tell you how to recognize when you've fallen into *recovery traps,* obstacles that may require outside help in order for you to move forward.

At the end of each section, where relevant, I include notes for people who aren't parents but live with or have an ongoing relationship with someone with an eating disorder.

Letting Go and Ending the Food Wars

When you and your child agreed she'd go into treatment for her eating disorder, the agreement included putting her in charge of her own recovery. This is not an arrangement someone drew out of a hat; rather, it's the only arrangement that can work. Your job with respect to the eating disorder is to pull out of your child's frontline struggle with food and weight so she can find her own way. This is a time when you can go back to being mom or dad instead of therapist or food police. In this section I discuss why that's so important, what makes it so hard, and how you can actually go about doing it.

Understanding why letting go is so hard

After your child has begun treatment, you still may have a strong parenting urge to step in and "help." If this urge is really strong, ask anyone who's ever tried to stop drinking for an alcoholic friend or relative how well that went. You can't do it for them. Putting your child in charge of her own recovery is easier said than done. But it is absolutely the right thing to do.

In fact, you may actually find it helpful to read some Al-Anon literature (Al-Anon is a support organization for families of people addicted to alcohol) or attend an Al-Anon meeting. The controls and ways of seeing herself that your child needs to get well can only come from inside her.

But powerful forces may be pulling you in the opposite direction. Understanding these forces and recognizing that they're normal equips you to resist them. It's natural to be plagued by thoughts like the following:

- **You're the parent, so it's your job to fix things:** Seeing her with her eating disorder makes you feel, by turn, guilty, frightened, angry, frustrated, and helpless. Not only is it human nature to want to fix these feelings, but you also want to make *her* do something to fix them! You're used to being in charge of working out problems that come up in your family and helping your kids when they're in trouble. However, the eating disorder is now being worked out between your child and the therapist. This means you are now free to truly be a parent.

- **You feel that the consequences of the eating disorder are too great to simply stand by:** Visible signs of the disorder are a stab in any parent's heart, especially if the child has anorexia. But you aren't just standing by. You took the initiative to have "the talk," and you are providing the means for your child to be in recovery. Besides, you don't want to get pulled back in because becoming re-engaged in struggling over what she eats and weighs takes the focus off of her recovery. You may feel like you're helping, but you're not.

Does this mean there's nothing you can do? Absolutely not! Your child still needs you in all the usual ways children need their parents. I talk about how important that is later in this chapter. You may also find it reassuring to recognize that you actually are doing something — something *helpful* — by disengaging from the frontlines of her fight with her eating disorder. You're sending a powerful signal that you believe she's capable of handling it (even if sometimes you have to do it by sitting on your hands with your fingers crossed!). That's *huge* to a child who feels inadequate so much of the time. It means more to her coming from you than from anybody else on the planet. P.S. It's perfectly fine to put this message of faith in your child's ability to handle her eating disorder into words. Some parents even choose to write cards or letters conveying such a message to their children.

Disengaging from your child's disorder

When any kind of crisis involves a family member, everyone naturally focuses on the problem at the beginning. Family members feel frightened, lack information, and want to know how they can help. In the long-haul situation presented by an eating disorder, this initial period of intense activity and involvement needs to give way to the period of disengagement. *Not disengagement from your child, but from her eating disorder.*

There seems to be a fork in the road where some families are able to move more-or-less successfully into disengagement. (I say "more-or-less" because families, so far as I know, are still made up of imperfect people, and nothing about eating disorder recovery goes smoothly and simply.) How can you recognize whether you're still engaging with your child's eating disorder? If you're making statements similar to any of the following, you're still engaged:

- **Threatening:** "If you don't stop purging, I'm going to have you put away."

- **Pleading:** "If you only eat a little of this, it will make your dad so happy."

- **Cajoling:** "You can take a bite of this. I know you can do it."

- **Bargaining:** "If you gain five pounds, you can quit seeing the nutritionist."

- **Bribing:** "I'll give you $10 for every pound you gain."

- **Cheerleading:** "I see you've lost a few pounds. You look great in your jeans now. Keep up the good work!"

Did you hear yourself in any of these statements? If so, even though you feel like you're helping, you're actually not. In reality, pulling back from trying to manage your child's recovery sends an important message of confidence in her capabilities. Here are four more reasons to commit to disengagement:

- **When you get into a power struggle with your child over the eating disorder, you lose.** Eating disorders are a lesson in humility. The strength of the survival energy your child focuses through them is awesome.

- **By struggling with the eating disorder, you give it more prominence and power.** The more you make it a showdown between your will and the eating disorder, the more you give it center stage.

- **The more you focus on the eating disorder, the more other family members resent the person with the eating disorder.** She's robbing them of air time and negating the family's other interests.

- **All the patterns of engagement I just listed (threatening, bribing, and so on) suggest your child can just turn off the eating disorder if she wants to.** This is actually a very American idea: If you just put in enough incentive, you can make the change you want happen. But the motivation for eating disorder behavior actually has to do with desperately hanging onto feelings of personal control and worth. Threats, bribes, and the rest don't mean very much compared to these values.

Coming to terms with letting go

Many parents find the realization that *they* can't fix their child's eating disorder extremely hard to digest. The reality of being powerless over your child's eating disorder may stir up feelings of guilt, failure, or other negative emotions. The good news is that this is a normal reaction, and you can reason yourself out of the emotion and into the truth. The following examples begin with the negative emotional expression of a parent, and proceed to debunk the fallacy by replacing it with the truth, or reality:

- **"I don't matter in my child's life anymore."** Of course you do! Your child is more than her eating disorder. She will always need you in one way or another. The *way* she needs you will change, just as the way you needed your own parents changed over time.

The all-hands-on-deck Maudsley exception

In Chapter 12 I describe a family approach for the treatment of children and young adolescents who have anorexia that's the opposite of everything I just said. The Maudsley approach puts the family in charge of getting their child to eat and gain weight. It's completely hands-on in comparison to the hands-off recommendations I make in this chapter. What you need to know about Maudsley is that

1. The hands-on work is done under highly specific guidelines.

2. The hands-on phase ends when the child's weight takes her out of jeopardy. Then recovery reverts to the hands-off prescription for the family when it comes to eating disorder symptoms.

- ✔ **"I'm a failure as a parent."** Normal parenting doesn't include the treatment of eating disorders — as if you're a therapist! Keep in mind that children are independent beings who can and do make choices parents don't like. Other powerful influences in your child's life may contend with your best parenting.

- ✔ **If I can't control a problem in my child, can I control anything?** It's normal to feel like everything is falling apart in the middle of a crisis. Even the tiniest problem looms larger than it is. For reassurance, focus your efforts on other parts of your life that are not in crisis and not tied to the eating disorder.

Letting go is a good and positive act, and a natural part of all good parenting. Coming to terms with your inability to make your child get better means these three things are happening:

- ✔ **You and your child are moving on to a different kind of relationship:** Both of you are entering a stage of development in which "help" is more about moral support and example than trying to fix another person.

- ✔ **You're willing to change yourself to supply what your child needs most:** Remember when she needed you to help steer her bike? Remember the moment when she needed you to let go instead? Her eating disorder is just like that. The time comes when what your child needs most is for you to let go.

- ✔ **You're "getting it" about the eating disorder:** You're beginning to see your child's fight for identity and worth, which is tied up with the eating disorder. This is a sign of respect for your child's struggles.

If you find you're unable to make behavioral changes around control or you can't come to terms with this change of role in your child's life, you may want to talk it over with a counselor or therapist. Often the question of control can be very loaded with issues from your own history. It can be helpful to disentangle historic issues from the present.

You can't guarantee that your child will use the space and confidence you offer her to work toward an effective recovery. You can only be sure you'll block her efforts if you step in and try to manage her eating disorder yourself.

Taking "Fat Talk" Off the Table

"Fat talk" is your child's obsessive preoccupation with her own body weight and shape. You may start to wonder if she thinks about anything else. (Answer: Not much.) In this section I go over some important things to keep in mind when deciding how to interact with "fat talk."

Refusing to acknowledge "fat talk"

Engaging you in "fat talk" is one of the ways your child draws you in to her eating disorder. She may do this if you're being particularly effective at disengaging and she doesn't know how else to reassure herself you're still there. Or she may do it to test whether she can trust you to *really* back off. Or she may just do it because this is what somebody with an eating disorder does. How many times have you heard her ask

- ✔ "Do I look fat?"
- ✔ "Does this dress make me look fat?"
- ✔ "Have I gained weight?"
- ✔ "Are my thighs too big?"

My advice when you hear any of these? Run! It's a trap! Well, even if you don't run, you still need to know it's a trap. Someone with an eating disorder digests *anything* you say about weight and size badly. She doesn't trust the good stuff and she hammers herself with any negative stuff. You need to stake out your turf clearly with her: Tell her you're not going to respond to these questions precisely because they are no-win for her — and then remind her of that each time she asks again.

The dinner table version of "fat talk" is "calorie talk." The family meal shouldn't be dominated by eating disordered thinking. If your child still can't stop herself from counting every calorie, she at least needs to do it on her own time and not pull the family meal down with her. You can't make her better by reassuring her you used bouillon instead of fat, no matter how anxious she seems.

Cheering nonfat positives

Cheerleading involves making positive statements about developments in your child's weight as she progresses in recovery. For a person with anorexia, weight gain is progress. For someone with bulimia or BED, it may be weight loss. This kind of cheerleading is exactly what your child *doesn't* need. It's counterproductive.

The idea that cheering on her weight gain (or loss) is bad may be puzzling for you. What's wrong with supporting and complimenting progress? This is where it gets tricky with your child with an eating disorder. She simply can't engage in talk about size and weight in a healthy way, no matter what your intentions. What's more — and this is the most important point — she's convinced that size and weight are all that matter about her. The more you

---

Just say no to monitoring

People with eating disorders often ask partners, friends, or roommates to monitor their eating or purging behavior. Resist! It never works. You can't be with the person 24/7, which is what the operation requires. Besides, the only way the person you love is going to get better is by finding out how to install her own internal monitor. When you collude in a plan that suggests somebody else can do the work of recovery for her, you only help her put off the day when she has to come to terms with the need to do it herself.

---

comment on them, the more she believes you think the same thing. (She also notices how much you focus on your own size and weight and on those of other people.)

The most healing kind of support you can offer her right now is to notice progress that has nothing to do with her weight. Cheer on positive growth and maturity in every other area of accomplishment. For example:

- ✔ Her pursuit of a sport
- ✔ Her success on the debate team
- ✔ Her cleaning up her room
- ✔ Her helping a sibling with his homework

While you need to keep a hands-off approach with the eating disorder, you can be totally hands-on by providing nonfat-related sincere, positive, encouraging messages. This is an example of how you can really contribute to your child's recovery. After all, who doesn't like to hear positive encouragement!

Insisting on Accountability

An eating disorder isn't brain death. Adolescence isn't either. But people get confused about both. For the sake of both your family and your child with the eating disorder, you need to hold her accountable for her behavior, just like everybody else.

Eating disorder behaviors can affect other members of the family in a lot of ways. Not good ways. You may be allowing these negative behaviors to stand with no consequence because they're part of your child's disorder. Maybe you think if you can't control the disorder, you can't control anything related to it. Maybe you're accustomed to treating your child with the eating disorder with kid gloves, or maybe you're a little intimidated by her ability to get angry and withdraw.

These reactions on your part, especially a failure to set limits on the effects of eating disorder behaviors on others, have negative effects of their own. For example:

- ✔ Letting others be harmed without consequence makes the eating disorder a bigger and bigger part of family life.

- ✔ Allowing your child with the eating disorder to run roughshod over everyone else's rights just makes your other kids resent her.

- ✔ Not holding your child with the eating disorder to account for what she does tells her you think she can't control herself — something she's already afraid is true.

Paying for wrong behavior

If you can't just tell your child to cut it out with the eating disorder behaviors, what can you do? Try not to let the fact that the behaviors are based on an eating disorder negate your skills as a parent. You've been handling misbehavior in your kids for a long time. What do you do if one of your kids takes a toy or a book from another sibling? If it can't be returned, she has to find a way to pay for it, probably out of her allowance, right?

Food taken for bingeing is no different. Depending on how your family divvies up food, you may have to do some fancy footwork to figure out exactly what fine to assess. *But doing it is crucial.* It allows everybody else to feel they're living in a fair family, and it keeps the child with the eating disorder within the fairness fold. Other common examples in families include insisting that someone who binges clean up the kitchen after a binge and that someone who purges clean up the bathroom after she purges.

Making rules with roommates or spouses

You can't levy fines on a spouse or a roommate. But you can negotiate the effects of eating disorder behavior just the way you negotiate anything else in your relationship, like leaving dirty clothes on the bathroom floor or dishes in the sink. You may have to go to greater lengths than you like to divvy up food or figure out how to handle the situation when she binges her way through your favorite stuff while she's still symptomatic. But successful negotiating always strengthens relationships.

If a roommate with an eating disorder can't stick to rules you and she have agreed on, you may have to figure out your own bottom line for continuing to live with her. If this is your partner, you need to let her know how her failure to respect your agreement is harming the relationship.

Focusing Outside the Eating Disorder

This chapter is full of don'ts. *Don't* try to control the eating disorder. *Don't* comment on your child's weight. *Don't* let her run roughshod over the family with eating disorder behavior. With so many don'ts, is there anything positive you *can* do? Yes, actually, plenty! You can focus on other aspects of your child and other parts of family life that don't involve the eating disorder.

Seeing beyond the eating disorder

Just because you can't fix your child's eating disorder doesn't mean she doesn't need you anymore. Your child has wandered off into an obsession with food and weight. She's lost her way with growing up and engaging in the world, and seeing what matters most in life. Your steady focus on the bigger picture contributes to your child's recovery.

Putting the eating disorder in perspective

Think of your child as having different parts to her personality. Actually, she's just like everyone else this way. For instance, the demands of your workplace probably bring forward different aspects of yourself than a casual evening with your friends. Though your child may be leading with the eating disorder part of her personality right now, other aspects or parts are within her than can be drawn forward. What can you do to help bring forward the non-eating disorder parts of your child?

You can ask for normalcy. Keep expecting your child to do her share to help make the family run. Unless she needs hospitalization, she can do her chores. The eating disorder part of her may be behaving in a very young way. Insisting that she do her share for the family tells her you see another part of her that can be responsible and be a contributor like other kids her age.

You can emphasize enjoyable activities you two can share that have nothing to do with food and weight. What else have you two enjoyed doing in the past? Do you love to go antiquing? Do you both knit? Sail? Walk in the neighborhood to see what's new? Volunteer at the women's shelter? There's no guarantee that if you reach out to a part of your child that can enjoy such activities, your child will be able to reach back — at least not all the time. But by reaching out, you deliver the message that you see more to her than the eating disorder. The message isn't lost on her.

Taking recovery in phases

You can think of getting better from an eating disorder as having two phases. One involves reducing the acute symptoms of the disorder — dieting, restricting, bingeing, purging. The other involves building up an inner arsenal of personal strengths and qualities that help prevent relapse. This phase includes increasing self-esteem and developing a sense of identity and worth that doesn't depend on weight.

I say pretty clearly earlier in this chapter that your child has to be the one who takes control of her symptoms. When all is said and done, she's also the one in charge of her longer-term recovery. But you can be an important contributor. (You can read more about recovery skills in Chapters 8 and 14.)

The following is a list of milestones your child needs to achieve for a solid recovery. You can't force-feed any of them to her, any more than you can force-feed her food. But you can challenge your child's eating disordered way of thinking. And here's a suggestion that can have the most impact on her: You can do your best to model a healthier version in yourself. Important recovery milestones include

- **Knowing that worth doesn't depend on weight:** Even though your child has forgotten that other things matter about her besides her weight, you haven't. I mention earlier that you can specifically choose these other qualities to praise and support (see the section "Cheering nonfat positives"). Notice how much emphasis you give to your own weight versus other qualities, especially in your child's presence.

- **Living with imperfection:** You don't have to jump on board with your child's position that only perfection is good enough. You can cultivate a problem-solving approach to mistakes to replace her catastrophic one. Keep in mind that she gleans the most from how she sees you handle your own mistakes and imperfections.

- **Graying up black-and-white thinking:** Your child thinks things are all one way or another. If she makes a mistake, she's ruined everything. If you criticize her, everyone is against her. If she didn't make class delegate, high school is over for her and nobody likes her. You can challenge whether these extremes are actually the only possible responses. She needs help seeing that gray area exists between these extremes. You may want to talk out loud when you're looking for gray areas that don't involve your child: a compromise in a dispute, a number of possible ways to solve a dilemma, a moral situation that can be seen from different points of view, and so on.

- **Tolerating emotions:** Your child needs to discover that she can tolerate difficult feelings instead of trying to diet or binge her way out of them. You can help her by being available to talk about her feelings and making it clear that you're okay with those feelings, even if they're intense. You can also help by expressing feelings your child brings up in you. You can say, "That's making me angry" (or scared, or warm and fuzzy, or annoyed). The trick is to make sure your child knows you don't expect her to fix your feelings. Your child also picks up plenty from situations that don't involve her — when she sees that you're coping with difficult feelings, rather than hiding them or losing control.

✔ **Honoring relationship boundaries:** You don't read her mail. You don't ask what she said in therapy. You don't need to know the secrets between her and her sister (assuming they're safe and legal). You let her finish her thoughts. You don't assume her feelings and opinions are the same as yours. All of these are ways you convey that you see your child as a separate person and that's fine by you. People with eating disorders want to please others by agreeing. Your child may find it hard to believe that she's entitled to privacy or even has her own point of view. You can help!

Bringing "normal" back to family life

There's more to your child than her eating disorder. And there's more to your family than having a child with an eating disorder. Shifting all the focus to the eating disorder during a period of acute crisis is normal. (Usually this covers the time of intensifying symptoms, the initial talk, and the period of finding treatment.) But eating disorder recovery is a long-term project. Taking steps to move out of crisis mode and reclaim as much normal family life as possible is important for everyone.

The return to normal doesn't happen automatically. Instead, families typically start by simply reorganizing themselves around the requirements of the member with the problem. That's true whether the problem is an eating disorder, some other psychological disorder (like substance abuse or a phobia), or a chronic physical illness. Either due to guilt or exhaustion, other aspects of family life or the needs of other family members become secondary — which means they often get dropped altogether. Mealtimes and leisure times get particularly disrupted in families where a member has an eating disorder.

Enjoying mealtimes at home and dining out

Mealtimes are important times for coming together in many families. Family members who have gone their way during the day get to catch up with each other. People share fun, facts, ideas, and stories. When you have a child with an eating disorder, a lot of this may disappear. Mealtimes may become so tension-filled that other family members drift away to find a more peaceful place to eat. Or the menu may cater so much to eating disordered worries that nobody else wants to eat what's on the table. Or the person with the eating disorder may refuse to join the rest of the family.

How do you start to get life back to normal? Tell yourself, here and elsewhere, that as much as possible you're going to move the eating disorder off center stage. You've gone a long way in this direction if you've quit trying to control your child's eating and have taken "fat talk" off the table (suggestions I make earlier in the chapter). Next you need to promise yourself that the food preferences and phobias of the child with the eating disorder don't get to dictate everything you do around the dinner table. Here are a few guidelines for putting that promise into action:

- ✓ **Make what you normally make for family meals:** You have one child with an eating disorder, not an entire family. Plan meals for the healthy family, not the unhealthy eating disorder.

- ✓ **Don't make special meals for her:** She needs to be the one to take responsibility for her eating disorder. The more you move the effects of the disorder off your shoulders and onto hers, the more you help her grow up.

- ✓ **Negotiate her presence at the table:** This is especially important if meals serve that social gathering and sharing purpose in your family. If she can be there for the main course, but not dessert, then that's your deal. If she can't tolerate being there for any food right now, ask her to come at coffee time after dinner. Or arrange for everyone to be at the table for ten minutes before you serve the meal.

- ✓ **Don't go to eating disorder restaurants:** She gets her place in the rotation of restaurant choices only if she chooses places at least the majority of the family likes.

Having fun with leisure activities

Leisure activities — the fun, relaxing times — usually go overboard first with an eating disorder diagnosis. And they're usually last in line to return. The sad thing is that the family especially needs them after weathering such a crisis. Like mealtime, shared leisure is a chance for family members to feel a sense of being valued by each other, of belonging and well-being.

The child with the eating disorder is better off in a family that's gotten back to some shared leisure times, whether she can participate or not. Why is that true? Here are a few reasons:

- ✓ **She can always jump in:** She needs ways to practice being something other than eating disordered. And she needs to connect to her family in ways that have nothing to do with her eating disorder.

- ✓ **She gets reassurance that she hasn't ruined the family:** Family members with eating disorders carry around a lot of guilt for what they've put their families through.

- ✓ **She gets reassurance that she's not the queen of the family or the family bully:** The presence of other activities helps move the eating disorder off center stage. Kids aren't well-served by feeling they have the power to run their families, either directly or indirectly.

- ✓ **She gets some breathing room to take ownership of her eating disorder:** When everyone in the family isn't hovering over her eating disorder because they have other things to focus on, she's more likely to take responsibility for it herself.

> ✔ **She's being provided with a model of balance in life:** Most people with eating disorders aren't very good with the idea of living in a balanced way (for example, a balance of work and play). Perfect discipline is more what they have in mind as a model of the good life. Remember: She learns more from what you do than what you say.

You can't make your child's life better by sandbagging the rest of family life in the name of her eating disorder. You help her more by restoring sanity and health to the rest of your family. Rejuicing your family's shared leisure life is a way for you to put your instincts to *do* something to effective work.

Breaking through Recovery Traps

A *recovery trap* is anything that presents an obstacle to following through with the guidelines for recovery. Obstacles can come from inside you, such as feelings, beliefs, or fears. They can also be reactions you encounter in the person with the eating disorder.

Recovery traps are serious. They can stop a person's recovery in its tracks or slow it down to a trickle. They can also interfere with a family's recovery. (After all, you've been through plenty, too.) Don't wait to address them! Your situation will only get worse if you do.

In Chapter 11, I go over some common reasons families with eating disordered members seek out family treatment. If you're already in family treatment, this can be a great place to work out any of the recovery traps I list in this section. If you're not in family treatment, getting it can provide just the help you need to break through any recovery traps you may be stuck in.

Consider yourself in a recovery trap if you or other key family members

- ✔ Can't surrender efforts to control your child's weight or eating.
- ✔ Can't stop commenting on your child's weight gains and losses. (Not counting emergency situations where you think weight loss may require hospitalization or some different level of intervention than the current one.)
- ✔ Can't ask your child with the eating disorder to take responsibility for the effects of her behaviors on others.
- ✔ Can't follow through even when you set up such expectations.
- ✔ Can't ask your child with the eating disorder to do her share of family chores.
- ✔ Can't stop arranging meals to suit the child with the eating disorder.

✔ Can't bring yourself to arrange leisure activities for yourself or the rest of the family.

✔ Can't find anything to think about or talk about besides the eating disorder.

You may also be stuck in a recovery trap if

✔ Your entire relationship with your child with the eating disorder focuses on her eating disorder.

✔ Your family life revolves around the eating disorder.

✔ The child with the eating disorder doesn't comply with any of the expectations you set.

✔ The child with the eating disorder continues to boycott all aspects of family life (not counting adult children).

✔ The child with the eating disorder is seriously disrupting family life, for instance, with temper tantrums or stealing.

Your family therapist can help you in a number of ways. For instance, she may help you

✔ Discover fears or beliefs that block more appropriate recovery behavior

✔ Address your fears or beliefs in ways that don't harm your child's recovery

✔ Figure out rules and expectations that work for your family

✔ Explore ways to make your family life feel more satisfying

Families who use family treatment often find they get more out of it than resolution of their problems. In the process of solving problems, they usually gain insights and skills that make them stronger than when they started. Family members often feel they understand each other better and can solve problems on their own more effectively in the future.

Chapter 24

Finding Support for Yourself While Supporting Another's Recovery

* *

In This Chapter

▶ Recognizing the need for counseling or support for yourself

▶ Making decisions for yourself, independent of your child's treatment decisions

▶ Identifying treatment and support options and how to find them

* *

*T*he person with the eating disorder isn't the only one in need of support! Eating disorders inflict a lot of wear-and-tear on everyone in the family. Parents of children who relapse or who have long-term struggles with their disorders get hit particularly hard.

You may have been drawn into such a worried or angry battle with the eating disorder that you barely know how to focus on yourself anymore. The rest of your family life may be in tatters. You may not recognize some of your own behaviors or reactions. You may worry that sometimes when you're trying to help, you're hurting instead. Your relationships with other people may be suffering. You may be literally sick from worry, grief, anger, or exhaustion.

All of these effects on caregivers can be normal and temporary. How do you recognize when these or other negative effects are taking root and require more attention? What type of support can help prevent you from getting to that stage in the first place? If your child is stonewalling treatment for herself, does it make any difference what you do for yourself? How do you identify the right kind of services for the trouble you're having? How do you find those services? These are the kinds of questions I take up in this chapter.

I address this material to parents (and others) involved in long-term care-giving and treatment decisions for a child (or other loved one) with an eating disorder. Although the decision-making responsibilities are different in a partnership, much of the chapter applies to couples' relationships as well.

Knowing When to Seek Treatment for Yourself

When you have such an important role as caregiver and support person, everything you do and every reaction you have to your child has a magnified effect. (But no pressure!) You feel the effects of the eating disorder more than others. And your child is more affected by your responses to it.

As your child's recovery develops, taking care of yourself becomes part of taking care of her. This includes recognizing when living with an eating disorder is taking too much of a toll and is affecting your ability to be supportive. You may need to come to terms with personal problems that jeopardize your role as caregiver. You also want to be aware of ways in which your reactions to the eating disorder interfere with your child's recovery. In this section I go over the warning signals of a potential caregiver meltdown, and I discuss why seeking treatment is a useful option.

Contributing to family recovery traps

In Chapter 23 I identify *recovery traps* as obstacles that prevent the kinds of behaviors necessary for your family to support your child's recovery. Usually, recovery traps are fueled by some internal fear, doubt, or misgiving about how the appropriate recovery behavior may change things. For instance, some parents worry that they aren't needed anymore if they can't fix the eating disorder. Or that they're inadequate if a professional helps in a way they can't. Or that their child may change in ways they can't relate to as she gets better. Most fears like these operate outside conscious awareness, so it can be hard to get a handle on them.

Here are some signs that you're stuck in a recovery trap and may need some help becoming unstuck:

- You can't stop trying to manage the behavior of your child with the eating disorder.
- You can't focus on anything but the eating disorder with your child.
- You find it difficult to engage in parts of life that don't involve the eating disorder.

In Chapter 23 I suggest family therapy as a good option for getting unstuck from recovery traps. However, it may seem to you that your own strong feelings are the biggest obstacle in a particular trap. In that case, you may appreciate some individual work to sort out what's getting in your way and figure out how you can move through it more comfortably.

Having difficulty managing your emotions

A child's eating disorder turns your life upside down and leaves you feeling unskilled as a parent and often as if you no longer know your child. Under circumstances like these, any of the following reactions are normal:

- ✔ Guilt, feelings of failure
- ✔ Anger, outrage
- ✔ Fear
- ✔ Mistrust

Such feelings will probably come and go throughout your child's recovery. The more you can accept them as normal, the less disruptive and upsetting they're likely to be to you. And the more likely they are to pass on through.

But how do you know when such feelings have become more than a normal response? The key is that our usual mechanisms for digesting emotion shut down when an emotion feels like too much to handle. Instead of passing through, the emotion gets stuck inside. Here are some signals that one or more of your emotions may have hit the *too much* point and gotten stuck:

- ✔ **You've become paralyzed and can't take necessary action:** Guilt or fear of anger (hers or yours) stops you from setting appropriate limits on your child's behavior.

- ✔ **You don't feel like you can be close with your child:** Your feelings are causing you to distance yourself from your child.

- ✔ **You're too close with your child:** You've gotten *too* involved as a way to "make up" for negative feelings.

- ✔ **The relationship with your child feels fake or lifeless:** You can't let spontaneous or honest feelings come through for fear they'll be the negative ones.

If you look at the preceding list of warning signals, you notice a common thread. Stuck emotions usually result in a stuck way of interacting with the other person. When the other person is your child with the eating disorder, it means you've lost some of your flexibility for responding to her because of the way your feelings are affecting you.

Feeling despair and hopelessness

Eating disorder recovery tends to be a long road, filled with potholes, wrong turns, and standstills. It's nearly inevitable that at one time or another you're going to throw up your hands and believe things will never get better.

You're especially vulnerable when your child suffers her own setbacks. It can also occur when you've just run out of steam for one reason or another. For example, you may be ill, too many other problems may have piled up in the family at the same time, or you may be feeling criticized about how you handle things. Normally, the rough patch ends, and the feelings of despair lift along with it.

But sometimes a rough patch can hang around for a little too long. Or there can be too many rough patches. Maybe you're juggling too much with too little support. Or maybe your personal history makes you especially vulnerable to these kinds of feelings (for example, you had a depressed or anxious parent or one who responded to adversity with doom and gloom). These or other features of your particular situation can make it difficult to keep bouncing back throughout your child's recovery.

Sometimes feelings of despair and hopelessness develop to a point where they become dangerous. If any of the following apply to you, you should seek out help as soon as possible:

- **Feelings of despair and hopelessness are paralyzing you:** You feel helpless to act in the face of such overwhelming odds. Or you wonder why you should bother.

- **Once-in-a-while feelings of despair or hopelessness are gelling into a state of steady depression:** At some point, your ability to bounce back disappeared. Not only are you feeling pessimistic about your child's recovery, you're feeling pessimistic about everything. You've probably slipped into a clinical depression. (You can read more about depression in Chapter 7.)

- **You feel suicidal:** Despair and hopelessness are often triggers for suicidal feelings. If you have suicidal impulses and aren't sure you can manage them, immediately call 911 or head for a hospital emergency room. If you're having thoughts and feelings without immediate urgency to act, this is a definite signal to get support or treatment. (Read more about sizing up suicidal feelings in Chapter 7.)

Putting your problems on hold

If only eating disorders had the courtesy to wait until all other problems in the family were under control! Your may have sent your own problems to the back of the line when the eating disorder hit. But of course this is an arrangement that can't work for very long, especially if your own problems get in the way of your leadership role in the family. When you're not okay, it affects everybody (not the least of whom is you!) in a big way.

Some kinds of problems can take a big bite out of your own well-being and the well-being of your family. These problems include

> ✔ Depression
>
> ✔ Anxiety, panic
>
> ✔ Alcohol or substance abuse
>
> ✔ Low self-worth
>
> ✔ Anger management problems

These kinds of problems don't tend to get better on their own. In fact, they often tend to get worse. (You can read more about recognizing and treating depression, anxiety, and addictions in Chapter 7.) Putting yourself last when it comes to choosing a movie or naming the new puppy is one thing. Putting yourself last when your problems impair your ability to parent is definitely not a good idea.

Turning Your Attention to Your Needs

Many times parents get paralyzed when a child digs in her heels and refuses treatment for an eating disorder. The logic seems to be that the child with the eating disorder is the only gateway to the entire community of treatment for her family. Nothing could be farther from the truth.

More and more services — although still not nearly enough — are developing for families of people with eating disorders. None of these services require that your child be in treatment for you to get their benefits. In this section I review the circumstances that may lead you to seek services without your child's participation or cooperation. Then I discuss some effects you can expect to see, even if your child boycotts treatment.

Seeing a therapist even if your child won't

Even if your child refuses to go to therapy, you (and other members of your family) have more than enough reasons to go ahead without her. You may be mostly in need of support and reassurance. Maybe you need to hear how other parents who've been down this road have coped or handled similar situations — and survived! (See the section "Support groups for families and parents" later in this chapter for more on how to find them.)

Treatment for you as a parent often addresses how your child's eating disorder is affecting you. But your concerns may also have to do with how issues of yours are affecting your child. (My discussion of recovery traps in Chapter 23 and in the section "Contributing to family recovery traps" earlier in this chapter provides some good examples.) You don't need your child's cooperation to do some soul searching on issues that may affect your support for her recovery.

You may be surprised to learn that your family can also go to family therapy, even if your child with the eating disorder boycotts (assuming the child is old enough to boycott). Of course, this arrangement isn't ideal. But that shouldn't deprive the rest of your family from a therapy experience and the support and advice you may need. Besides, the therapist may have some ideas for helping you bring the holdout in. Or she may find it too hard to keep holding out when everyone else keeps going.

Setting an example with your treatment

You can't cure your child's eating disorder. But you can help your family create an environment that supports her recovery. The helping environment of her family is one more resource your child can draw on as she faces getting better. Some of the changes you can bring about in therapy, even without your child's participation, can have a big impact. For example:

- **You can get assistance with personal problems that make it hard to parent:** This helps both you and your child.

- **You can desensitize buttons your child is pushing:** Things quiet down and you make better choices about how to respond when your child isn't getting under your skin so much with her behavior.

- **You can stop engaging in recovery trap behavior:** When you can figure out what's keeping you stuck in behavior that blocks your child's recovery, her chances of moving forward are that much better.

- **Your family can change in ways that no longer support an eating disorder but instead support recovery:** Families usually have to change something about the way they do business to help a child with an eating disorder get better. Maybe your family needs to communicate more openly. Or share feelings. Or put less emphasis on appearances. All of this can happen with or without the presence of the child with the eating disorder in treatment. And all of it helps.

Sending a positive message

Your children learn more from what you do than what you say. A child can learn some important things when she won't go to treatment but you go anyway. Some of the most helpful messages you send by doing so include

- **Caring:** When you go to therapy or a support group to talk about your child's eating disorder, regardless of what she's doing about treatment, you send a powerful message of your caring and concern. You don't allow her boycott to be the last word on the subject of getting help.

✔ **Modeling:** When you go for your own treatment, you model some important lessons, such as

- This is one way a responsible person can step up and deal with her problems.

- This is something that you can do to help. (Of course, this message works best when your child sees you are getting better!)

- You don't have to be crazy to go to a therapist.

✔ **Taking care of yourself:** Many children with eating disorders get caught up in trying to take care of their parents' emotions. They do so at the expense of their own needs and recovery. When you find other help, you make it clear to your child that she can retire from this inappropriate caretaking and focus on herself.

✔ **Taking charge:** Children with eating disorders often feel too central to and too much in charge of what happens in their families. They can actually find it a relief (though they probably can't admit it) for you to take back your rightful place in making decisions that affect you and the family.

Finding the Help That's Right for You

Finding the kind of help that's right for you involves knowing what to look for and where to look. Knowing what to look for means knowing what your goals are. For example, maybe you want to change something about yourself that has surfaced while dealing with your child's eating disorder, or maybe you just want more information about your child's disorder. In the first part of this section, I help you match up your needs with the kinds of services that can best meet them. In the second part of the section, I tell you where to look for providers of these services.

Knowing what choices are available

You can go in any one of several directions to get help for yourself. The direction you choose depends primarily on the kind of help you need. It also depends on finding the right format at a price you can afford. The main options include

✔ Individual therapy

✔ Couples therapy

✔ Parent counseling

✔ Family support groups

✔ Online resources

✔ Psychoeducational groups

I describe each of these options in the following sections and discuss what may make you choose one over another. I also go over online options.

Individual therapy

Therapy aims at changing something about you. (This is different from *support*, which aims at helping you cope with a difficult situation.) Maybe the change you want is to get rid of a symptom, like anxiety or depression. Or maybe you want to change the way you think or feel about something, like constantly doubting or criticizing yourself. Or you may want to change a behavior, like allowing others to take advantage of you or flying off the handle too easily.

If you have a child with an eating disorder, two situations can make you think about changing something about yourself. The first is when you suspect that something you're doing or saying is interfering with your child's recovery. Examples of this are the recovery traps I discuss earlier in this chapter (see the section "Contributing to family recovery traps") and in Chapter 23, like trying to control your child's eating or commenting on her weight.

The other thing you may want to change is your reaction to your child's eating disorder, and the effect it's having on you. This includes the emotional reactions I discuss earlier in this chapter, such as anger, fear, depression, guilt, and hopelessness. Remember, all these reactions are normal. You're most likely to seek therapy when you get stuck in one or more of them and support isn't enough to help you get unstuck.

Individual therapy comes in many shapes and sizes. Some types of therapy are set up to be short term, say 12 to 20 sessions. Others take as long as they take. Some, like cognitive-behavioral therapy, focus only on the present. Others, like psychodynamic psychotherapy, assume current problems are rooted in the past, so they include exploration of your childhood. (You can read about individual therapy approaches in greater detail in Chapter 10.)

Couples therapy

A child with an eating disorder can expose the fault lines in any marriage — or produce new ones. Signs that your child's eating disorder is taking too big a bite out of your marriage and some couples counseling may be in order include

✔ Your relationship with your partner has gotten ragged from the eating disorder wear-and-tear (for instance, you feel too distant or too exhausted to connect).

✔ You can't agree on how to handle your child.

✔ You fight constantly.

✔ Other aspects of your relationship have gone out the window (sex, hobbies, vacations, and so on).

In couples therapy you work on how you operate as a couple. You discover how to change some steps so you can both feel more satisfied with the way things go between you.

Parent counseling

Parent counseling doesn't aim at changing or improving you. Rather, it aims at educating you and supplying you with ideas about how to help a child with an eating disorder. It's likely to provide support as well. Parent counseling may be part of a larger package in which you alternate the parent counseling with sessions with the entire family. Conversely, you may seek out parent counseling separate from any treatment your child is in.

Support groups for families or parents

Those who live with someone with an eating disorder have specific needs. These needs include

✔ Information

✔ Guidance

✔ Emotional support

Family and parent support groups have developed to respond to these needs. Groups are an effective, efficient way to get information to lots of people. More importantly, they draw on the power of people going through similar experiences to understand, validate, comfort, and, when necessary, challenge each other.

Some support groups are open to all concerned others, while other support groups are just for parents. Some are facilitated by an eating disorder professional who supplies information and/or keeps an agenda on track. Other support groups are led by a volunteer, usually somebody who's been in the group for awhile. Some groups are time-limited, and you are expected to attend every session. Others are ongoing and you can attend whenever you want to.

A support group meeting may feature an invited speaker who gives a presentation on some eating disorder topic. This is likely to be followed by a question-and-answer period. Other support groups may discuss a subject introduced by the group leader at each meeting. For example: How should you handle insurance problems? What should you do when your child asks, "Am I fat?"

How can you cope with long-term emotional exhaustion? Still other groups allow members to bring up whatever is on their minds at meetings.

Support groups can supply useful places to

✔ **Discover you're not the only one:** Having an eating disorder in the family takes you off the known path. Sometimes what you go through feels extreme and confusing. It can be a great relief to find out that other people have had similar experiences or shared similar reactions. It can also be quite a comfort to know you're not in this alone.

✔ **Talk about all the reactions and feelings you're having that aren't so helpful to share with your child:** For example, your desire to ship her to Patagonia or your impulse to run away or your fears that she won't make it.

✔ **Lean on and confide in other adults instead of your child:** Your child will try to be your friend if you ask her to. But this interferes with her development and with her recovery.

✔ **Get ideas and support for handling new or tough situations:** In a group, other parents have faced what you're facing. You can call on the collective wisdom and experience of members who've already been through it.

✔ **Get backup when you're taking unpopular positions with your child:** Your child isn't going to reassure you that you're doing the right thing. But you can have a whole chorus of grownups who will!

✔ **Receive congratulations for your successes, and commiseration and suggestions when your plans don't work out so well:** When you're trying to grow and do hard things, it can be really helpful to have witnesses for your efforts, people who understand how much courage they take.

Online support

Online support for parents and families has been increasing, just like all the other services available on the Internet. Online forums fill an important need for people who don't have support groups or other eating disorder services where they live (usually rural areas). Many people who can't bring themselves to participate in groups face-to-face also find that online services provide a solution.

Online support can take place in forums like the following:

✔ **Chat rooms:** Conversation can take place in real time in text or by voice hookup. This allows formation of online support groups with ongoing membership, just like face-to-face groups. Or you can chat with whoever is in a chat room whenever it's convenient for you to enter.

✔ **Newsgroups:** Postings on a particular topic are e-mailed to subscribers. You can read them or not, respond or not, or ask for input for yourself — or not.

> ✔ **Message boards:** A Web site-sponsored message board posts questions and comments from participants, just like a bulletin board in an office. You are free to comment on a posting or just read what others post. The arrangement allows you to come and go according to your own schedule.

Any of these groups may or may not have a professional moderator. Studies find that a fair amount of misinformation gets slung around online, so your safest bet is to stick with a moderated group. A number of reputable eating disorder Web sites are beginning to host professionally-moderated groups.

Psychoeducational groups

Imagine a class (with no exams or homework!) called "Everything You Need to Know About Your Child's Eating Disorder and How to Handle It." Would you take such a class? If so, a psychoeducational group may be for you.

Psychoeducational groups are usually run as a series of lectures. Topics in the series may include nutrition, medication, psychological issues, family relations, and so on. You have a chance to ask questions. Most psychoeducational groups aim at helping you cope better with having someone with an eating disorder in the family.

Finding what you need

Okay, you've figured out what kind of help you need. Now where do you find it? Your most likely sources are word-of-mouth, local institutions, and the Internet.

Asking locally

The best way to find resources right in your own community is to ask other professionals or consumers who live or work there. This way you also get a recommendation. For example:

> ✔ **For an individual or couples therapist or parent counselor:** Ask any member of your child's professional team. Ask school counselors. Try your family doctor. Ask friends, neighbors, or parents of your child's friends.
>
> ✔ **For support groups or psychoeducational groups:** Call local universities, hospitals, and clinics that have eating disorder programs.

Looking it up

A boatload of resource information is available on the Internet. A number of reputable eating disorder sites maintain lists of therapists throughout the country who specialize in eating disorders. Some of the same sites list for-fee and free support groups for families. If you dig through them, you also find listings of online groups, message boards, and the like.

A good place to start your search is the "Resource Guide" at the end of this book. There you find the major Web sites listing the professional and support resources you're looking for.

Part V
The Part of Tens

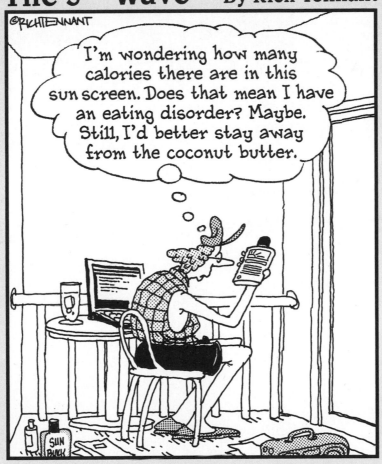

In this part . . .

In the best *For Dummies* tradition, I end with "The Part of Tens." My "Part of Tens" is dedicated to your recovery. Check in here as often as you like to keep yourself on track or draw a little inspiration.

First I give you ten "don'ts" — a list of behaviors and thought habits guaranteed to keep an eating disorder going or to interfere with getting better. Next I offer up a list of ten "do's." The do's are thoughts and practices to help your recovery process keep moving along successfully. Finally, I provide a list of benefits you can expect from sticking with it in recovery, advantages you may not have thought of, but will probably be happy to know.

Chapter 25

Ten Don'ts: Behaviors and Thoughts to Avoid

. . . .

*P*eople with eating disorders typically have certain behaviors and ways of looking at things that keep the disorder going and interfere with recovery. This chapter gives you a quick rundown of some of the most important behaviors and ways of thinking to avoid.

Don't Diet

Dieting is part of your eating disorder. You can't even diet a little without risking relapse. Not for your cousin's wedding. Not to fit into your bathing suit. Not to take off a few pounds you gained on vacation. Not to "jump start" weight loss before you start eating sensibly. If you have binge eating disorder (BED) or bulimia, you're too likely to end up bingeing. If you have anorexia, you're too likely to just keep going.

Besides increasing the risk of relapse, dieting distracts you from focusing on recovery behaviors. You can't really do both. Furthermore, dieting reinforces any ideas you have about your weight coming before your health or well-being.

Don't Try to Fix Your Eating Disorder by Yourself

You already believe you're the only one you can rely on. Or that putting yourself in others' hands means giving up self-control. Those ideas helped create your eating disorder. You'll be tempted to apply them again when it comes to getting better. Fight the temptation!

Although a percentage of people whose eating disorders aren't severe can work successfully with self-help programs (books or online), even they are using expert guidance. Eating disorders are the kinds of problems for which you need expert guidance! If you have other complications, such as drug or alcohol abuse, bipolar disorder, a trauma history, or medical dangers from starving, in-person expert intervention is a must. Most people find they also need the human touch that comes along with it — support, compassion, and feeling understood — to help them get better.

Professional helpers can be a source of more than expert guidance. They can be a starting point for discovering a world of people who are reliable and support your independence. Developing the ability to trust in others is an important part of your recovery.

Don't Look for a Quick Fix

Many people come to treatment hoping that in a few weeks, or a few months at most, their eating disorder will be history. A number of these people leave in disappointment when they find out this is mostly fantasy. They often go from treatment to treatment, hoping to find the one that will make recovery quick and painless.

Often the people who spend their time searching for quick-fix treatment believe they aren't able to tolerate the awareness and discomfort that go with longer-term recovery work. This same kind of self-doubt led to your eating disorder behavior in the first place. If these kinds of doubts apply to you when you think of eating disorder treatment, remember: You don't start with the heaviest lifting in therapy any more than you do at the gym. Part of getting stronger is pacing yourself according to what you can handle at the time. Good treatment includes careful collaboration with your therapist about the pace of treatment.

Don't Do Anything that Feels Extreme

Although the behaviors and beliefs associated with your eating disorder probably feel normal to you, they actually represent extremes. You're either bingeing or starving. You're exactly the right weight or you're totally gross. Your feelings are completely under wraps or you're overwhelmed and out of control.

You're drawn to dramatic remedies because they match the way you think and live. What you need now is less drama and more practice with being in the middle. In that middle territory, things don't happen in the blink of an eye, and you're called upon to tolerate a lot of imperfections. Being in the middle involves doing things a little bit at a time instead of avoiding them altogether or jumping in and drowning. Avoiding extremes and finding the middle is the opposite of your eating disorder. It's one more way you can help your recovery.

Don't Believe Your Weight Determines Your Worth

Believing that your weight determines your worth is central to eating disordered thinking. Many people think they're going to find out what they're worth when they get on the scales each day. (One more reason to throw out those scales!)

One of the most important things you do in recovery is begin to value yourself in other ways besides your weight. While you're working toward that goal, you may find it useful to stop and think of people you know and love or admire. Does *their* worth in your eyes depend on their weight? Can you imagine, just for a minute, applying the same standards to yourself?

Don't Avoid Your Negative Feelings

One of the biggest jobs your eating disorder has is to protect you from feelings you think you can't manage. The more you discover you can actually face your feelings without being overwhelmed, the less you need your eating disorder to rescue you from them. Of course, this can be a tall order. Discovering how to manage difficult emotions will probably be a big focus of your recovery work — and well worth it. In the meantime, you may want to practice just stretching yourself a little more than you're used to. Can you stay with that feeling just one minute longer?

Don't Ignore Signs of Relapse

Responding to signs of relapse requires a bit of a Goldilocks touch. You don't want to over-respond, as if a slip is a catastrophe and ruins everything. But, on the other hand, you need to make sure you're not under-responding, or maybe even using a little denial by telling yourself something like "This doesn't mean anything. I can fast (binge) (purge) just for now and it won't hurt anything. I'll get right back on track after the weekend."

Your best bet is to acknowledge a slip right away as an early warning sign. Talk with your professional helpers or support group members. Get a handle on what happened. The slip was an attempt to fix something that upset or threatened you. In recovery, you can find fixes that don't involve your eating disorder.

Don't Nurture Your Fascination with "Thin"

"Thin" has become an obsession for you. It's part of your eating disorder. In recovery, you need to make sure you're not fueling your thin obsession further. With that in mind, you want to avoid

- ✔ Poring over fashion magazines
- ✔ Putting photos of your favorite model or skinny celebrity on the fridge
- ✔ Talking calories with your friends or family
- ✔ Asking others if you look fat
- ✔ Spending endless time in front of the mirror rating body parts for fat

Don't Put Things Off Until You're "Thin Enough"

Many people have a list of things they're only allowed to do when they're "thin enough": go to the beach, wear shorts, eat at a party, have sex, go to a gym, date, go to a restaurant, or eat ice cream in public. Whatever is on your list, every time you deprive yourself, you reinforce the idea that pleasures in life have to be earned by being "thin." Even worse, this thinking reinforces the belief that you're only worthy when you're thin.

As an exercise to combat this eating disordered thinking, I invite you to list all your "thin only" activities and begin challenging yourself to include them in your life *now*. You're allowed to use whatever kind of support you see fit.

Don't Stop Treatment Too Soon

You may be very tempted to stop treatment once you've gained enough weight to get out of the hospital or you've finished that cognitive behavioral therapy (CBT) program and aren't bingeing and purging so much. You want to put it all behind you. Unfortunately, this is a lot like surviving Hurricane Katrina and ignoring the need to rebuild the levees. For most people, it's a recipe for relapse.

Recovery work involves building strong skills and thinking processes that can help you weather any storm. The more you accomplish in recovery, the less likely you are to turn to eating disorder behaviors in distress.

Chapter 26

Ten Do's: Ways to Enhance Your Recovery

. . . .

*O*nce you decide you want to get better, you have a lot on your plate. You not only want to get a handle on your acute eating disorder symptoms — dieting, starving, bingeing, and/or purging — but you also need to get started with a recovery process. Recovery includes building the skills and ways of thinking that help buffer you from relapse.

In this chapter I give you a list of practices that can help you make your way through the recovery process. They include activities for building recovery skills and habitual ways of thinking you can cultivate. Touch base with this list from time to time, just to help keep yourself on track.

Do Practice Being Imperfect

One of the hardest things you need to do in recovery is make peace with being an imperfect human being — one who, like everyone else, makes mistakes, has flaws in her body and personality, and can't do everything perfectly every time. Your job in recovery is to lay down that impossible burden of holding yourself to perfection. Instead you need to work on finding approaches that help you accept the times you don't get it right or the things about yourself you don't like but can't change. You can put a positive spin on your mistakes or flaws by thinking of them as opportunities to practice being imperfect!

Do Nurture Your Social Network as Part of Your Healing

An eating disorder is often a vote of no-confidence in other people. Discovering how to connect to others in healthy ways is part of your "medicine." This includes

✔ Discovering you can distinguish reliable from unreliable people, or people who are accepting from people who are judgmental

✔ Choosing to place your trust only in reliable, accepting people

✔ Committing to showing up rather than withdrawing or "flaking"

✔ Taking risks with letting yourself be known

✔ Reaching out for support

The more you develop your ability to get emotional and spiritual nurturance from other people, the less you need to turn to food and dieting to try to fill the void.

Do Speak Up!

Eating disorder behaviors are well-known ways of "swallowing" or "stuffing" your feelings. In order to get better, you need to stop doing that and start speaking up! (Of course, this takes time, practice, and support.) Finding ways to speak up about what you feel, what you think, or what you need gives you another recovery asset as a side effect. You can't help but develop the view, or at least the suspicion, that what you feel, think, and need actually matters. And that is a valuable contribution to your self-esteem.

Do Be Truthful with Your Treatment Team

You're used to keeping things to yourself — partly out of a desire for control, and partly out of shame. You may feel that nobody ever listens to you or takes you seriously. Ending the secrecy and coverup of your eating disorder is a very big turnaround, but it's necessary for your recovery. And it may just be a big relief. When you're not busy covering up, you're not waiting to get found out. And you're not carrying everything alone.

Do Experiment with Ways to Enjoy Being in Your Body

You've made your body the enemy for too long. That's part of your eating dis-order story. Part of your recovery story needs to include finding things your body can help you do that give you enjoyment or a sense of peace. This is, of course, a very individual matter. It requires some exploration. But imagine how different it will be to ask your body what feels most enjoyable instead of what burns the most calories!

If you're recovering from anorexia, keep in mind that you need to coordinate your activity level with your treatment team. Engaging in too much activity may be counterproductive to the higher-priority goal of regaining and stabilizing your weight.

Do Use "Feeling Fat" as a Call to Awareness

You may think of "feeling fat" as one of your biggest problems, but you can turn it into one of your best friends. "Feeling fat," after all, is where your eating disorder takes you when other unpleasant feelings are lurking, feelings you aren't so sure you know how to handle. In recovery, you commit to being aware of difficult feelings, and you discover how to cope with them. So when "fat" feelings pop up, you can use them as a signal that something's up you need to be aware of. You now know that even more challenging feelings are hiding behind them. Knowing this, you have the opportunity to stop and think about what they may be and how you want to handle them.

Do Appreciate that Improvement Often Proceeds in Baby Steps

Once you commit to getting better, you want it all done yesterday! Yet recovery often involves changing some very fundamental things about yourself, including how you manage your emotions, how you view yourself, and how you relate to other people. Nobody ever changes such basic patterns overnight. What's more, many of the changes you need to make may feel scary or overwhelming at first. Even a tiny step can feel humongous.

Try to appreciate the significance of those first tiny steps. They change your direction, no matter how small they are. They show that you understand and respect the limits of what you can do at a particular moment. And they often signal the way to bigger steps down the line as your experience and confidence grow.

Do Keep Track of Your Accomplishments

If you only focus on what you still have to accomplish, you get too discouraged. Find ways to remind yourself of what you've already achieved. It's okay to let others help you with this!

Do Talk with Other Women about Social Pressures to Be Thin

Dangerous and destructive cultural messages can be so commonplace that you fail to notice them or the effect they have on you. Instead, you may tend to internalize the message and think it defines how things are supposed to be. This is what happens to most women (and some men) when it comes to messages that say you have to be thin to be accepted and loved. Counteracting these messages is an uphill battle. Thin keeps getting rewarded and overweight keeps getting ridiculed or excluded.

If you want change, at least in your own life, you need to speak up and disagree. You need to talk to others about the tyranny of thin and protest, even when you can't totally free yourself from the effects! In the 1960s and '70s, this was called *consciousness raising*. When you're aware, you're conscious. You have the possibility of making better choices. You can't single-handedly change the culture, but you can at least help and encourage others to think in healthier ways about their bodies.

Do Remember that People Can and Do Recover from their Eating Disorders

Recovery from an eating disorder can be a lengthy, frustrating process — one in which you often can't see the end or believe that getting better is a possibility for you. Doubt and discouragement are normal feelings during recovery. Frequently they show up when you're on the verge of the next big change.

The majority of people who hang in there through recovery get better. By "better," I mean they leave their eating disorders essentially in the past and go on to focus on other things in life — only now with increased strength and confidence.

Resource Guide

Web Sites for Eating Disorder Information

*F*or all general and specific information about eating disorders, treatments, online support, and so on, start your search with the Web sites in this section. If you don't find what you need, check out the Web sites listed in the other sections as well.

National Association of Anorexia Nervosa and Associated Disorders (ANAD)
www.ANAD.org

Anorexia Nervosa and Related Eating Disorders, Inc. (ANRED)
www.anred.com

Bulimia.com
www.bulimia.com or www.gurze.com

Eating Disorders Awareness and Prevention (EDAP). Also known as National Eating Disorders Association (NEDA)
www.edap.org

Something Fishy
www.something-fishy.org

My ED Help
www.myedhelp.com/treatment_finder_state_listings.htm

National Eating Disorder Association (NEDA)
www.nationaleatingdisorders.org

Web Sites for Finding Treatment

These sites help you get started in your search for the experts and facilities you need for a winning therapy team. You can find out about each specialty in Chapters 9, 10, and 11.

Individual, family, couples, and group therapists specializing in eating disorders

Academy for Eating Disorders (AED)
www.aedweb.org
Click on For the Public, and then click on Find an ED Professional

The Eating Disorder Referral and Information Center
www.edreferral.com

Gürze Books Therapist Directory
www.gurze.com or www.bulimia.com

International Association of Eating Disorder Professionals (IAEDP)
www.iaedp.com

Finding specialized forms of treatment

Cognitive-Behavioral Therapy (CBT)
The Association for Behavioral and Cognitive Therapies, Referral directory
www.aabt.org/members/Directory/Find_A_Therapist.cfm

Dialectical Behavioral Therapy (DBT)
The Association for Behavioral and Cognitive Therapies, Referral directory
www.aabt.org/members/Directory/Find_A_Therapist.cfm
Click on Dialectical Behavioral Therapy under therapist specialty areas

EMDR
The EMDR International Association (EMDRIA)
www.emdria.org

Emotional Freedom Techniques (EFT) Practitioners
www.emofree.com/

Feminist therapists
There is no centralized directory of feminist therapists. You'll need to ask a prospective therapist whether she uses feminist principles in her work.

Maudsley approach
Maudsley Parents Treatment Finder
www.maudsleyparents.org/providerlist.html

Psychodynamic therapies
There is no centralized directory of psychodynamic therapists. You'll need to ask a prospective therapist what his treatment orientation is.

Sensorimotor Psychotherapy
Sensorimotor Psychotherapy Institute
www.sensorimotorpsychotherapy.org
Click on Find an SP Therapist

Somatic Experiencing (SE)
The Foundation for Human Enrichment
www.traumahealing.com

Thought Field Therapy (TFT)
Association for Thought Field Therapy (ATFT), Membership Directory
www.atft.org

Music therapists

American Music Therapy Association, Inc.
8455 Colesville Rd., Suite 1000
Silver Spring, MD 20910
Phone: 301-589-3300
Fax: 301-589-5175
E-mail: findMT@musictherapy.org

Dance/movement therapists

The American Dance Therapy Association
www.adta.org
Click on About Us, and then scroll down to Members Directory

Finding other experts who specialize in eating disorders

Physicians

American Medical Association (AMA)
AMA Doctor Finder
http://webapps.ama-assn.org/doctorfinder/home.html

Dieticians

American Dietetic Association (ADA)
www.eatright.org
Or speak to a dietician and get local referrals at 800-366-1655

Web Sites for Finding Local Support Groups

In Chapter 11 you can read about support groups to supplement eating disorder treatment. In Chapter 24 I discuss support groups for families and friends. Here are ways you can find a support group in your area.

For people with eating disorders

National Center for Overcoming Overeating
Local support groups for people using the Overcoming Overeating approach
www.overcomingovereating.com/groups.html

Overeaters Anonymous
www.oa.org

Poppink.com
www.poppink.com/supportgroups/supportgroups.php

For family and others

Maudsley support groups
Something Fishy
www.something-fishy.org/treatmentfinder/

Web Sites for Size Acceptance and Self-Esteem

Body Positive
Promotes positive body image for people of all sizes
www.bodypositive.com

International Size Acceptance Association (ISAA)
An activist organization that fights size discrimination
www.size-acceptance.org/

National Association to Advance Fat Acceptance (NAAFA)
Local chapters
http://naafa.org/

Largely Positive
Information and support for people of size
www.largelypositive.com

SelfMatters
Focuses on issues of body image, shame, and self-esteem for women who struggle with weight and eating disorders. You can sign up for their online newsletter.
www.SelfMatters.org

Self-Help Books

Agras, W. Stewart, and Robin F. Apple. *Overcoming Eating Disorders: A Cognitive-Behavioral Treatment for Bulimia Nervosa and Binge-Eating Disorder* (workbook). New York: Oxford University Press, 1997.

Andersen, A. E., L. Cohn, and T. Holbrook. *Making Weight: Men's Conflicts with Food, Weight, Shape & Appearance.* Carlsbad, CA: Gürze Books, 2000.

Bryant-Waugh, Rachel, and Bryan Lask. *Eating Disorders: A Parent's Guide.* Philadelphia: Brunner-Routledge, 2004.

Cash, Thomas F. *The Body Image Workbook: An 8-Step Program for Learning to Like Your Looks.* Oakland, CA: New Harbinger, 1997.

Dellasega, Cheryl. *The Starving Family: Caregiving Mothers and Fathers Share Their Eating Disorder Wisdom.* Fredonia, WI: Champion Press, LTD, 2005.

Fairburn, Christopher G. *Overcoming Binge Eating.* New York: Guilford, 1995.

Goodman, Laura J., and Mona Villapiano. *Eating Disorders: The Journey to Recovery Workbook.* New York: Brunner-Routledge, 2001.

Hall, Lindsey, and Leigh Cohn. *Bulimia: A Guide to Recovery.* Carlsbad, CA: Gürze Books, 1998.

Hall, Lindsey, and Monika Ostroff. *Anorexia Nervosa: A Guide to Recovery.* Carlsbad, CA: Gürze Books, 1998.

Hamilton, Linda H. *Advice for Dancers: Emotional Counsel and Practical Strategies.* San Francisco: Jossey-Bass, 1998.

Katzman, Debra K., and Leora Pinhas. *Help for Eating Disorders: A Parent's Guide to Symptoms, Causes & Treatments.* Toronto: Robert Rose, 2005.

Lock, James, and Daniel le Grange. *Help Your Teenager Beat an Eating Disorder.* New York: Guilford, 2005.

Michel, Deborah M., Susan G. Willard, et al. *When Dieting Becomes Dangerous: A Guide to Understanding and Treating Anorexia and Bulimia.* New Haven: Yale University Press, 2003.

Natenshon, Abigail H. *When Your Child Has an Eating Disorder: A Step-by-Step Workbook for Parents and Other Caregivers.* San Francisco: Jossey-Bass, 1999.

Sherman, Roberta Trattner, and Ron A. Thompson. *Bulimia: A Guide for Family and Friends.* San Francisco: Jossey-Bass, 1990.

Sherman, Roberta Trattner, and Ron A.Thompson. *Helping Athletes with Eating Disorders.* Champaign, IL: Human Kinetics Publishers, 1992.

Siegel, Michelle, Judith Brisman, and Margot Weinshel. *Surviving an Eating Disorder: Strategies for Family & Friends.* New York: HarperCollins Publishers, Inc., 1997.

Walsh, B. Timothy, and V. L. Cameron. *If Your Adolescent Has an Eating Disorder: An Essential Resource for Parents.* New York: Guilford, 2005.

Zerbe, Katheryn J. *The Body Betrayed: A Deeper Understanding of Women, Eating Disorders, and Treatment.* Carlsbad, CA: Gürze Books, 1995.

Index

BUSINESS, CAREERS & PERSONAL FINANCE

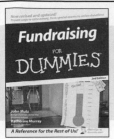

0-7645-9847-3

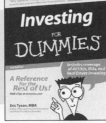

0-7645-2431-3

Also available:
- Business Plans Kit For Dummies
  0-7645-9794-9
- Economics For Dummies
  0-7645-5726-2
- Grant Writing For Dummies
  0-7645-8416-2
- Home Buying For Dummies
  0-7645-5331-3
- Managing For Dummies
  0-7645-1771-6
- Marketing For Dummies
  0-7645-5600-2

- Personal Finance For Dummies
  0-7645-2590-5*
- Resumes For Dummies
  0-7645-5471-9
- Selling For Dummies
  0-7645-5363-1
- Six Sigma For Dummies
  0-7645-6798-5
- Small Business Kit For Dummies
  0-7645-5984-2
- Starting an eBay Business For Dummies
  0-7645-6924-4
- Your Dream Career For Dummies
  0-7645-9795-7

HOME & BUSINESS COMPUTER BASICS

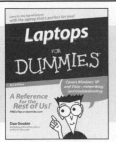

0-470-05432-8

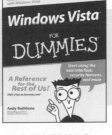

0-471-75421-8

Also available:
- Cleaning Windows Vista For Dummies
  0-471-78293-9
- Excel 2007 For Dummies
  0-470-03737-7
- Mac OS X Tiger For Dummies
  0-7645-7675-5
- MacBook For Dummies
  0-470-04859-X
- Macs For Dummies
  0-470-04849-2
- Office 2007 For Dummies
  0-470-00923-3

- Outlook 2007 For Dummies
  0-470-03830-6
- PCs For Dummies
  0-7645-8958-X
- Salesforce.com For Dummies
  0-470-04893-X
- Upgrading & Fixing Laptops For Dummies
  0-7645-8959-8
- Word 2007 For Dummies
  0-470-03658-3
- Quicken 2007 For Dummies
  0-470-04600-7

FOOD, HOME, GARDEN, HOBBIES, MUSIC & PETS

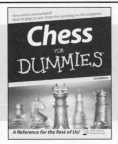

0-7645-8404-9

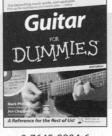

0-7645-9904-6

Also available:
- Candy Making For Dummies
  0-7645-9734-5
- Card Games For Dummies
  0-7645-9910-0
- Crocheting For Dummies
  0-7645-4151-X
- Dog Training For Dummies
  0-7645-8418-9
- Healthy Carb Cookbook For Dummies
  0-7645-8476-6
- Home Maintenance For Dummies
  0-7645-5215-5

- Horses For Dummies
  0-7645-9797-3
- Jewelry Making & Beading For Dummies
  0-7645-2571-9
- Orchids For Dummies
  0-7645-6759-4
- Puppies For Dummies
  0-7645-5255-4
- Rock Guitar For Dummies
  0-7645-5356-9
- Sewing For Dummies
  0-7645-6847-7
- Singing For Dummies
  0-7645-2475-5

INTERNET & DIGITAL MEDIA

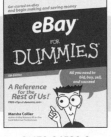

0-470-04529-9

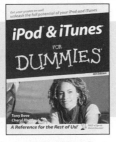

0-470-04894-8

Also available:
- Blogging For Dummies
  0-471-77084-1
- Digital Photography For Dummies
  0-7645-9802-3
- Digital Photography All-in-One Desk Reference For Dummies
  0-470-03743-1
- Digital SLR Cameras and Photography For Dummies
  0-7645-9803-1
- eBay Business All-in-One Desk Reference For Dummies
  0-7645-8438-3
- HDTV For Dummies
  0-470-09673-X

- Home Entertainment PCs For Dummie
  0-470-05523-5
- MySpace For Dummies
  0-470-09529-6
- Search Engine Optimization For Dummies
  0-471-97998-8
- Skype For Dummies
  0-470-04891-3
- The Internet For Dummies
  0-7645-8996-2
- Wiring Your Digital Home For Dummie
  0-471-91830-X

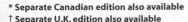

* Separate Canadian edition also available
† Separate U.K. edition also available

Available wherever books are sold. For more information or to order direct: U.S. customers visit www.dummies.com or call 1-877-762-2974.
U.K. customers visit www.wileyeurope.com or call 0800 243407. Canadian customers visit www.wiley.ca or call 1-800-567-4797.

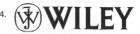

SPORTS, FITNESS, PARENTING, RELIGION & SPIRITUALITY

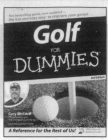

0-471-76871-5

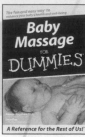

0-7645-7841-3

Also available:

- Catholicism For Dummies
  0-7645-5391-7
- Exercise Balls For Dummies
  0-7645-5623-1
- Fitness For Dummies
  0-7645-7851-0
- Football For Dummies
  0-7645-3936-1
- Judaism For Dummies
  0-7645-5299-6
- Potty Training For Dummies
  0-7645-5417-4
- Buddhism For Dummies
  0-7645-5359-3

- Pregnancy For Dummies
  0-7645-4483-7 †
- Ten Minute Tone-Ups For Dummies
  0-7645-7207-5
- NASCAR For Dummies
  0-7645-7681-X
- Religion For Dummies
  0-7645-5264-3
- Soccer For Dummies
  0-7645-5229-5
- Women in the Bible For Dummies
  0-7645-8475-8

TRAVEL

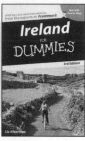

0-7645-7749-2

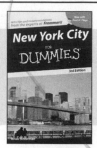

0-7645-6945-7

Also available:

- Alaska For Dummies
  0-7645-7746-8
- Cruise Vacations For Dummies
  0-7645-6941-4
- England For Dummies
  0-7645-4276-1
- Europe For Dummies
  0-7645-7529-5
- Germany For Dummies
  0-7645-7823-5
- Hawaii For Dummies
  0-7645-7402-7

- Italy For Dummies
  0-7645-7386-1
- Las Vegas For Dummies
  0-7645-7382-9
- London For Dummies
  0-7645-4277-X
- Paris For Dummies
  0-7645-7630-5
- RV Vacations For Dummies
  0-7645-4442-X
- Walt Disney World & Orlando
  For Dummies
  0-7645-9660-8

GRAPHICS, DESIGN & WEB DEVELOPMENT

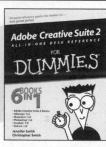

0-7645-8815-X

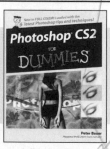

0-7645-9571-7

Also available:

- 3D Game Animation For Dummies
  0-7645-8789-7
- AutoCAD 2006 For Dummies
  0-7645-8925-3
- Building a Web Site For Dummies
  0-7645-7144-3
- Creating Web Pages For Dummies
  0-470-08030-2
- Creating Web Pages All-in-One Desk
  Reference For Dummies
  0-7645-4345-8
- Dreamweaver 8 For Dummies
  0-7645-9649-7

- InDesign CS2 For Dummies
  0-7645-9572-5
- Macromedia Flash 8 For Dummies
  0-7645-9691-8
- Photoshop CS2 and Digital
  Photography For Dummies
  0-7645-9580-6
- Photoshop Elements 4 For Dummies
  0-471-77483-9
- Syndicating Web Sites with RSS Feeds
  For Dummies
  0-7645-8848-6
- Yahoo! SiteBuilder For Dummies
  0-7645-9800-7

NETWORKING, SECURITY, PROGRAMMING & DATABASES

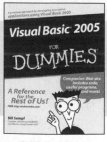

0-7645-7728-X

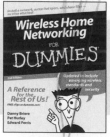

0-471-74940-0

Also available:

- Access 2007 For Dummies
  0-470-04612-0
- ASP.NET 2 For Dummies
  0-7645-7907-X
- C# 2005 For Dummies
  0-7645-9704-3
- Hacking For Dummies
  0-470-05235-X
- Hacking Wireless Networks
  For Dummies
  0-7645-9730-2
- Java For Dummies
  0-470-08716-1

- Microsoft SQL Server 2005 For Dummies
  0-7645-7755-7
- Networking All-in-One Desk Reference
  For Dummies
  0-7645-9939-9
- Preventing Identity Theft For Dummies
  0-7645-7336-5
- Telecom For Dummies
  0-471-77085-X
- Visual Studio 2005 All-in-One Desk
  Reference For Dummies
  0-7645-9775-2
- XML For Dummies
  0-7645-8845-1

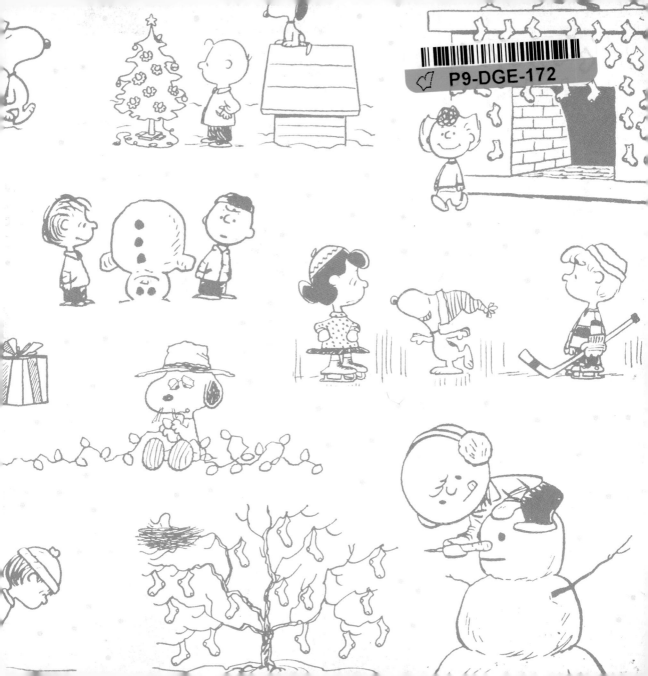

THE JOY OF
A PEANUTS CHRISTMAS

50 Years of Holiday Comics!

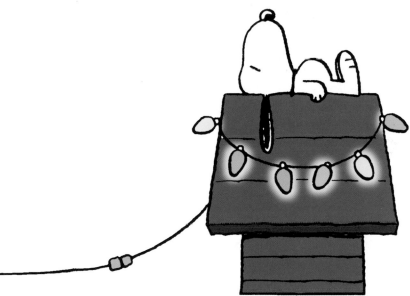

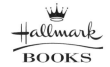

Hallmark
BOOKS

The Joy of a PEANUTS Christmas published in 2000 by Hallmark Cards, Inc.

Hallmark logo and Hallmark Books logo are trademarks of
Hallmark Cards, Inc., 2501 McGee, Kansas City, MO, 64141.

http://www.hallmark.com

http://www.unitedmedia.com

Designed and produced by book soup publishing, inc., Philadelphia, PA,
with Running Press Book Publishers, Philadelphia, PA.

Cover and interior design by Susan Van Horn.

Edited by Erin Slonaker and Megan Bossuyt.

Printed in the United States.

10 9 8 7 6 5 4 3 2 1

CONTENTS

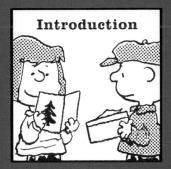
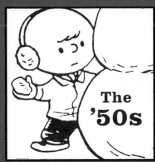
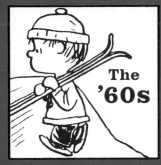
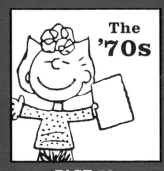
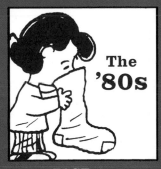
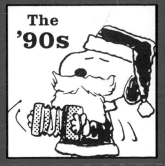

INTRODUCTION

Charles Schulz is the cartoon champion of all time. . .
He is a magician with a pencil.

—JOYCE C. HALL, FOUNDER, HALLMARK CARDS, INC.

In some way, we can all relate to the trials and tribulations,
the fun and foibles of the PEANUTS gang.

—DONALD J. HALL, CHAIRMAN, HALLMARK CARDS, INC., AND SON OF JOYCE C. HALL

PEANUTS and Hallmark have been playing on the same team for more than forty years, but unlike the ill-fated baseball team Charlie Brown valiantly captains, ours has always been a winning combination. Together we've created over one hundred different products—cards, ornaments, address books, yo-yos and even a Hallmark Hall of Fame production. Together we've shared in the joys and sorrows, the laughter and loves of the whole PEANUTS gang: Charlie Brown and Snoopy, Lucy and Linus, Sally and Schroeder, Peppermint Patty and Marcie, Franklin and Pig-Pen, Woodstock and Spike. We've seen them grow up (sort of), fall in and out of love (in a manner of speaking) and set off on adventures and journeys from Snoopy's Red Baron flights to Linus's relentless quest for the Great Pumpkin.

And we're proud to have been a part of it all.

For us, it all began on May 16, 1960, when Charles Schulz agreed to create four greeting cards for our company. Forty years and more than one hundred products later, the Schulz family and my own have become both great business partners and great friends. Sparky and I shared a love of golf, and, like Charlie Brown, we always hoped that the next game would be better.

I think PEANUTS and Hallmark get along so well because we have so much in common. We're both known for a dedication to quality. We share a commitment to family and community. And we both bring good feelings—warmth, joy, happiness and love—into the daily lives of millions. We're a perfect match. "They think a lot of times of things I wish I had thought of myself," Charles Schulz once said of our family business. "I frequently look at their cards and think, 'I wish I'd used that in my strip.'" Believe me, the feeling is mutual.

A cartoon strip, after all, tells a story—much like a card. And one of the truly magical things about PEANUTS is the way that the characters so truthfully share their emotions. Maybe that's why they work so well in greeting cards.

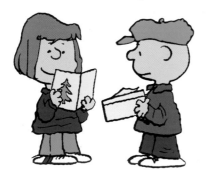

We've learned a lot of things about Charles Schulz and his PEANUTS gang over the years. We've learned that all PEANUTS characters are right-handed (one of our artists accidentally drew Peppermint Patty writing with her left hand). We learned that Schroeder only listens to

Beethoven (one of our designers once mistakenly drew rows and rows of music by a different composer). We learned that despite their cartoony nature, each PEANUTS character actually has a human hand (another designer once drew a character with only three fingers and a thumb).

But mostly, we've learned what millions of people around the world already know about PEANUTS—that it simply, honestly and beautifully teaches us about life. After all, despite all the gang's quarrels, trials and tribulations, they always come together when it's really important.

When Charles Schulz died in February of 2000, the world lost more than a brilliant artist, a creator of cultural icons and a national treasure. We lost a man who loved his work, who loved his family, who loved his country. We lost a man who spoke his message clearly through his beloved characters and taught us that we can all win the game if we work together, if we love, if we laugh and if we keep on trying.

Somehow, it doesn't matter that Charlie Brown never did kick that football. That he kept trying was enough.

I hope you enjoy this look back at the PEANUTS gang over the years—from the '50s through the '90s. We at Hallmark are delighted to be publishing this one-of-a-kind collection of Charles Schulz's classic Christmas strips, in honor of *The Joy of a PEANUTS Christmas*.

—DON HALL

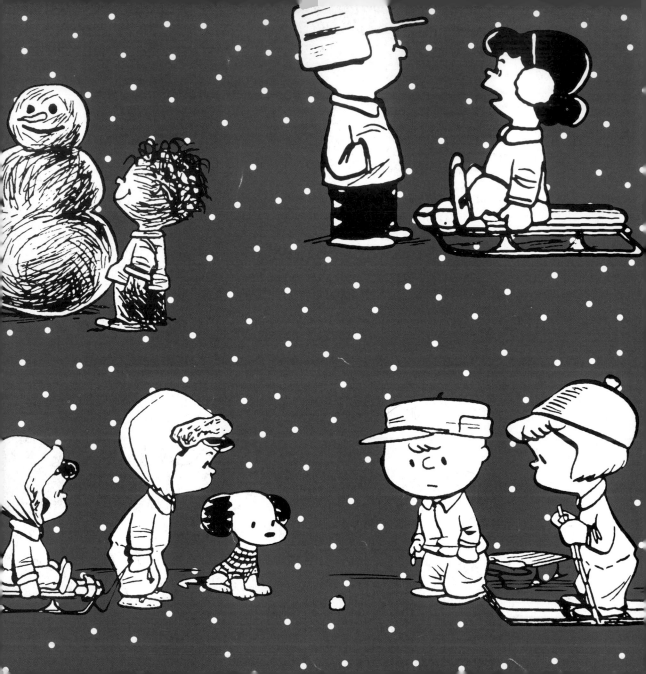

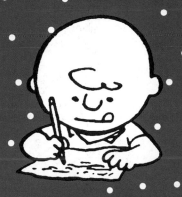
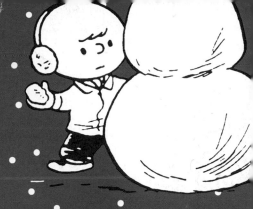

THE '50s

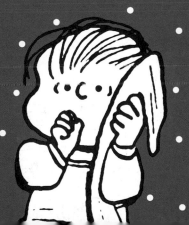
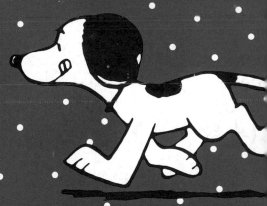

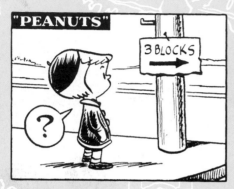
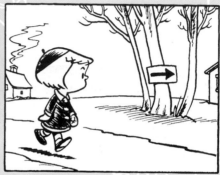
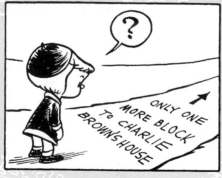
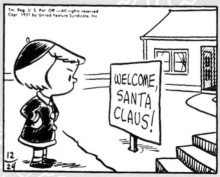

December 24, 1951

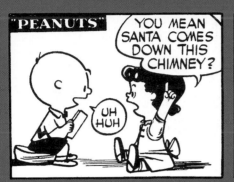
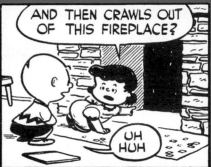
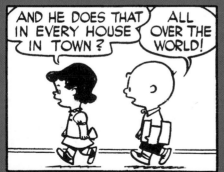
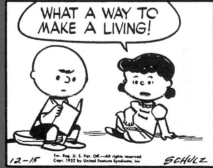

December 15, 1952

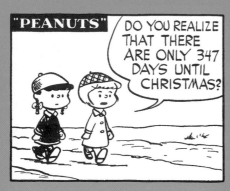

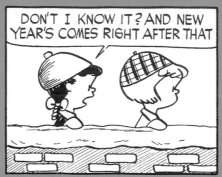

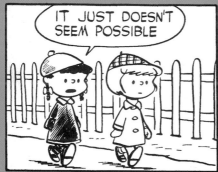

January 12, 1953

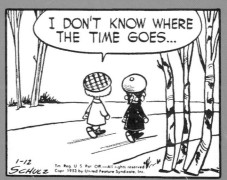

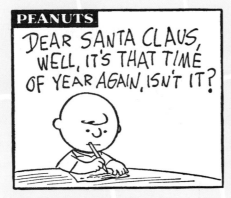

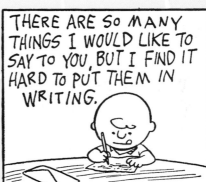

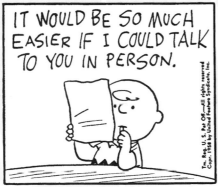

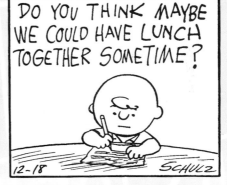

December 18, 1958

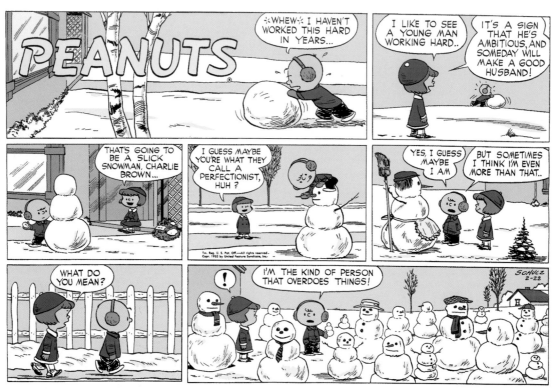

February 22, 1953

CHARLIE BROWN

His dog calls him "that round-headed kid" and his friends sometimes call him "blockhead," but everyone knows him by his full name. He is Charlie Brown, the occasionally tarnished star of the gang, a born loser who

"CHRISTMAS EVE IS MY FAVORITE DAY OF THE YEAR. IT MAKES ME FEEL GOOD ABOUT EVERYTHING."

never loses hope. Even though his baseball team always loses, Lucy always pulls the football away, and his friends ridicule his Christmas tree, Charlie Brown keeps trying and always faces the coming holiday or sport season with optimism.

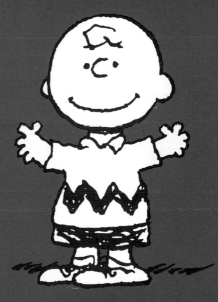

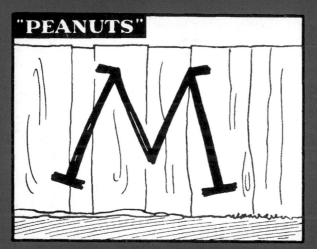

"PEANUTS"

December 25, 1953

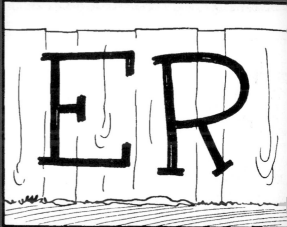

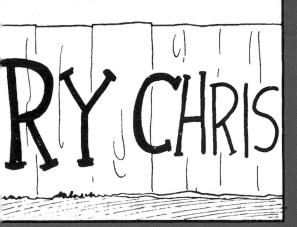

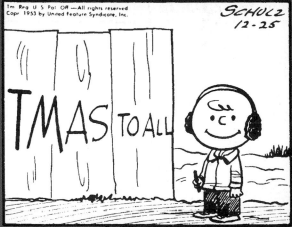

SCHULZ
12-25

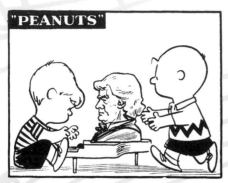
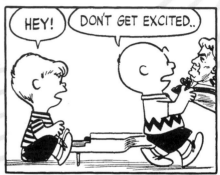
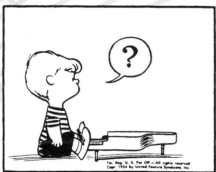
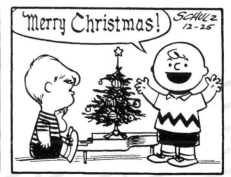

December 25, 1954

PIG-PEN

Pig-Pen always wanders around in a cloud—of dirt. And he leaves dirt on everything in his path. But Pig-Pen has accepted his dirtiness and is happy that way. His Christmastime snowmen may not be the cleanest snowmen in town, but at least they've got character—just like Pig-Pen.

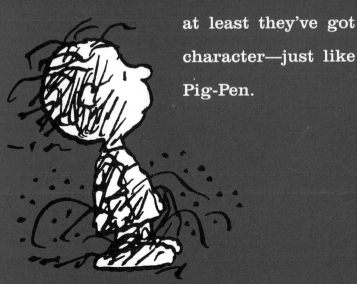

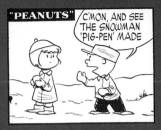

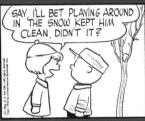

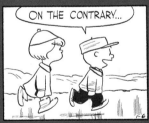

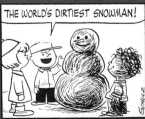

January 6, 1955

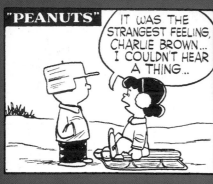

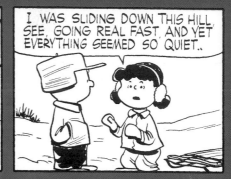

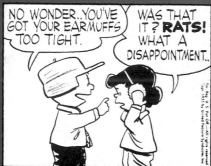

January 13, 1955

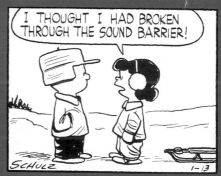

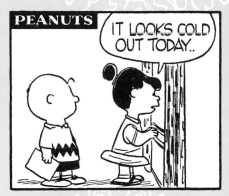
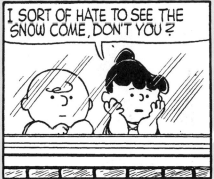
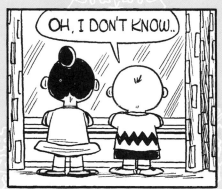
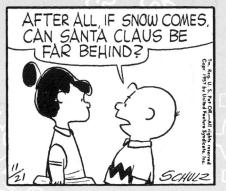

November 21, 1957

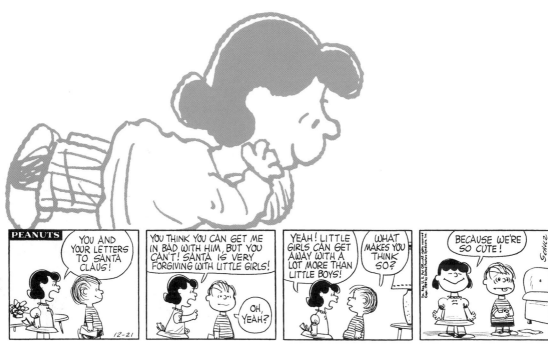

December 21, 1959

LUCY

Lucille Van Pelt is crabby, loud, often angry, and proud of it. She makes no attempt to hide her emotions or her opinions and can be just plain mean to her brother Linus, her friends and even the neighborhood dog. She always knows the answers (she's the neighborhood psychiatrist), she's always right (no matter what the facts say), and she is always in charge (whether or not anyone wants her to be). Despite resistance from Schroeder, she continues to pursue him by hanging mistletoe at Christmas or leaning seductively on his piano.

"I JUST NOTICED SOMETHING ABOUT THIS ROOM. THERE'S AN APPALLING LACK OF MISTLETOE."

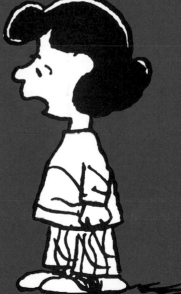

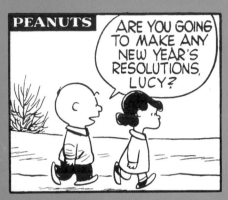
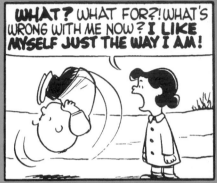
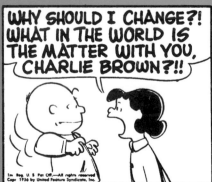
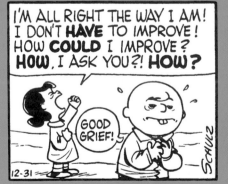

December 31, 1956

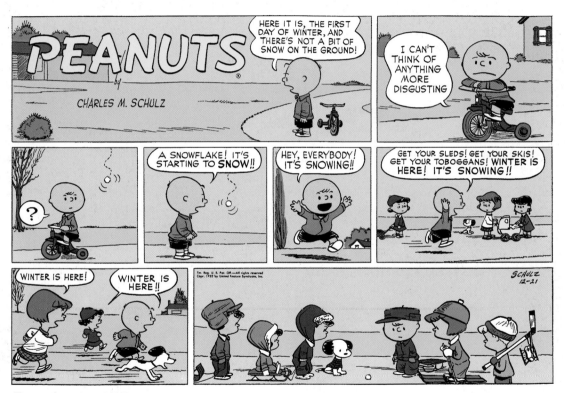

December 21, 1952

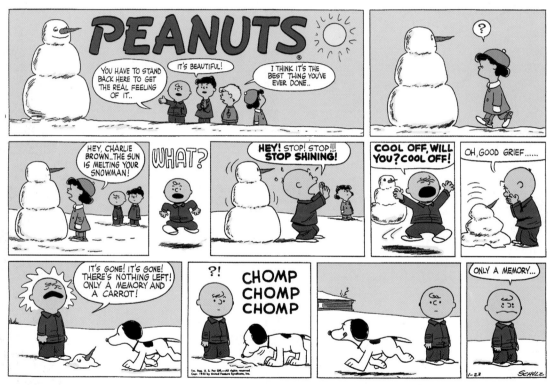

January 23, 1955

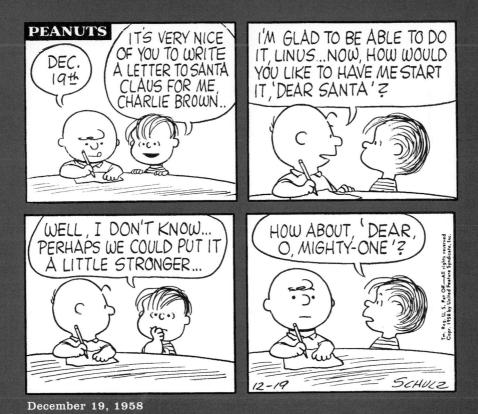

December 19, 1958

LINUS

Sucking his thumb and gripping his powder-blue blanket, Linus Van Pelt taught us about the meaning of Christmas and convinced us that the Great Pumpkin would bring us presents on Halloween. The deep thinker, he solves problems for all of the PEANUTS gang. His older sister Lucy

"DEAR SANTA, I AM NOT SURE WHAT I WANT FOR CHRISTMAS THIS YEAR. PERHAPS YOU SHOULD SEND ME YOUR CATALOGUE."

can't stand him, but Charlie's little sister Sally is infatuated with him. Despite an ongoing rivalry with Snoopy for the blanket, Linus always comes out on top. He is clearly wise beyond his years.

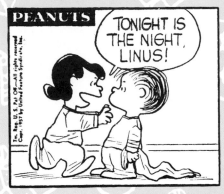
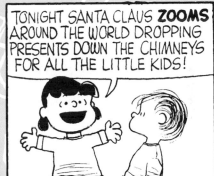
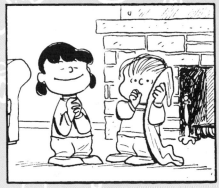
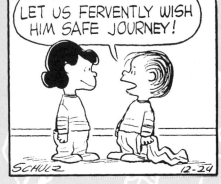

December 24, 1957

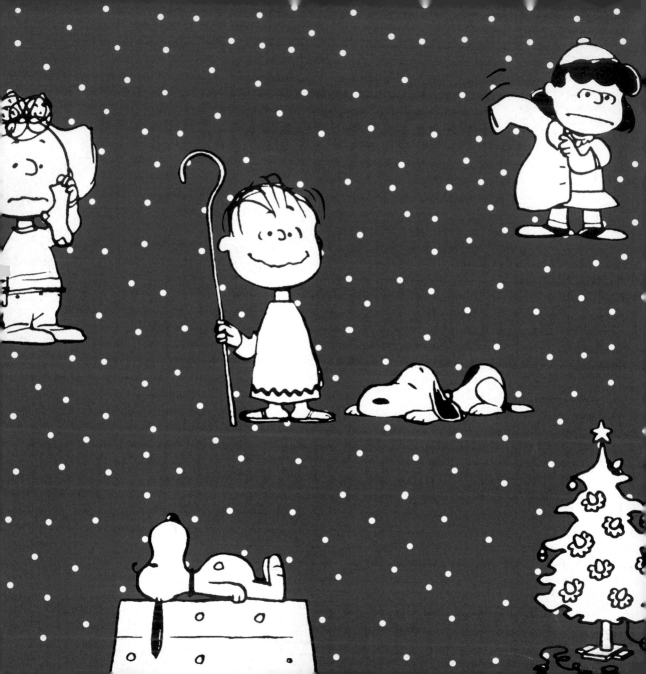

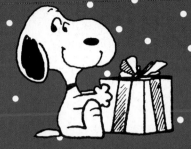

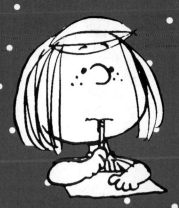

THE '60s

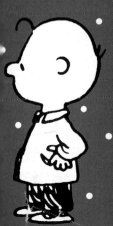

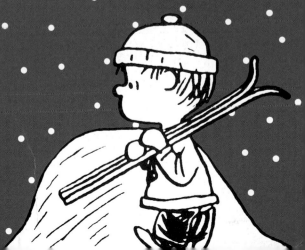

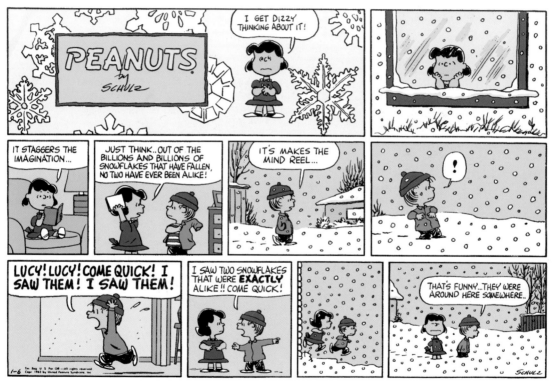

January 6, 1963

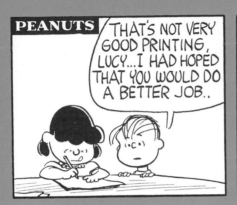
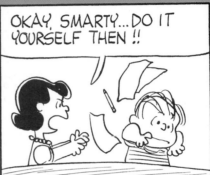
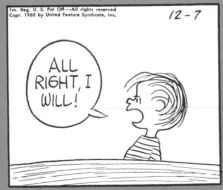
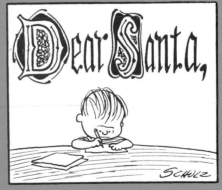

December 7, 1960

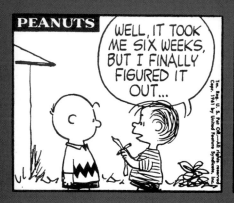

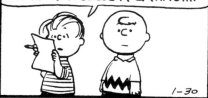

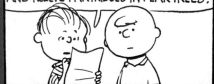

January 30, 1961

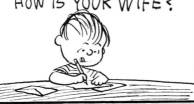

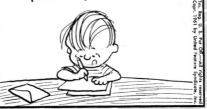

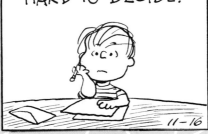

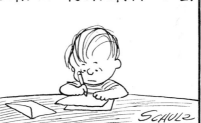

November 16, 1961

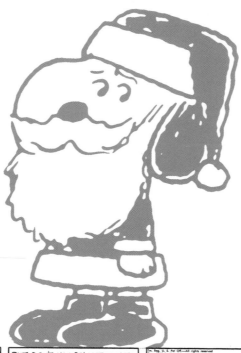

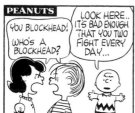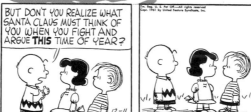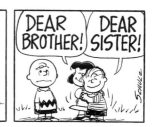

December 11, 1961

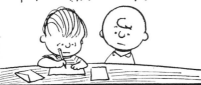

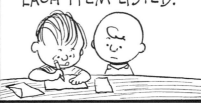

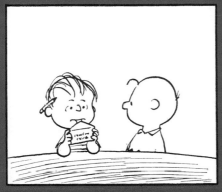

November 18, 1961

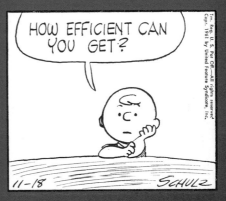

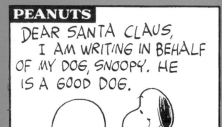

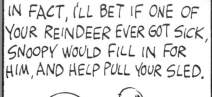

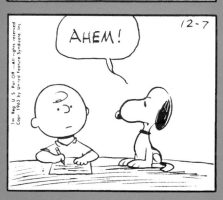

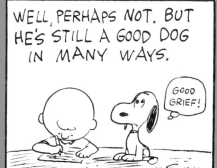

December 7, 1963

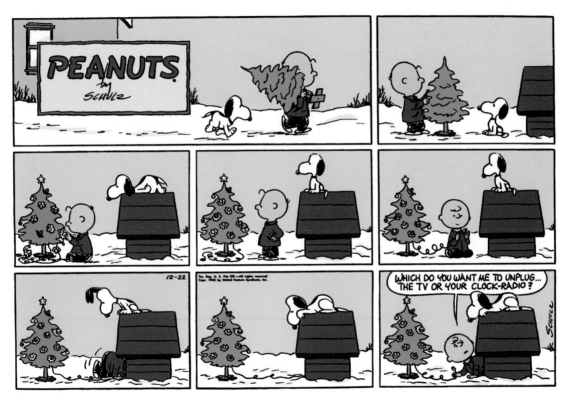

December 22, 1963

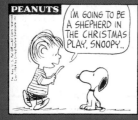**PEANUTS** I'M GOING TO BE A SHEPHERD IN THE CHRISTMAS PLAY, SNOOPY..

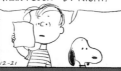THIS IS THE PIECE I HAVE TO MEMORIZE...

"AND THERE WERE IN THE SAME COUNTRY SHEPHERDS ABIDING IN THE FIELD, KEEPING WATCH OVER THEIR FLOCK BY NIGHT."

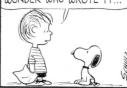THAT'S A GOOD LINE... I WONDER WHO WROTE IT...

December 21, 1964

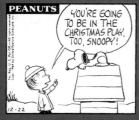**PEANUTS** YOU'RE GOING TO BE IN THE CHRISTMAS PLAY, TOO, SNOOPY!

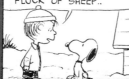I'M GOING TO BE A SHEPHERD, AND YOU'RE GOING TO BE MY FLOCK OF SHEEP..

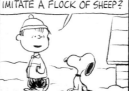DO YOU THINK YOU CAN IMITATE A FLOCK OF SHEEP?

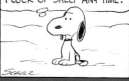NO TROUBLE AT ALL.... ONE BEAGLE IS WORTH A WHOLE FLOCK OF SHEEP ANY TIME!

December 22, 1964

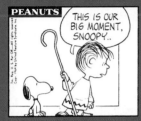
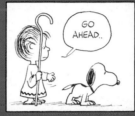
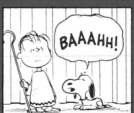
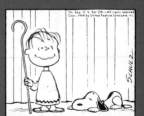

PEANUTS

THIS IS OUR BIG MOMENT, SNOOPY..

YOU GO OUT ONTO THE STAGE FIRST BECAUSE YOU'RE THE SHEEP...I'LL FOLLOW, AND PRETEND I'M GUIDING YOU...

GO AHEAD..

IF HE EVEN COMES **NEAR** ME WITH THAT SHEPHERD'S STAFF, I'LL GIVE HIM A JUDO CHOP!

December 23, 1964

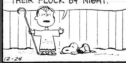
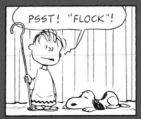
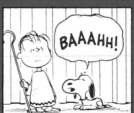
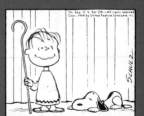

PEANUTS

"AND THERE WERE IN THE SAME COUNTRY SHEPHERDS ABIDING IN THE FIELD, KEEPING WATCH OVER THEIR FLOCK BY NIGHT."

PSST! "FLOCK"!

BAAAHH!

December 24, 1964

December 21, 1966

PEPPERMINT PATTY Captain

of her baseball and football teams, Peppermint Patty is a rough-and-tumble girl who would rather be on the playing field than in the classroom. She and her friends Marcie and Franklin attend a different school from Charlie Brown, but they all go to the same summer camp. Throughout the rest of the year, they see each other

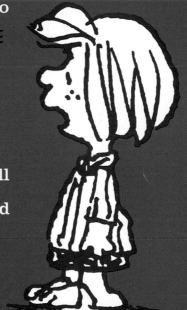

"DON'T SIGH LIKE THAT MA'AM. . . CHRISTMAS VACATION IS A LONG WAY OFF."

occasionally—for baseball and football games, as well as at Halloween and Christmas parties.

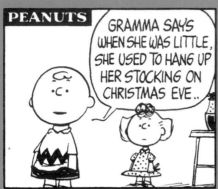
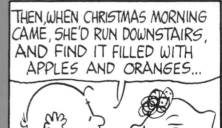
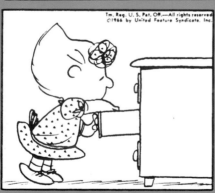
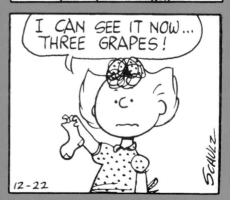

December 22, 1966

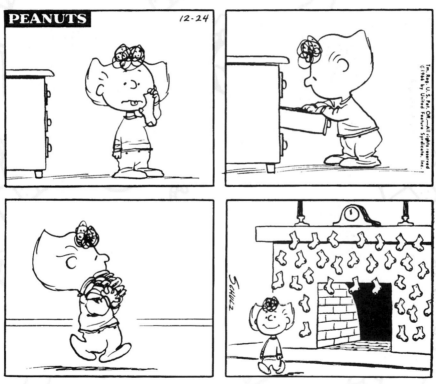

PEANUTS   12-24

December 24, 1966

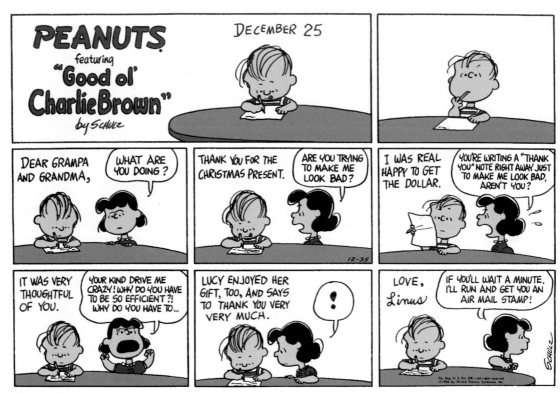

December 25, 1966

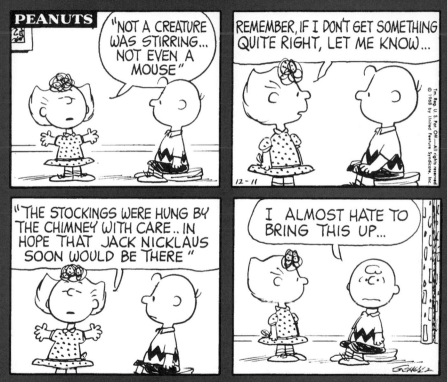

December 11, 1968

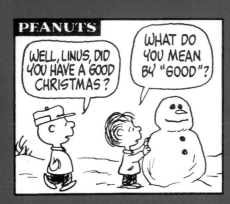

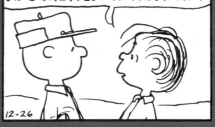

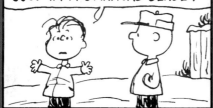

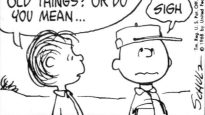

December 26, 1968

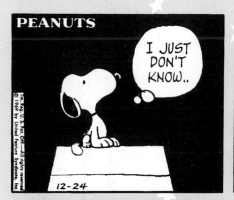

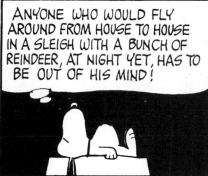

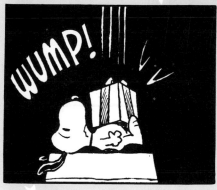

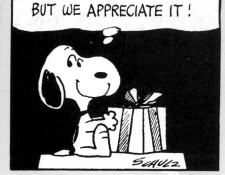

December 24, 1969

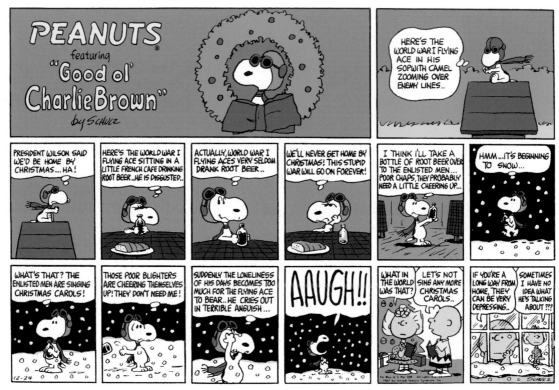

December 24, 1967

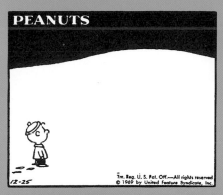

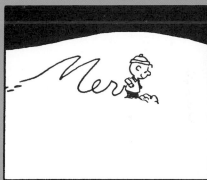

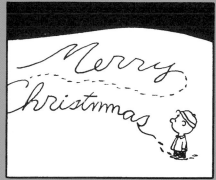

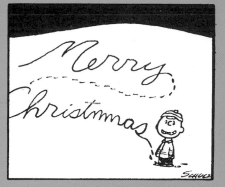

December 25, 1969

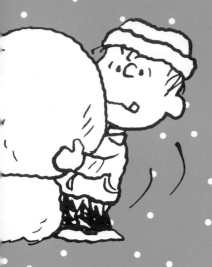
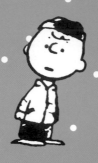
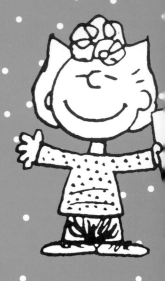
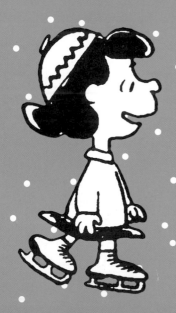
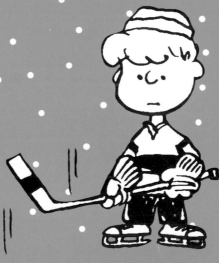

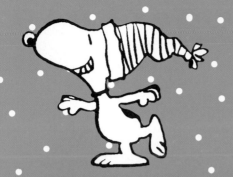
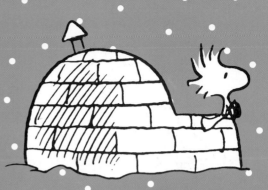

THE '70s

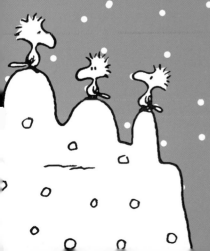
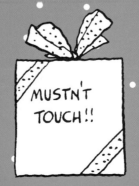

MUSTN'T
TOUCH!!

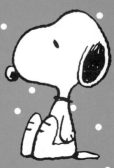

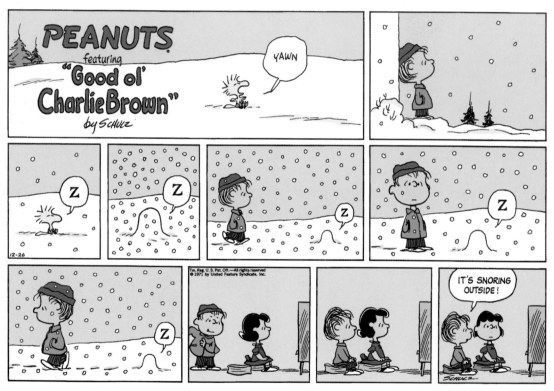

December 26, 1971

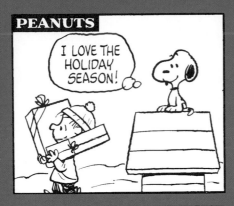

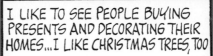

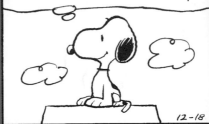

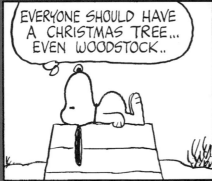

December 18, 1972

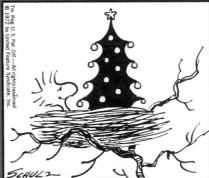

SALLY

Sally Brown is a silly little sister to Charlie Brown. She spends most of her time making

"THE STOCKINGS WERE HUNG BY THE CHIMNEY WITH CARE. . IN HOPE THAT JACK NICKLAUS SOON WOULD BE THERE."

up excuses to stay home from school for a day, coercing her big brother into doing her homework for her, or pursuing Linus, her unrequited love, her "Sweet Babboo." Easily confused, she once wrote a school report on "Santa Claus and his Rain Gear" and thanked the wrong grandmother for her Christmas presents.

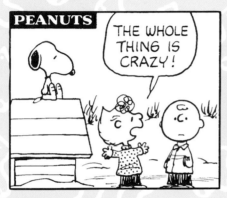
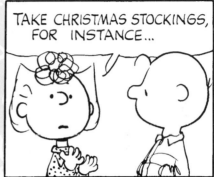
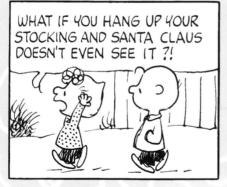
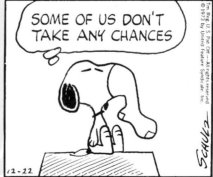

December 22, 1973

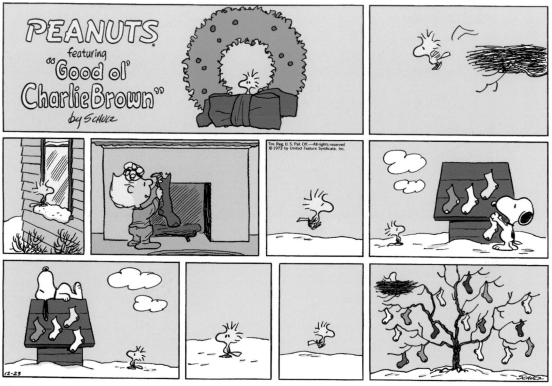

December 23, 1973

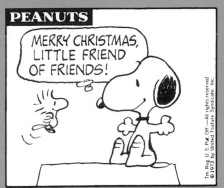
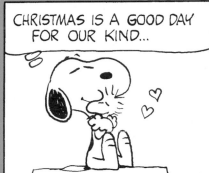
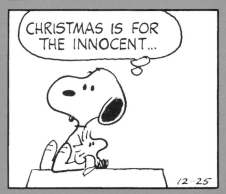
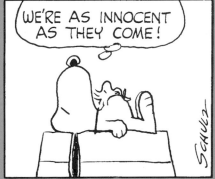

December 25, 1973

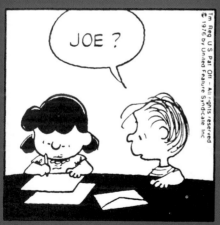
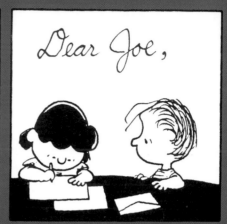
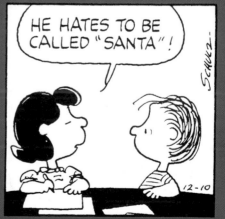

December 10, 1976

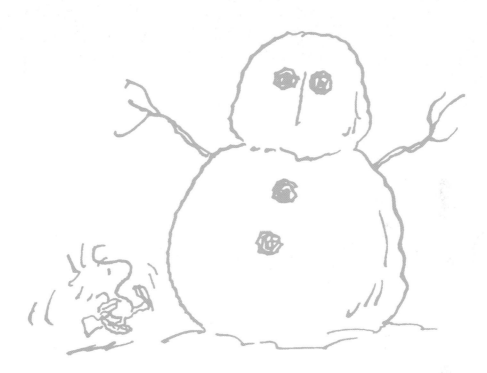

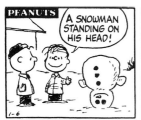
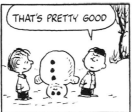
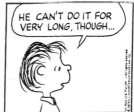
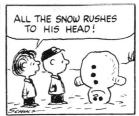

January 6, 1975

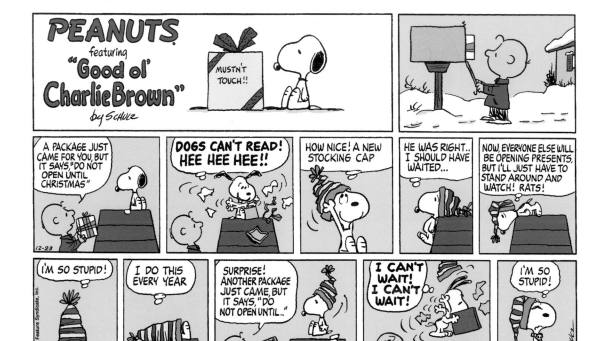

December 23, 1979

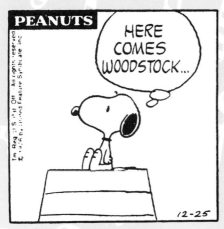

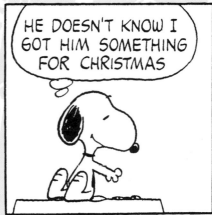

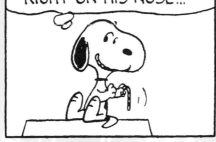

December 25, 1976

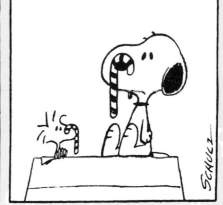

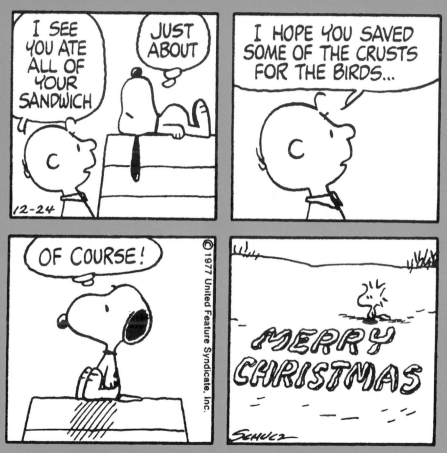

December 24, 1977

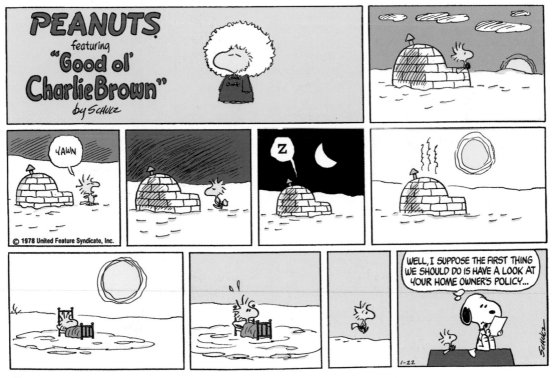

January 22, 1978

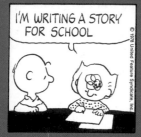

I'M WRITING A STORY FOR SCHOOL

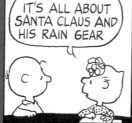

IT'S ALL ABOUT SANTA CLAUS AND HIS RAIN GEAR

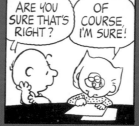

ARE YOU SURE THAT'S RIGHT?

OF COURSE, I'M SURE!

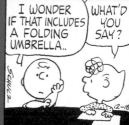

I WONDER IF THAT INCLUDES A FOLDING UMBRELLA..

WHAT'D YOU SAY?

December 18, 1978

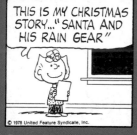

THIS IS MY CHRISTMAS STORY..." SANTA AND HIS RAIN GEAR"

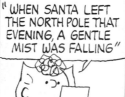

"WHEN SANTA LEFT THE NORTH POLE THAT EVENING, A GENTLE MIST WAS FALLING"

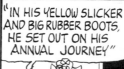
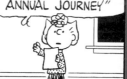

"IN HIS YELLOW SLICKER AND BIG RUBBER BOOTS, HE SET OUT ON HIS ANNUAL JOURNEY"

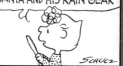

"IT WAS CHRISTMAS EVE, AND SOON CHILDREN AROUND THE WORLD WOULD BE HEARING THE SOUND OF SANTA AND HIS RAIN GEAR"

December 19, 1978

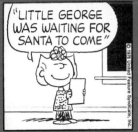

"LITTLE GEORGE WAS WAITING FOR SANTA TO COME"

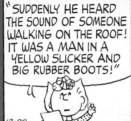

"SUDDENLY HE HEARD THE SOUND OF SOMEONE WALKING ON THE ROOF! IT WAS A MAN IN A YELLOW SLICKER AND BIG RUBBER BOOTS!"

12-20

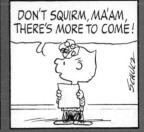

"'I SAW HIM!' SHOUTED LITTLE GEORGE..'I SAW SANTA AND HIS RAIN GEAR'"

DON'T SQUIRM, MA'AM, THERE'S MORE TO COME!

December 20, 1978

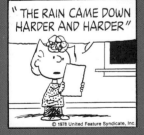

"THE RAIN CAME DOWN HARDER AND HARDER"

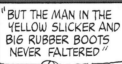
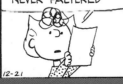

"BUT THE MAN IN THE YELLOW SLICKER AND BIG RUBBER BOOTS NEVER FALTERED"

12-21

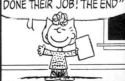

"ANOTHER CHRISTMAS EVE HAD PASSED, AND SANTA AND HIS RAIN GEAR HAD DONE THEIR JOB! THE END"

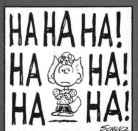

HA HA HA! HA HA! HA HA!

December 21, 1978

WOODSTOCK

Whether his hockey team is playing on the birdbath or he's typing letters on Snoopy's behalf, Woodstock is a busy little bird. He speaks only in birdspeak, a complex language of apostrophes and gestures, and he can just as easily express his happiness as his anger. He has been known to give Snoopy birdseed for Christmas and often becomes little more than a mound of snow if he sits still too long in a snowstorm. Above all, he's Snoopy's best friend and has more love and heart than anyone else his size.

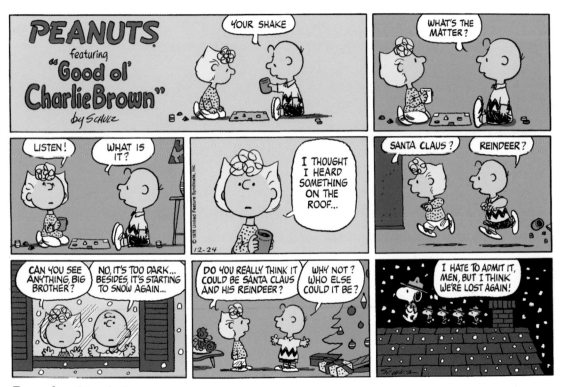

December 24, 1978

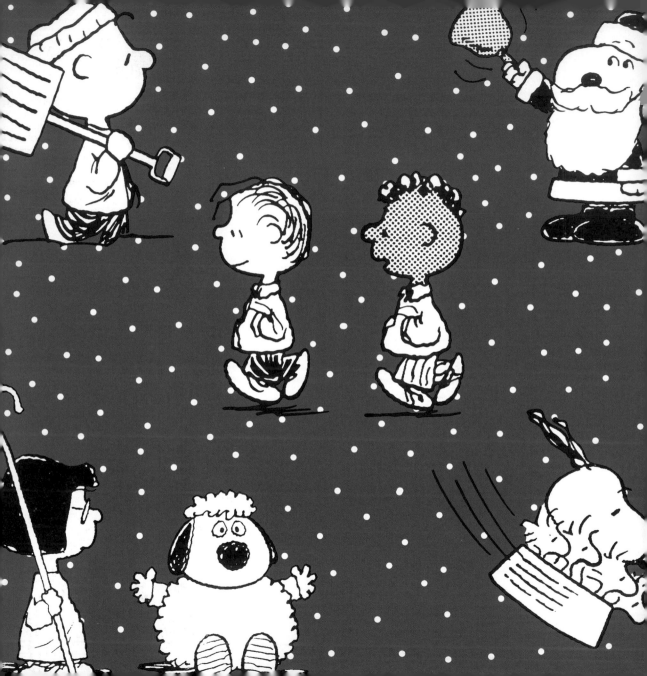

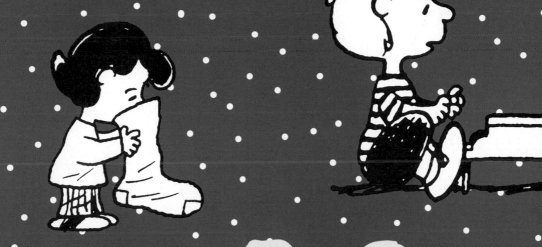

THE '80s

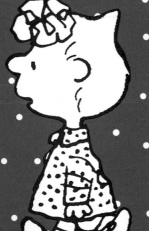

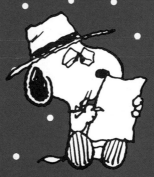

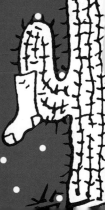

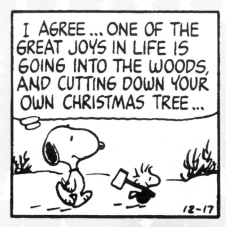

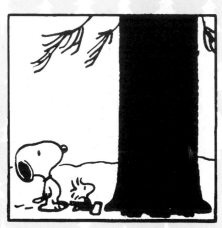

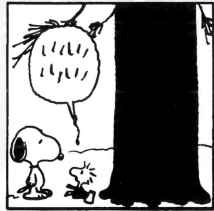

December 17, 1980

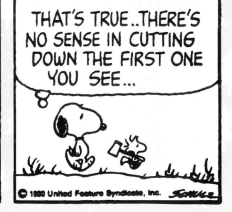

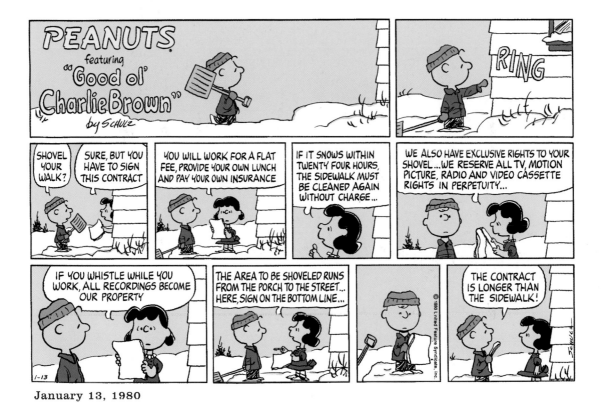

January 13, 1980

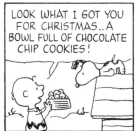
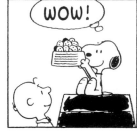
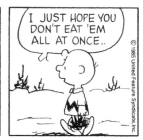
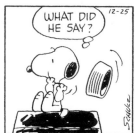

December 25, 1985

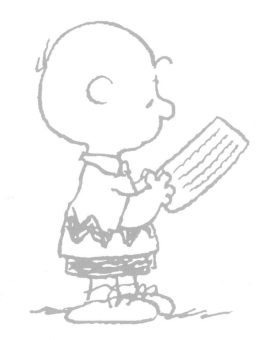

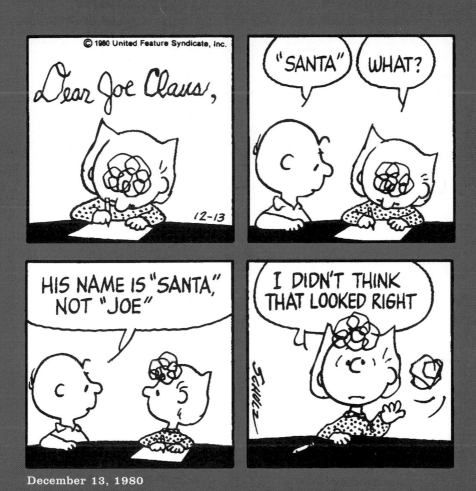

December 13, 1980

SCHROEDER

A prodigy with a toy piano, Schroeder idolizes Beethoven and cannot be bothered with much else. Much of his Christmas season is spent avoiding Lucy and mistletoe; he much prefers his favorite holiday, Beethoven's birthday. He can

"I'VE BEEN READING UP ON WINTER."

always be counted on for his musical talents, however, and is always a part of any school production.

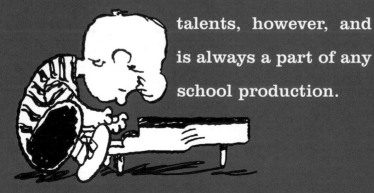

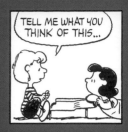

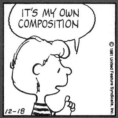

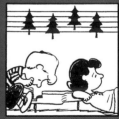

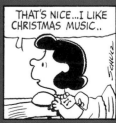

December 18, 1981

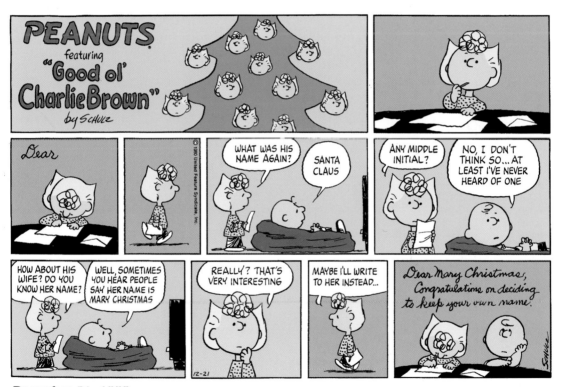

December 21, 1980

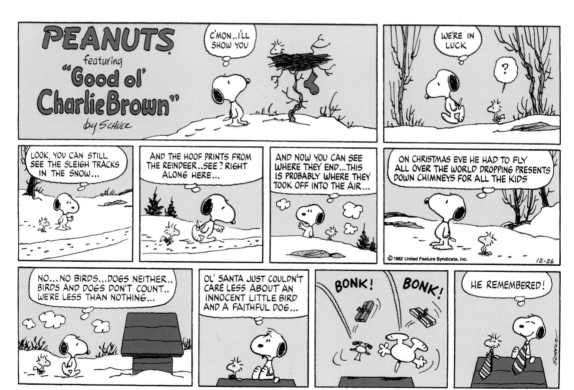

December 26, 1982

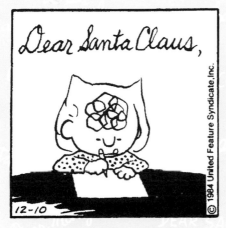

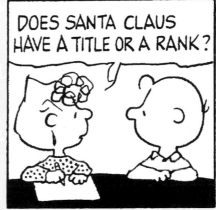

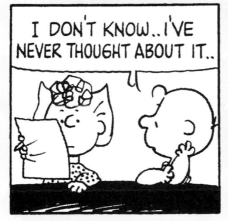

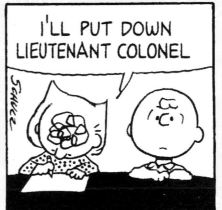

December 10, 1984

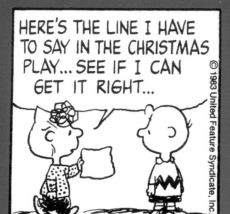

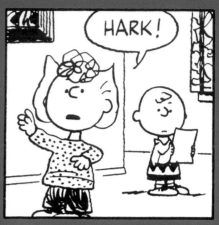

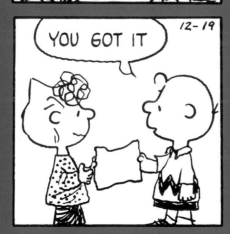

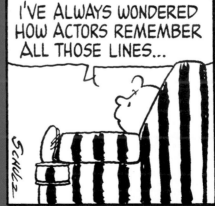

December 19, 1983

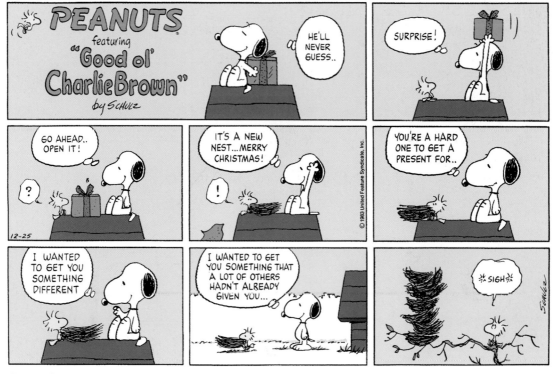

December 25, 1983

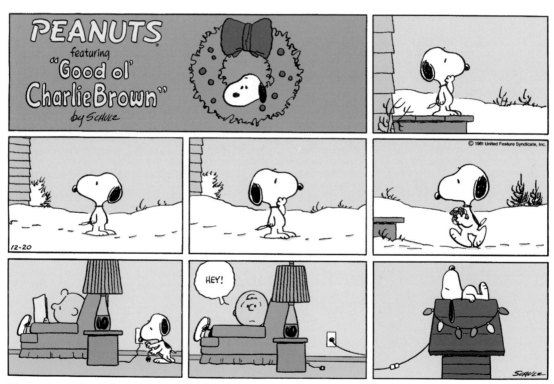

December 20, 1981

SNOOPY

Snoopy does it all—he's everything from a World War I Flying Ace to an accomplished writer to a tennis champion to a trickster. He has a weakness for root beer and pizza, often consuming so much that he spends the night atop his doghouse listening to his stomach rumble.

"ANYONE WHO WOULD FLY AROUND FROM HOUSE TO HOUSE IN A SLEIGH WITH A BUNCH OF REINDEER HAS TO BE OUT OF HIS MIND!"

He is protective of his best friend, Woodstock, and the two make sure to exchange Christmas presents every year. Snoopy is a true Renaissance beagle.

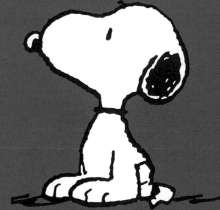

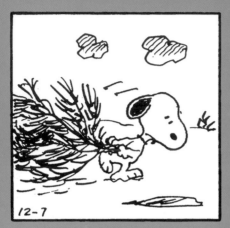

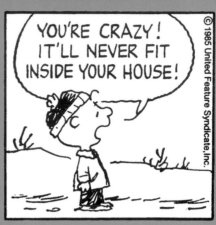

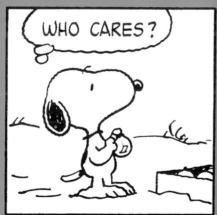

December 7, 1985

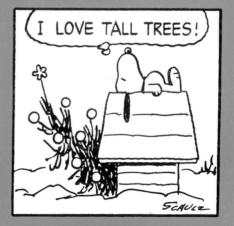

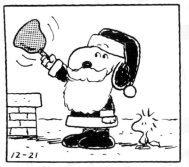

December 21, 1989

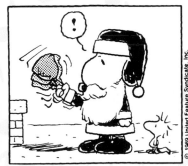

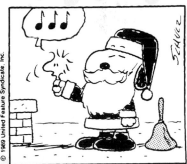

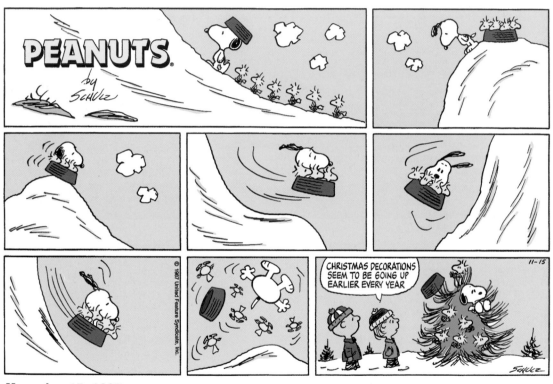

November 15, 1987

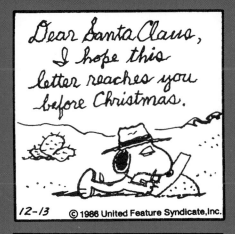

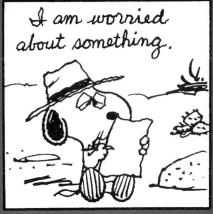

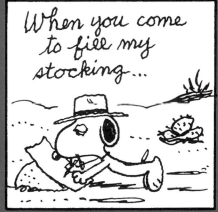

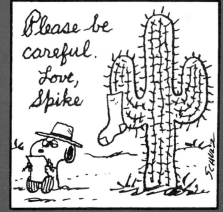

December 13, 1986

MARCIE

The complete opposite of her best friend, Peppermint Patty, Marcie has both book smarts and common sense—but she is completely inept at sports. She insists on calling Peppermint Patty "Sir" in the face of all Patty's protests and is always nearby if Peppermint Patty's around. Even though she's not confident on the baseball diamond, she always participates and finds areas in which she can excel; she was Mary in the Christmas pageant.

"MY FAMILY SAID IT'S ALL RIGHT TO BELIEVE IN SANTA CLAUS, BUT NOT THE GREAT PUMPKIN."

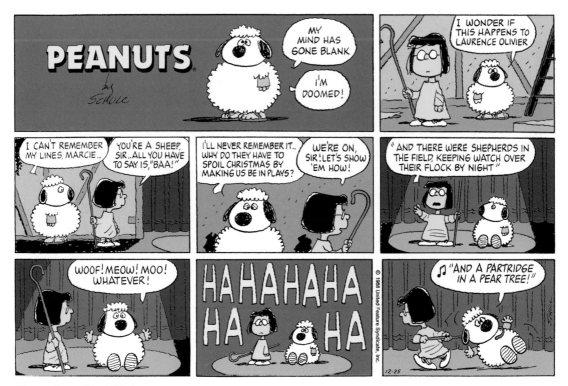

December 25, 1988

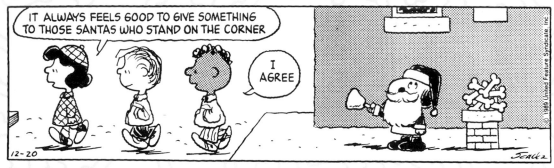

December 20, 1989

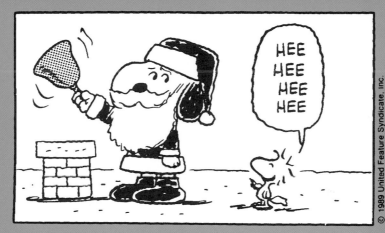

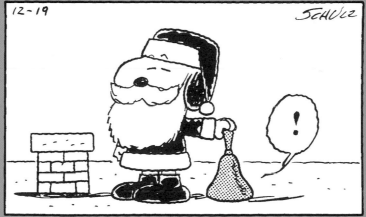

December 19, 1989

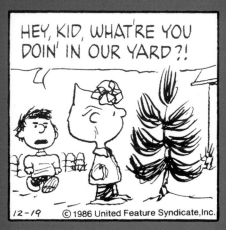
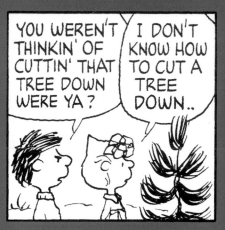
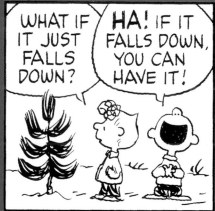
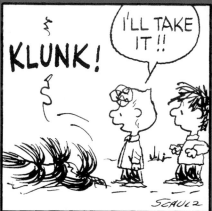

December 19, 1986

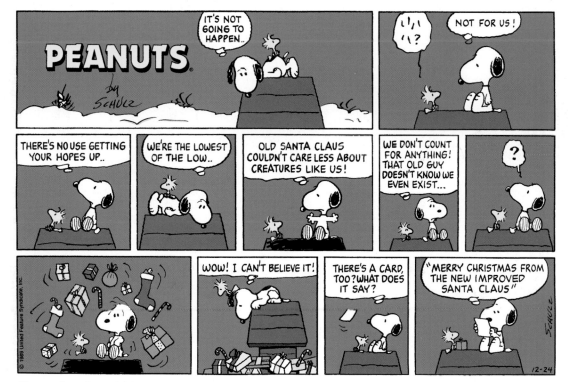

December 24, 1989

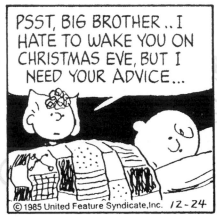

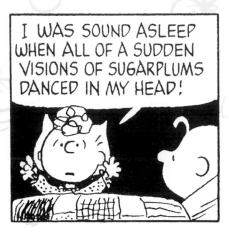

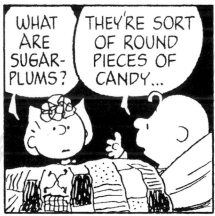

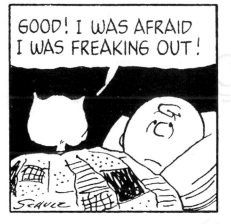

December 24, 1985

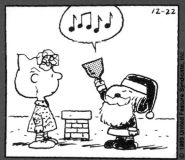

December 22, 1989

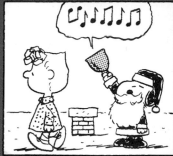

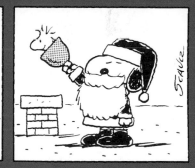

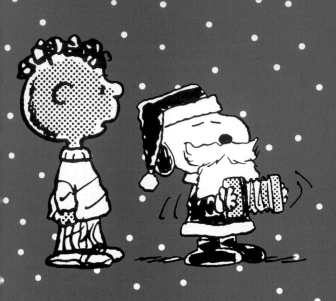
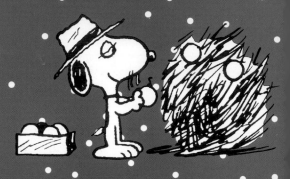
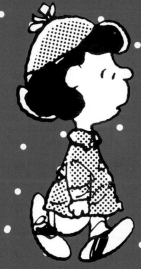
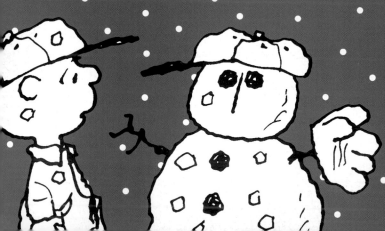

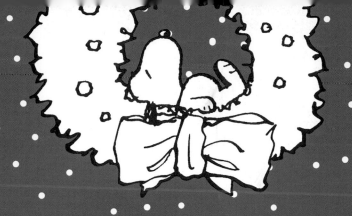
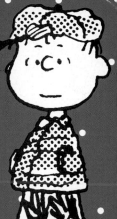
THE '90s
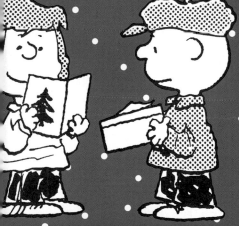
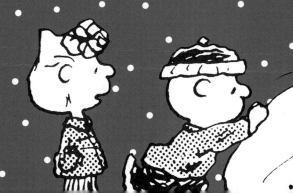

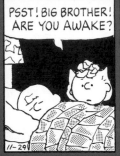
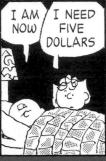
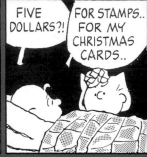
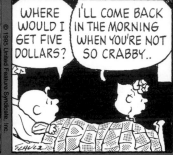

November 29, 1995

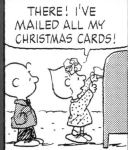
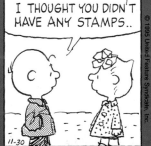
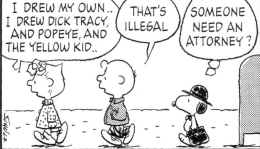

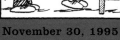

November 30, 1995

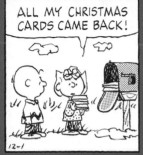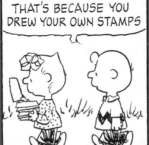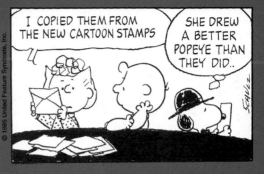

December 1, 1995

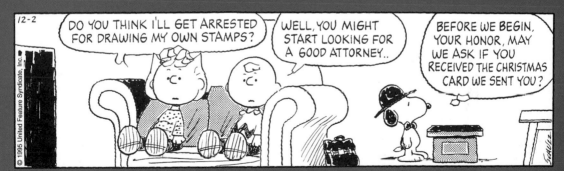

December 2, 1995

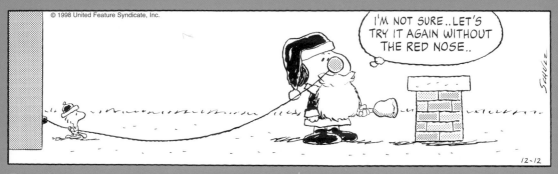

December 12, 1998

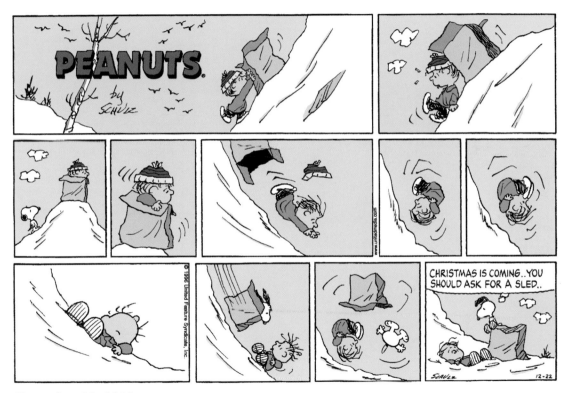

December 22, 1996

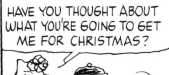

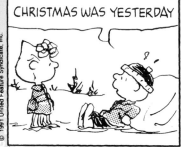

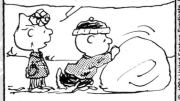

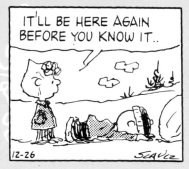

December 26, 1991

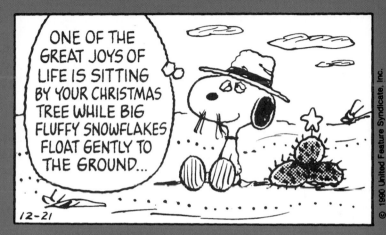

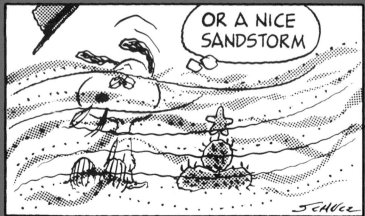

December 21, 1990

FRANKLIN

In 1968, Charlie Brown made a new friend at the beach. Franklin goes to a different school in town, where he is good friends with Peppermint Patty and Marcie. He plays against Charlie Brown on Peppermint Patty's baseball team, but the rivalry doesn't get in the way of their friendship— he is always invited to the Christmas party. During the year, Franklin goes to the movies with the rest of the PEANUTS gang and he and Charlie Brown have long talks about their grampas.

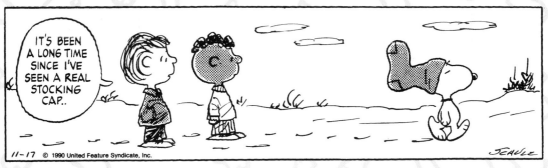

November 17, 1990

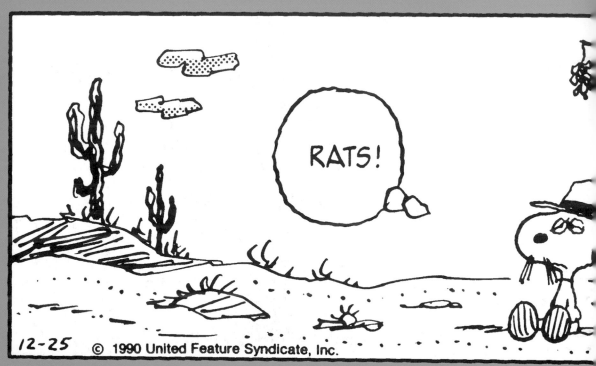

December 25, 1990

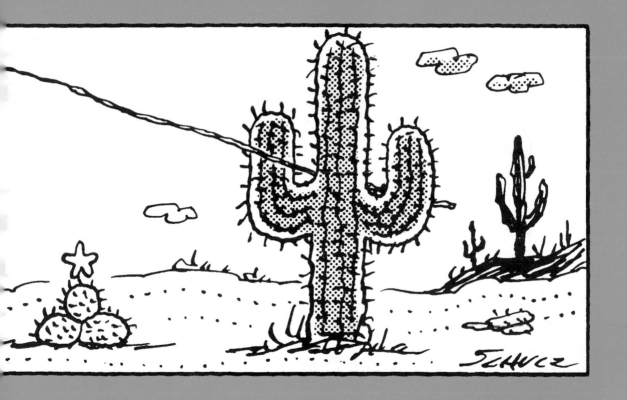

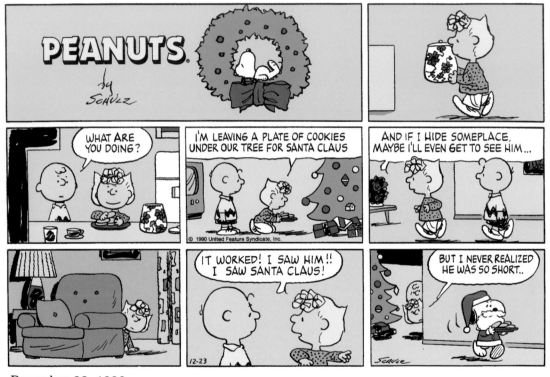

December 23, 1990

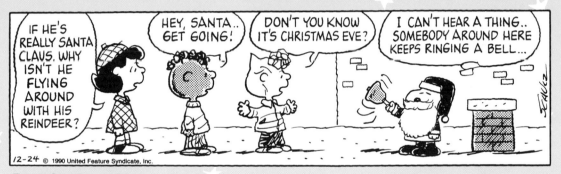

December 24, 1990

SPIKE

Snoopy and his brother Spike were separated as puppies at the Daisy Hill Puppy Farm. While Snoopy took the traditional path after graduation and went to live with Charlie Brown, Spike moved to the desert, where he gets along on his own with the company of "Joe Cactus" and several friendly tumbleweeds. Spike always celebrates Christmas, despite the distinct lack of snow in the desert and he and Snoopy exchange Christmas cards annually.

"ONE OF THE GREAT JOYS OF LIFE IS SITTING BY YOUR CHRISTMAS TREE WHILE BIG FLUFFY SNOWFLAKES FLOAT GENTLY TO THE GROUND . . . OR A NICE SANDSTORM."

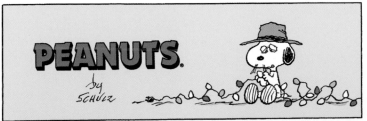
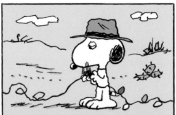
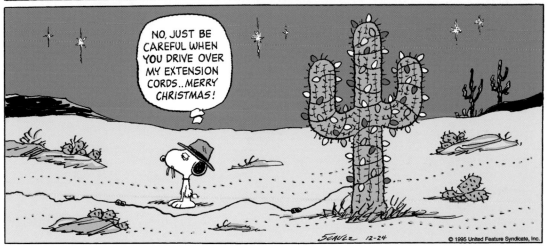

December 24, 1995

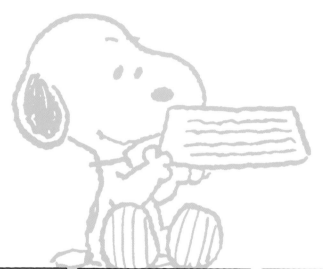

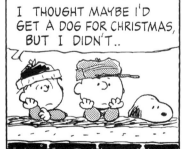

I THOUGHT MAYBE I'D GET A DOG FOR CHRISTMAS, BUT I DIDN'T..

January 2, 1996

OWNING A DOG IS A BIG RESPONSIBILITY, RERUN..THEY NEED LOTS OF CARE..

© 1995 United Feature Syndicate, Inc.

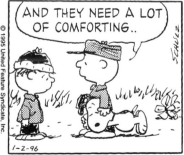

AND THEY NEED A LOT OF COMFORTING..

1-2-96

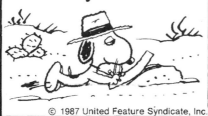

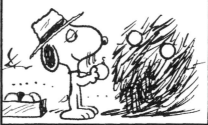

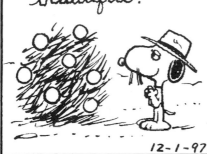

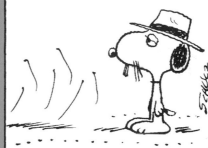

December 1, 1997

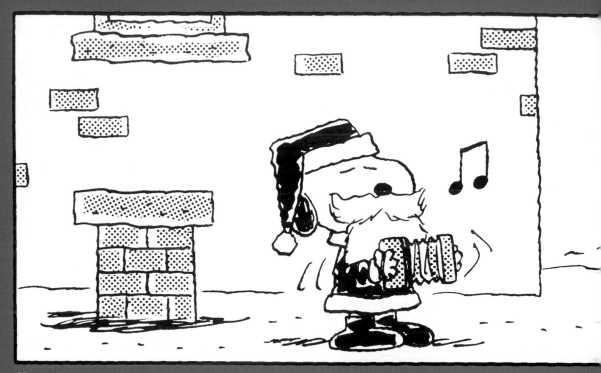

November 27, 1992

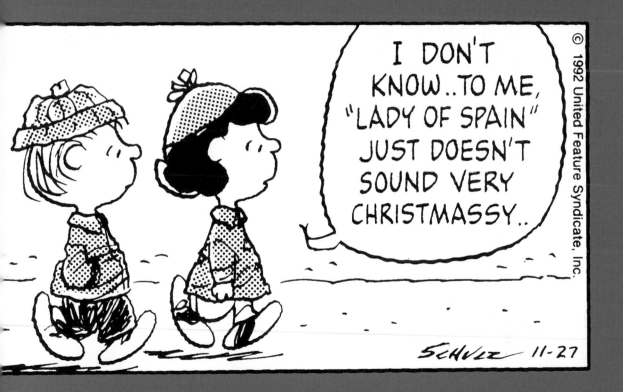

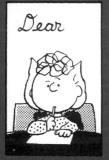
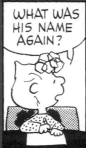
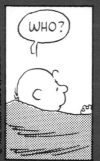
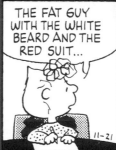
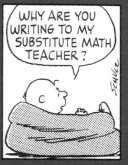

November 21, 1990

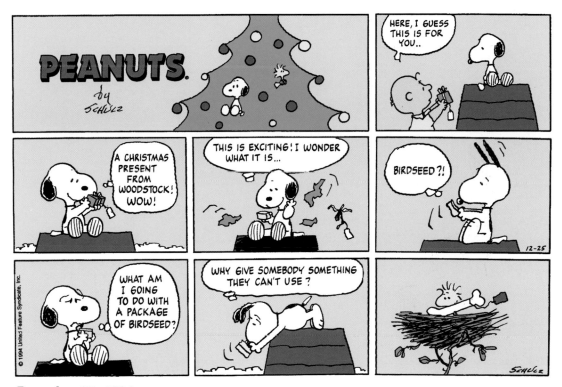

December 25, 1994

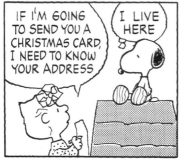
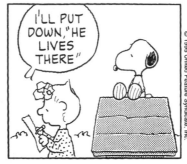
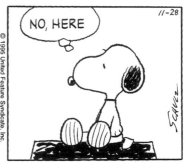

November 28, 1995

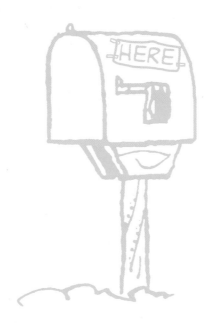

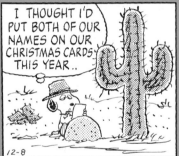
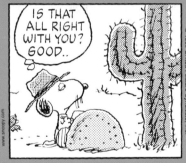
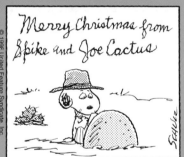

December 8, 1998

Charles Schulz (1922–2000)

"Someday, Charles, you're going to be an artist," his kindergarten teacher once told him. She probably didn't know how prophetic those words would be, but Charles "Sparky" Schulz grew up to become one of the most recognized names in comics.

Born to a barber in Minnesota, Charles Schulz grew up with dreams of writing his own comic strip. After admirable service in World War II, he returned to his passion, drawing, and he took a position as a teacher with his alma mater, Art Instruction Schools. While there, Schulz further honed his skills and met many of the people who would inspire his future work (including a friend named Charlie Brown and a girl with red hair who broke his heart).

Soon he was creating his own comic, which he called "L'il Folks" (it featured a younger Charlie Brown). The *Saturday Evening Post* printed several single comic panels, and the *St. Paul Pioneer Press* made it a weekly feature. "L'il Folks" became the focus of Schulz's career. After expanding it from a single panel to a strip format, he signed a five-year contract with United Feature Syndicate and began his lifelong dream: he was a full-time cartoonist. Because of legal issues surrounding the name "L'il Folks"—"Little Folks" and "L'il Abner" already existed—the strip was renamed PEANUTS, much to Schulz's displeasure.

Over the next fifty years, the world grew to love Charlie Brown, Snoopy, Linus and even Lucy. PEANUTS fans know the characters as well as they know their families, sharing in their losses as well as their triumphs. Every time Charlie Brown missed the football (thanks to Lucy's shenanigans), we missed it, too. When Linus awaited the arrival of the Great Pumpkin, we were out there in the pumpkin patch with him. As Snoopy flew through the air fighting The Red Baron, we flew right alongside him. By mixing humor, friendship, love and life, Charles Schulz made PEANUTS one of the longest-running, most popular comics of all time—and no one but Schulz himself ever drew a panel.

PEANUTS remained Schulz's focus throughout his life, and it became the most popular comic strip ever. It has been published in 21 languages, *in* more than 2,600 newspapers, and has spawned dozens of books, over 50 television specials and even a Broadway musical. *The Joy of a Peanuts Christmas* is Schulz's classic collection of holiday strips, a tribute Hallmark is proud to sponsor.

Charles Schulz died on February 12, 2000, in Santa Rosa, California at the age of 77—only hours before his last original PEANUTS strip was scheduled to appear in Sunday newspapers.

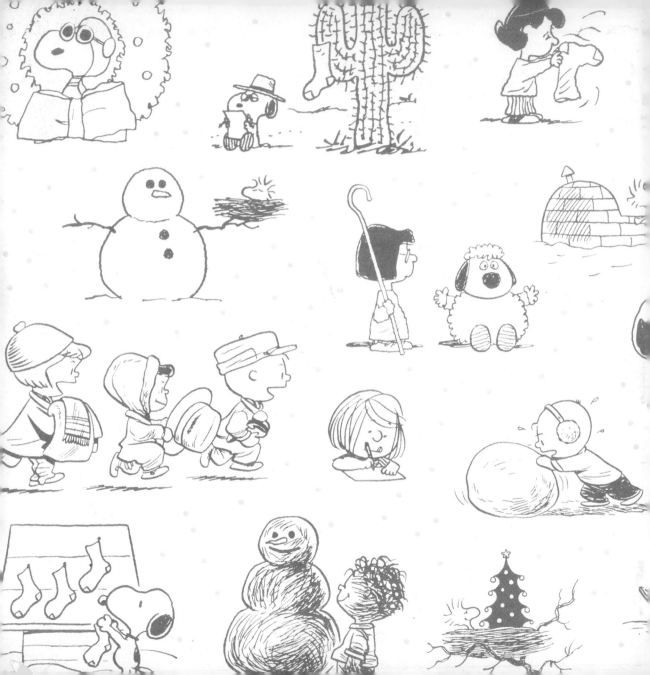